Shoulder Surgery Rehabilitation

Giovanni Di Giacomo • Silvia Bellachioma
Editors

Shoulder Surgery Rehabilitation

A Teamwork Approach

Springer

Editors
Giovanni Di Giacomo
Concordia Hospital for Special Surgery
Rome
Italy

Silvia Bellachioma
Concordia Hospital for Special Surgery
Rome
Italy

ISBN 978-3-319-24854-7 ISBN 978-3-319-24856-1 (eBook)
DOI 10.1007/978-3-319-24856-1

Library of Congress Control Number: 2016934463

Springer Cham Heidelberg New York Dordrecht London

Printed on acid-free paper

Springer International Publishing AG Switzerland is part of Springer Science+Business Media (www.springer.com)

To my mom, the most important person of my life, who was and still is able to make the impossible possible. Thank you for having believed in me, and for making every day of my life unique and special. With much love,

Silvia Bellachioma

To my friend Giovanni Danieli for his skill, professionalism, and passion for his work.

Giovanni Di Giacomo

Foreword

It is a pleasure to have the opportunity to write a foreword for *Shoulder Surgery Rehabilitation: A Teamwork Approach* on behalf of Doctors Di Giacomo and Bellachioma. Having worked personally with Doctors Di Giacomo and Bellachioma, I can attest to their skill and professionalism in what they do in their respective fields. Now they document how to work as an orthopedic surgeon-physiotherapist team. This text will enhance communication between treating healthcare professionals including orthopedic surgeons, non-orthopedic physicians, and physical therapists. It is well organized, provides excellent explanations of functional anatomy and biomechanics, discusses treatment options available and the rationale for decision-making, as well as possible complications.

With beautiful, meticulous illustrations of anatomy, pathology, and surgical procedures, and well-demonstrated rehabilitation techniques and exercises, this text will enhance the knowledge of what is involved in shoulder surgical procedures, and help physical therapists understand the rationale behind the recommended protocols and modification of protocols for each procedure, depending on the surgical variables. The importance of rehabilitation of the shoulder in the context of the kinetic chain, rather than in isolation is well supported, and is consistent with the way that Doctors Di Giacomo and Bellachioma have successfully worked together for many years. Each chapter clearly elucidates the roles of the orthopedic surgeon and physical therapist to insure a seamless recovery from injury whether or not surgery is involved.

Ben Rubin, MD
Orthopaedic Specialty Institute Medical Group of Orange County
Orange, CA, USA

Foreword

It is an exciting honor for me to help welcome the collaborative effort of this new textbook. The shoulder is a unique joint in that it is so dependent on soft tissue and muscular input, and this dependence is often underappreciated by orthopedic surgeons as we care for injuries around the shoulder joint. There has long been the need for our textbooks to approach the shoulder from a team-centered perspective. It is a pleasure to see this text and commend Doctor Di Giacomo and his team in capturing the collaboration between the surgeon and the therapist throughout the course of care. This textbook has captured the essence of multidisciplinary teamwork in the ideal approach to the shoulder. With a highly respected international group of authors, this text leverages the thought leaders from multiple nations, which gives it a worldwide relevance for surgeons and therapists wherever they live. I believe the reader will find this text extremely well illustrated, and with a combination of in-depth discussion with emphasis on key take-home points that will be valuable for readers at every level of training – from the young therapist to the seasoned orthopedic surgeon, there is something to be learned by all of us in this text. I believe it will become a well-referenced tool and a go-to reference for the entire shoulder team across the spectrum of care, and congratulate the editors on advancing our ability to care for the injured shoulder with this text.

John M. Tokish, MD
Steadman Hawkins Clinic of the Carolinas
Greenville, South Carolina, USA

Preface

Over the past decade, important advances in shoulder joint imaging and surgery have led to more accurate patient selection and constant updating of surgical procedures. On the rehabilitation front, too, functional anatomy and neurophysiology studies have combined with state-of-the-art biomechanics to improve rehabilitation protocols.

If positive postoperative outcomes are to be achieved, it is absolutely necessary that surgery and rehabilitation go hand in hand. Indeed, the recent acquisitions of know-how should ensure a seamless "cultural overlap" between orthopedics and rehabilitation. The physiotherapist must be familiar with indications for surgery, surgical techniques, and their possible complications in order to establish an appropriate rehabilitation protocol that caters for individual patient requirements and must also be able to interact effectively with the surgical team. Similarly, the orthopedic surgeon must be aware of the new rehabilitation possibilities that allow the achievement of better subjective and objective results.

The editors hope that this manual – developed together with surgical teams that have always attributed great importance to the rehabilitation phase – will meet the needs of physiotherapists, rehabilitation specialists, and surgeons and facilitate effective teamwork.

Rome, Italy — Giovanni Di Giacomo
Rome, Italy — Silvia Bellachioma

Contents

Proximal Humeral Fractures

1

Giovanni Di Giacomo, Silvia Bellachioma,
and Elena Silvestri

Contents

G. Di Giacomo (✉) • S. Bellachioma
Concordia Hospital for Special Surgery, Rome, Italy
e-mail: concordia@iol.it; sissybll@hotmail.it

E. Silvestri
fisiosmart, Rome, Italy
elena.silvestri@email.it

G. Di Giacomo, S. Bellachioma (eds.), *Shoulder Surgery Rehabilitation: A Teamwork Approach*,
DOI 10.1007/978-3-319-24856-1_1

1.1 Epidemiology

According to Horak and Nilsson 5 % of all fractures in the human body are fractures of the proximal humerus (PHF) [1].

In terms of frequency, PHF are the 7° in adults and 3° in patient over 65 following wrist and femoral neck fractures [4].

Majer et al. reported that, with respect to the incidence, 15 % of all PHF are complex 3-part and 4-part fractures [2–16].

Court- Brown et al. found that 70 % of all 3–4 part fractures are seen in patient aged over 60 years and 50 % in patients aged over 70 years [3].

These results conclude that poor bone quality and advanced osteoporosis will be found in the majority of patients with humeral head fractures.

PHF are more frequently osteoporotic fractures affecting women over 70 years of age.

The severity of the fracture increases proportionally with the age of the population (Table 1.1).

There are *two types of risk factors*:

- Fragile bones
- Patient-specific risk of falls

Roux reported that the mean age of PHF occurring was 70 (16–97), the fractured shoulder was on the right side 48 % and of the left 62 %, and the fracture affected dominant side in 48 % cases [4].

Analysis of the distribution of fractures through the year showed that the most of the fractures occurred during the cold season, with 60 % occurring between October and March.

Roux also reported that in 325 patients with 329 fractures, hospitalization was necessary in 43 % of the cases. In their study, displaced fractures made up 58 % of the total number and surgical management was necessary 21 % of the time [4].

The lack of relationship between the percentage of displaced fractures (58 %) compared to the percentage of surgically treated fractures (21 %) is a sign of the difficulties of managing this population, which is usually in poor general condition (Table 1.2).

Comorbid diseases increase the risk factors for PHF (Table 1.3).

The main cause of fractures in men 55 % of the time was due to a simple fall and 45 % of the time was from a high-energy kinetic trauma. In women the cause was a simple fall in 82 % of all cases (Table 1.4) [4].

High-energy injuries such as motor vehicle accidents usually produce significant associated injuries.

Moderate falls causing severe injury, such as a fall in the home, are suspicion of osteoporosis call for preventive measures.

Persistent pain after fall, even with an initially negative radiograph, should alert the physician to repeat the investigation with additional views.

Often hidden fractures of the tuberosities will be revealed (CT SCAN or MRI can help).

Adequate neurological and vascular investigation may also be necessary.

Palvanen and Kannus [5] found a threefold increase over a 33-year period in the incidence of PHF resulting from low-energy trauma in people aged 60 and above. The same author demonstrated an increase in the annual fracture rate of 13.7 % over the past every year.

The incidence is increasing, and these fractures tend to be more severe [6–8].

The management of these often debilitating injuries is based on various classification systems [8, 9].

Table 1.1

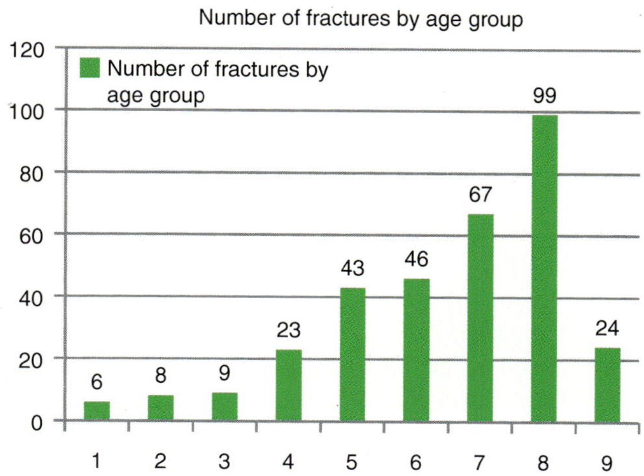

Table 1.2

Comorbidities	Number of patients	%
Diabetes	27	10
Epilepsy	7	3
Depression	53	21
Dementia	26	10
Parkinson's disease	4	1.6
Psychosis	8	3
Cardiopathy	21	8
HTA	10	4
History of stroke	8	3

Table 1.3

Risk factors for fractures	Number for patient	%
Osteoporosis	85	34
History of falling	82	33
Limited physical activity	75	30
History of femoral neck fracture in mother	31	12
Trouble walking	62	25
Pain in the lower limb	47	19
Trouble seeing	66	26
Trouble hearing	41	16
Alcoholism	37	15
Tobacco use	71	28

Table 1.4

Cause of fracture	Total	Men	Women
Falling from standing height	189	37	152
Road accident	34	18	16
Violent fall	17	7	10
Aggression	9	3	6
Suicide attempt	1	0	1

1.2 Classification

The proximal humerus can be divided into four anatomic areas: humeral head, greater tuberosity, lesser tuberosity, and shaft (Fig. 1.1) [9, 10].

The average humeral neck-shaft angle, that is, the angle between the neck of the humerus and the shaft, measures at approximately 140°. The humeral head version, on the other hand, is quite variable depending on which anatomic landmarks are used [11, 12].

Historically 30° of humeral head retroversion is considered normal.

The tuberosities, the diaphysis, and the humeral head are subjected to different compression and tractive forces, due to the muscles acting as lever. Following a fracture event, certain forces may determine different patterns and different degrees of displacement (Fig. 1.2a, b).

A fracture classification should aim to improve the understanding and therefore the management of fractures, based on the morphology, the biology, and mechanical behavior. It should also strive to provide therapeutic guidelines based on clinical outcomes and be comprehensive with all fractures types which are classifiable, and its application should lead to reproducible results [13].

The main criterion for a good classification system is that it addresses the clinically relevant questions.

Literature reports four *PHF classification systems* that are in use or have the potential for use:

- *The Neer system*, which groups each fracture by the number of fracture segments and describes the fractured anatomic segments as a part [9].
- *The AO system*, which describes each fracture as a being 1 of 3 types with 3 subdivisions each.

  Type A indicates extra-articular unifocal fractures, type B extra-articular bifocal fractures, and type C articular fractures. The 3 subdivisions are related to the pattern of the fractures [13].
- *The Codman-Hertel* binary fractures (the so-called Lego System of Hertel et al.) [7, 14].

  This classification corresponds to the four-part system of Codman with the option of 12 fractures types. There are 6 possible fracture combinations dividing the humerus in 2 parts, 5 possible fracture combinations dividing the humerus into 3 parts, and one fracture type dividing the humerus into 4 parts [15].
- *The 4° system, by Resch.* This is a proposed addendum of the Codman-Hertel classification system and addresses the fracture angulation and the pathomechanics of the injury.

It describes three biomechanical planes of injury classified by the observer [this distinction is crucial for reduction and fixation]:

1. *Impaction/Distraction*
   - *Impaction*: an impaction injury occurs when the length of the position of the fracture of the greater tuberosity is unchanged and the total length of the humerus is reduced due to the impact to the head [16].
   - *Distraction*: a distraction injury is defined as an increase in distance on the lateral side between shaft and head fragment (subcapital fractures) or between the shaft and the fractured greater tuberosity (subcapital fractures accompanied by a greater tuberosity fracture).
2. *Varus /Valgus/Neutral*
   - In *varus-type fractures*, the head is disrupted from the shaft and remains in the varus position as a result of the persisting attachment of the rotator cuff muscles. In the case of an additional fracture of the greater tuberosity, the head may follow the subscapularis muscle and rotate into an internally rotated position (3-part fracture according to Neer) [9]. An investigation of 200 consecutive cases showed that 2 varus types could be differentiated:
     – *Varus distraction type*: the head fragment is in varus position and completely separated from the shaft in an anteromedial position. The varus distraction with additional fracture to the greater tuberosity presents cute often with the head in an internally rotated position.
     – *Varus impaction type*: is characterized by the impaction of the head on the medial side, yet no distraction occurs on the lateral side. In the sagittal plane, the anterior angulation angle is increased, but in contrast to the distraction type, the shaft is not in a separated position. These fractures are characterized by residual primary stability, as a result of the periosteum steel being preserved on the lateral side. The calcar on the medial side has to be reduced (Fig. 1.3a, b).

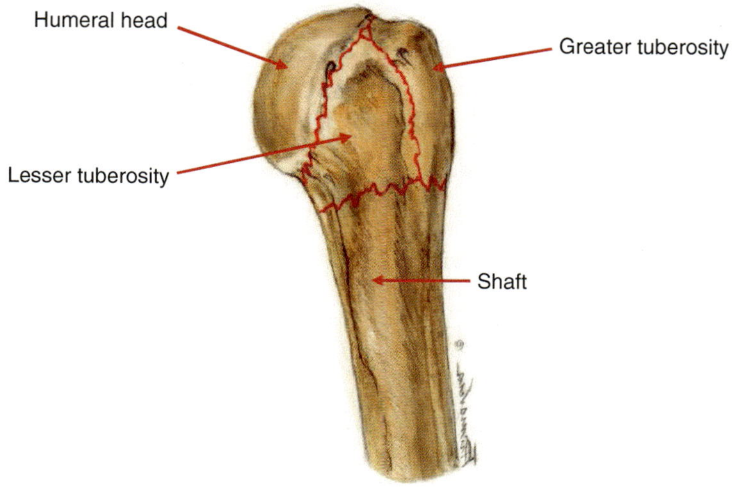

Fig. 1.1 Four anatomic areas of proximal humerus

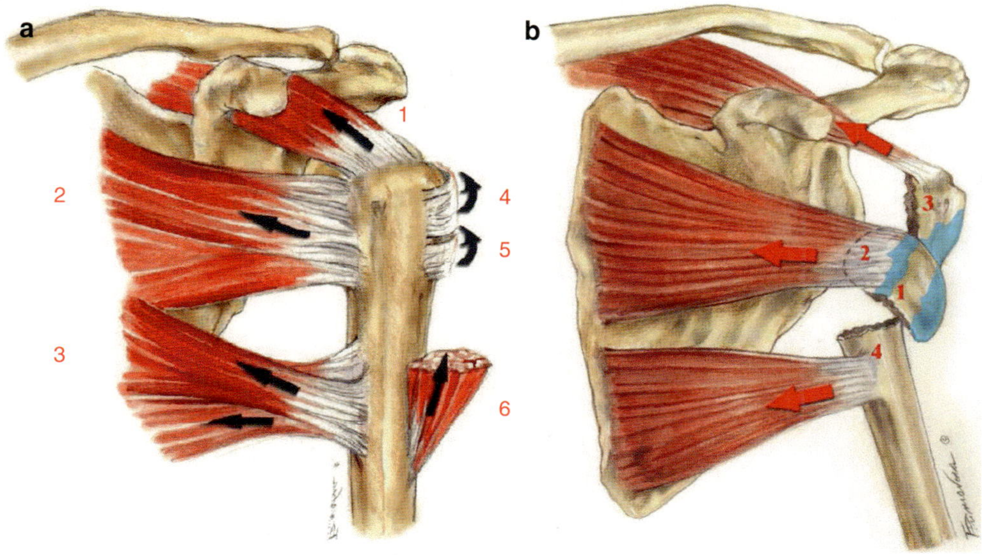

Fig. 1.2 (**a**) Displacement forces that occurs in the proximal humerus. (*1*) Supraspinatus, (*2*) Subscapularis, (*3*) Pectoralis major, (*4*) Infraspinatus, (*5*) Teres minor, (*6*) Deltoid. (**b**) Forces that can occur during PHF and increase the displacement of the different fragments. (*1*) Humeral head, (*2*) Subscapularis, (*3*) Greater tuberosity→supraspinatus, (*4*) Shaft →Pectoralis major

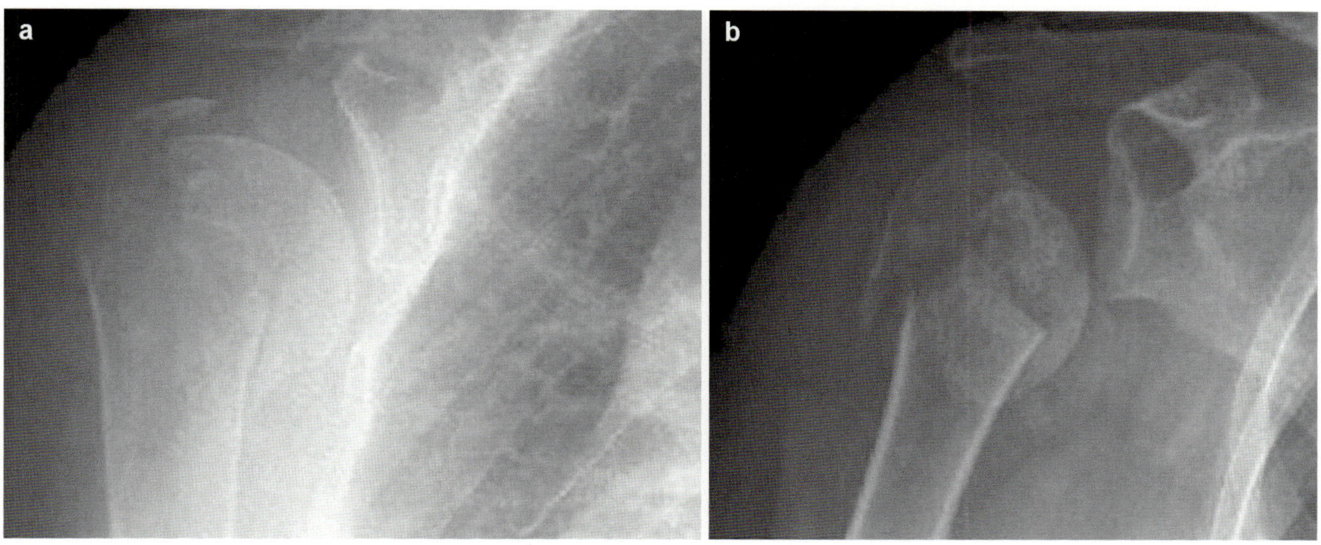

Fig. 1.3 (**a**) Varus impaction type fractures. (**b**) Varus impaction type fractures

– *Valgus type*: is characterized by the impaction of the head into the metaphyses of the shaft. The fracture of the tuberosity remains in the normal longitudinal position and is still relatively attached to the shaft by the undestroyed periosteum (Fig. 1.4).

This fracture without lateral displacement of the head in relation to the shaft is easy to reduce, because only the head has to be raised by an elevator that is introduced between the fractured tuberosities. The periosteum of the medial side serves as a mechanical hinge when performing this maneuver.

In the case of severe lateral displacement of the head in relation to the shaft, the mechanical hinge periosteum on the medial side is torn and the head fragment is very unstable and difficult to reduce (Fig. 1.5) [19].

Take-Home Message

From the study of Solberg et al. [17–19], the varus deformity of more of 20° should not be left uncorrected because this level of deformity is not be tolerated by the patient. In comparison to varus deformity, valgus deformity is better tolerated. Greater tuberosity displacement of more than 5 mm in any direction should not be accepted.

3. *Flexion/Extension/Neutral*

Finally the head-shaft angle in the trans-scapular plane is assessed and described as flexion, extension, or neutral. Thus addressing fracture angulation may also facilitate fracture reduction (Fig. 1.6).

Take-Home Message

Imaging: AP view, trans-scapular, and axillary views are the standard approach; anyway a CT scan with 3D reconstruction gives tri-planar excellent information (Fig. 1.7).

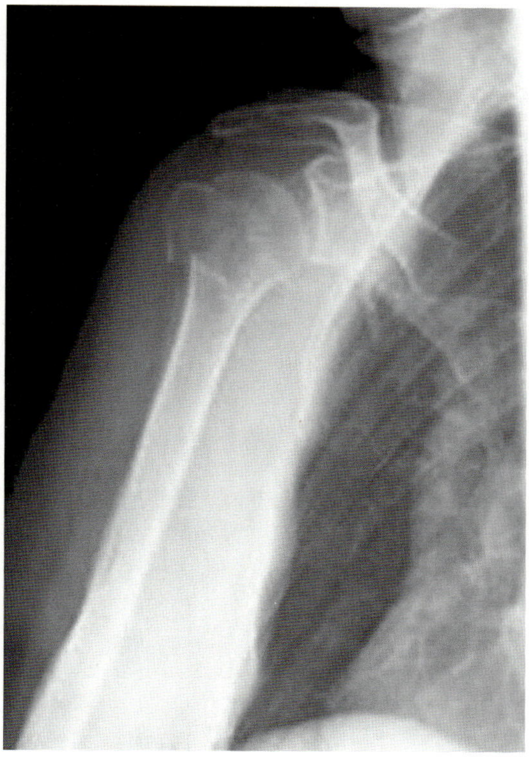

Fig. 1.4 Valgus impaction type fractures

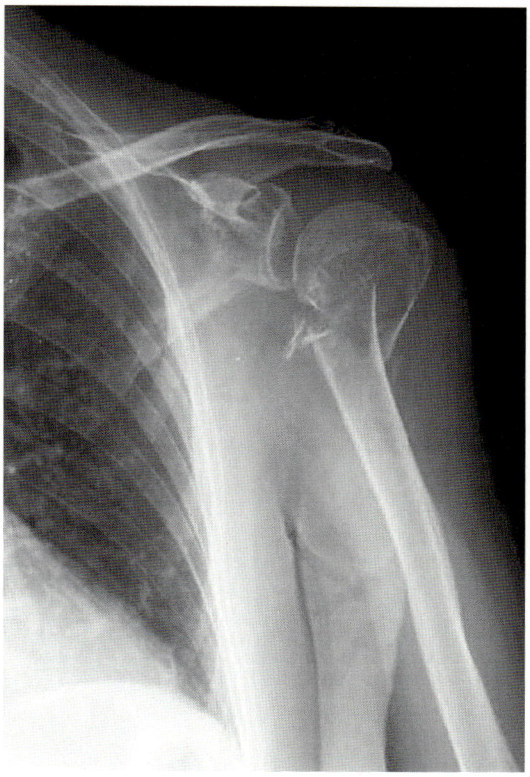

Fig. 1.5 Severe lateral displacement of the head in relation to the shaft

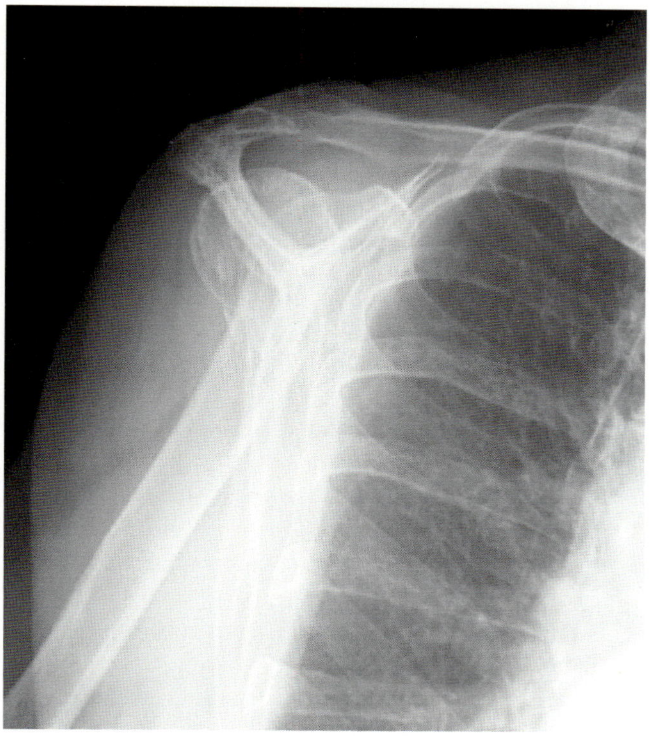

Fig. 1.6 Transcapular plane view

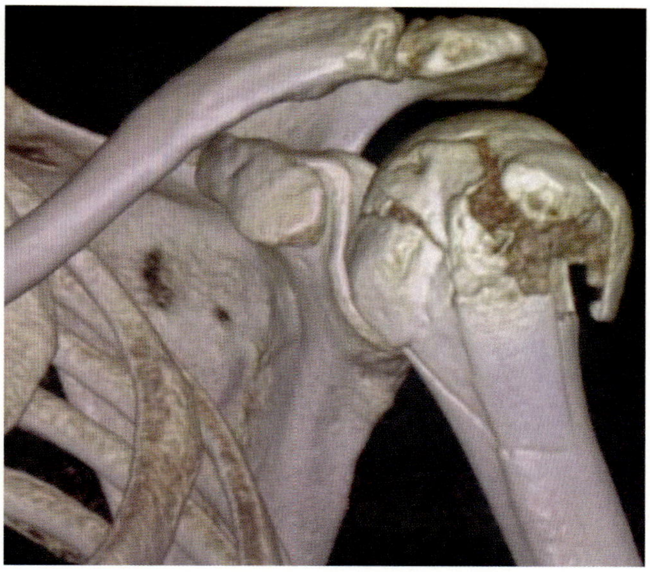

Fig. 1.7 3D reconstruction

The *Codman-Hertel* classification in our experience is comprehensive, easy to teach, and easy to learn. It has proved cogency because it provides clear-cut diagnostic subgroups, even if the residual difficulty, as with all classification systems, remained in actually recognizing the fracture lines. This requires adequate radiographs (anteroposterior and axillary view) and an experienced eye [7].

Codman-Hertel System:

The system describes *five basic fracture planes* that can be identified by answering the following questions:

1. Is there a fracture between the greater tuberosity and the head?
2. Is there a fracture between the greater tuberosity and the shaft?
3. Is there a fracture between the lesser tuberosity and the head?
4. Is there a fracture between the lesser tuberosity and the shaft?
5. Is there a fracture between the lesser tuberosity and the greater tuberosity?

This results in 12 basic fracture patterns (Table 1.5).

Evaluation criteria accessories are important additional considerations when deciding on the treatment of complex intra-articular fractures of the proximal humerus.

Accessory questions
6. How long is the posteromedial metaphyseal head extension (mm)?
7. How large is the displacement of the shaft with respect to the head (displacement measured between posteromedial edge of the head and posteromedial shaft fracture line "mm")? Medial or lateral displacement of the shaft?
8. How long is the displacement of the tuberosities with respect to the head (displacement measured of transition zone between the tuberosity and the cartilaginous fracture line "mm")?
9. Amount of angular displacement of the head (under consideration of the £-dimensional position)? Varus or valgus?
10. Is there a glenohumeral dislocation (Y/N)? Anterior or posterior?
11. Is there a head impression fracture (Y/N)? Anterior or posterior?
12. Is there a head split component (Y/N)? >20 % of the head involvement (Y/N)? With two intra-articular fracture planes (Y/N)? With one intra-articular fracture plane (Y/N)?

With the permission of Elsevier Saunders

Table 1.5 Codman- Hertel classification system

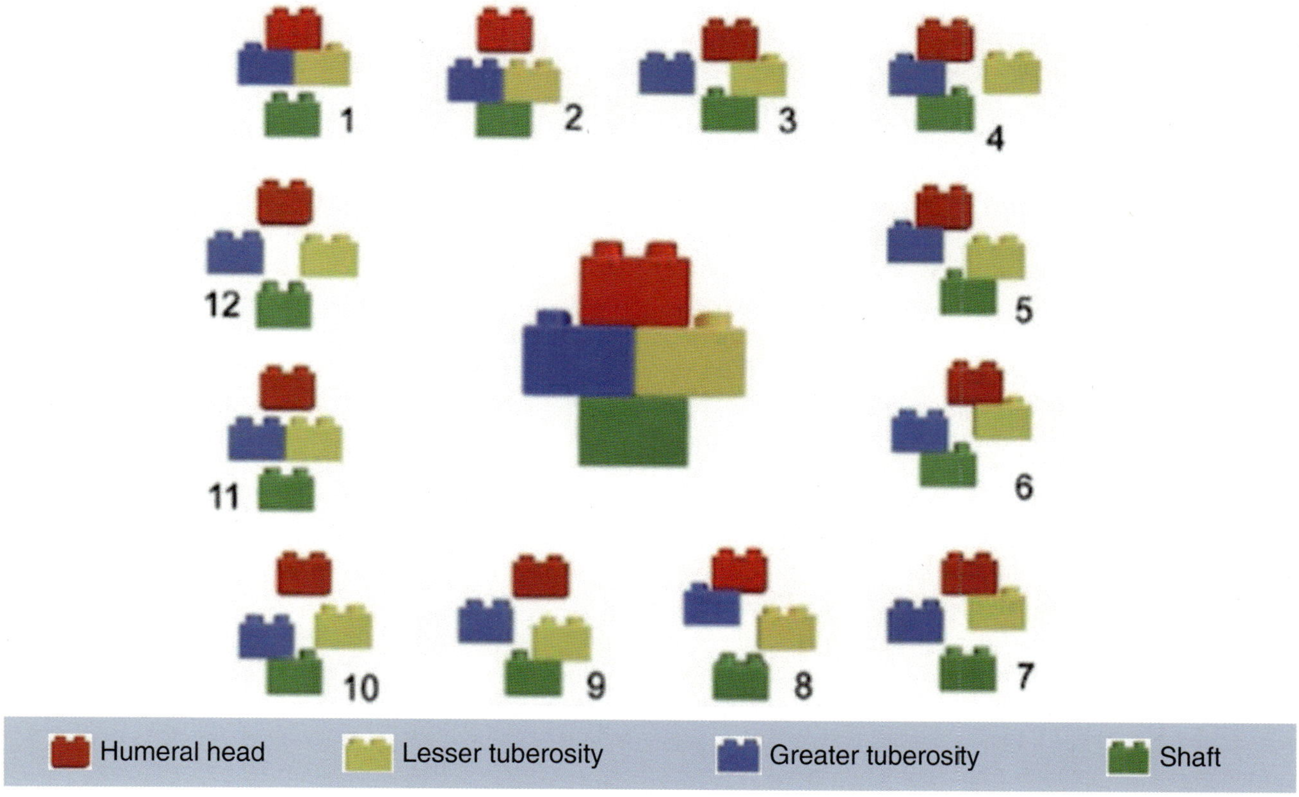

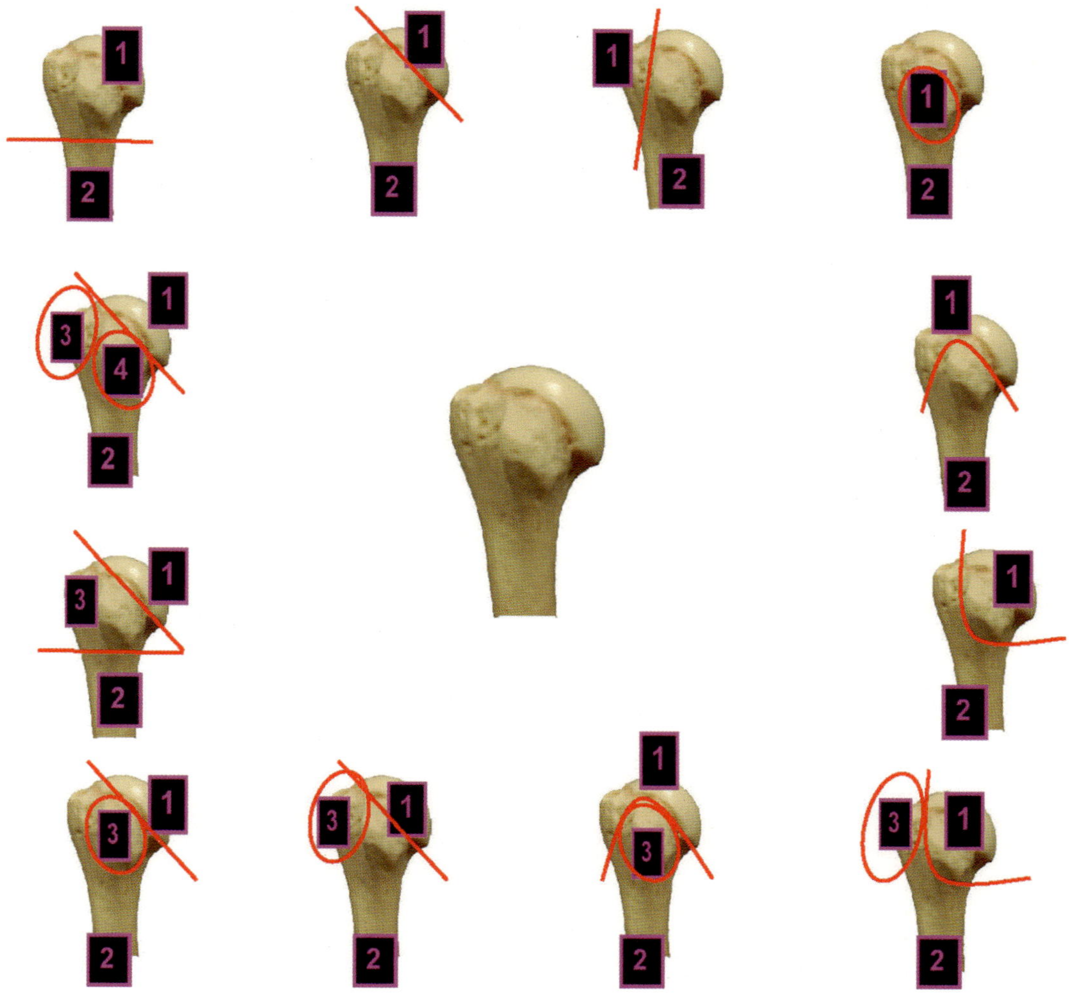

1.2.1 Vascular Supply

Vascularity of the proximal humerus is an important factor in assessing fracture pattern severity; thus a thorough knowledge of the vascular anatomy is important. Historically the anterior circumflex humeral artery and its terminal branch, the arcuate artery, have been noted as the preeminent sources of perfusion to the proximal humerus [20]. In a cadaver study, Brooks et al. [21] investigated the vascularity of the humeral head using a four-part fracture model. The authors noted that the primary source of perfusion to the proximal humerus was via the anterior circumflex humeral and arcuate arteries, with significant intraosseous anastomoses existing between the arcuate artery and the posterior circumflex humeral artery, the metaphyseal arteries, and the vessels of the greater and lesser tuberosities (Fig. 1.8).

The authors also reported that, in most cases, a four-part PHF disrupts perfusion to the humeral head. They also noted that the posteromedial vessels play a vital role in maintaining proximal humeral perfusion in certain fracture patterns.

However, debate continues regarding whether the anterior circumflex humeral artery is the dominant source of perfusion to the humeral head. Recent studies have demonstrated that the posterior circumflex humeral artery plays a greater role than the anterior circumflex artery does in supplying blood to the proximal humerus (Fig. 1.9a, b) [22, 23].

Duparc et al. [22] argued that the posterior and anterior circumflex humeral arteries are equally important in humeral head perfusion. Interestingly the authors noted that the posterior circumflex humeral artery was consistently larger in diameter than the anterior circumflex humeral artery. In a cadaver study, Hettrich et al. [23] quantitatively assessed the vascularity of the proximal humerus and found that the posterior circumflex humeral artery contributes 64 % of the blood supplied to the proximal humerus, whereas the anterior circumflex humeral artery contributes just 36 %.

The vascular supply to the greater tuberosity is provided through intraosseous connections between the arcuate artery, the posterior humeral circumflex artery, the metaphyseal vessels, and the vessels of the greater and lesser tuberosities. The arterial network provides a rich blood supply to the greater tuberosity which provides a good healing environment for greater tuberosity fractures. Unlike fractures of the anatomic neck of the humerus, isolated fractures of the greater tuberosity do not typically compromise the blood supply to the humeral head [21].

Take-Home Message

Note that in the metadiaphyseal region, the blue boundary (Fig. 1.9a, b) represents the "entry point" of the anterior and posterior circumflex.

In PHF, if this region remains in continuous with the fractured element of the head, the risk factors for aseptic necrosis are diminished. On the contrary, if no continuity exists between the head and the metadiaphysis, the risk factors for aseptic necrosis will be increase.

Fig. 1.8 Vascular supply of the proximal humerus. (*1*) Axillary Artery, (*2*) Thoraco Acromial Artery, (*3*) Subscapularis Artery, (*4*) Anterior Circumflex Artery, (*5*) Ascending branch of the anterior Circumflex, (*6*) Posterior Circumflex Artery, (*7*) Brachial Artery

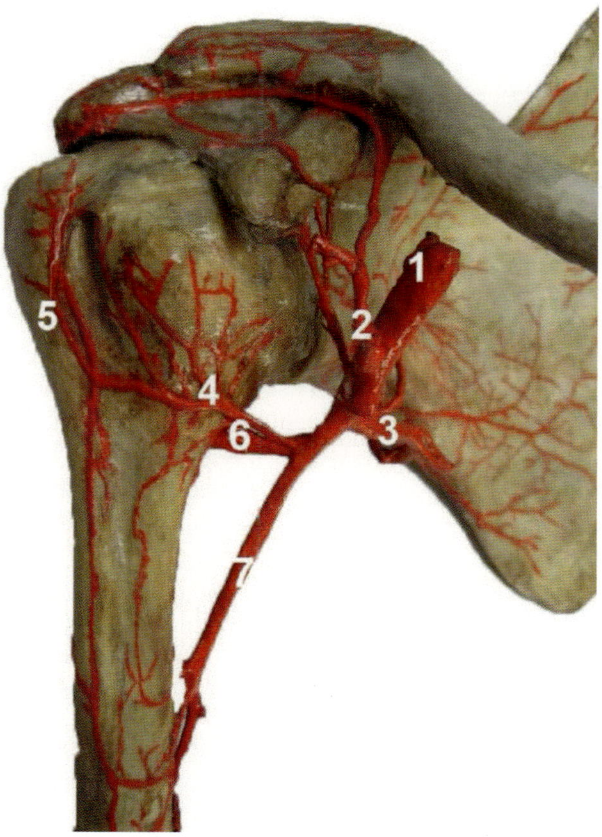

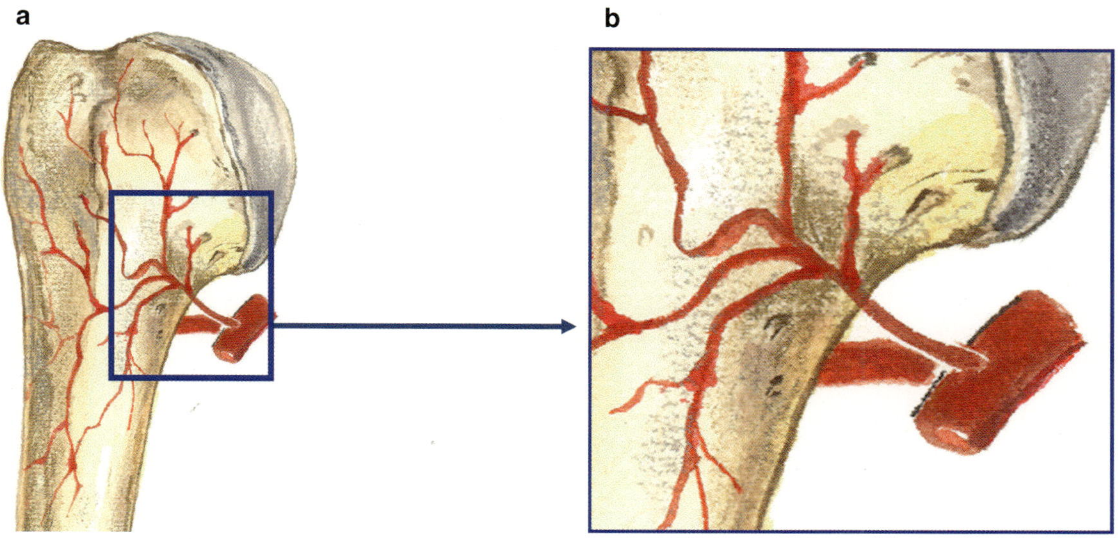

Fig. 1.9 (**a**) Anterior and posterior circumflex artery and its relationship with the medial hinge. (**b**) Magnification

1.2.2 Vascular Patterns

The perfusion of the fractured segments is the main problem to analyze the right decision-making of surgical program, if needed.

The classification systems give an important prospective view of the status of the fracture and help to decide what may be correct to do but at the same time is not enough.

To make a good prediction of the result, we must to consider the perfusion of the fractured segments and the real capacity of these to maintain a good biologic vascular response [24].

Preservation of proximal humeral vascularity is important when distinguishing between valgus-impacted and varus-angulated three- and four-part PHF. The valgus impacted fracture is characterized by intact medial soft tissue, which can potentially preserve the blood supply to the humeral head.

In the markedly displaced four-part PHF with significant varus malalignment, disruption of the medial soft tissue envelope can potentially compromise perfusion to the humeral head; at this purpose the Hertel classification is also to evaluate.

Hertel hypothesized that in the PHF, when a metaphyseal extension remained attached to the head, a degree of residual perfusion provided by the posterior circumflex humeral head vessels could be anticipated. It seems that one of the key points is to evaluate the impact of fracture morphology including the position and the size of the metaphyseal head extension of the humeral head perfusion (Fig. 1.10a, b).

The purpose of the Hertel classification is also to evaluate predicting factors of fractures that potentially could induce humeral head ischemia:

- Destruction of the medial hinge is a critical factor for fractures with a medial metaphyseal extension below 8 mm. Related to the vascular status, the integrity of the medial hinge is also an important hide in fracture reduction and stabilization. It is crucial for reduction and internal fixation.
- Another important element that is related as good predictor of ischemia besides the length of the metaphyseal head extension <8 mm and the integrity of the medial hinge is the basic fracture pattern for combined types 2-9-10-11-12 (fracture types with an anatomic head component) (Table 1.5).

Take-Home Message

- The metaphyseal head extension (also called calcar segment) part of the metaphysis remains attached to the head. The metaphyseal extension was most often located posteromedially (Fig. 1.10a).
- Medial hinge is defined as the pivot point of the head at the level of the posteromedial fracture line (Fig. 1.10b).

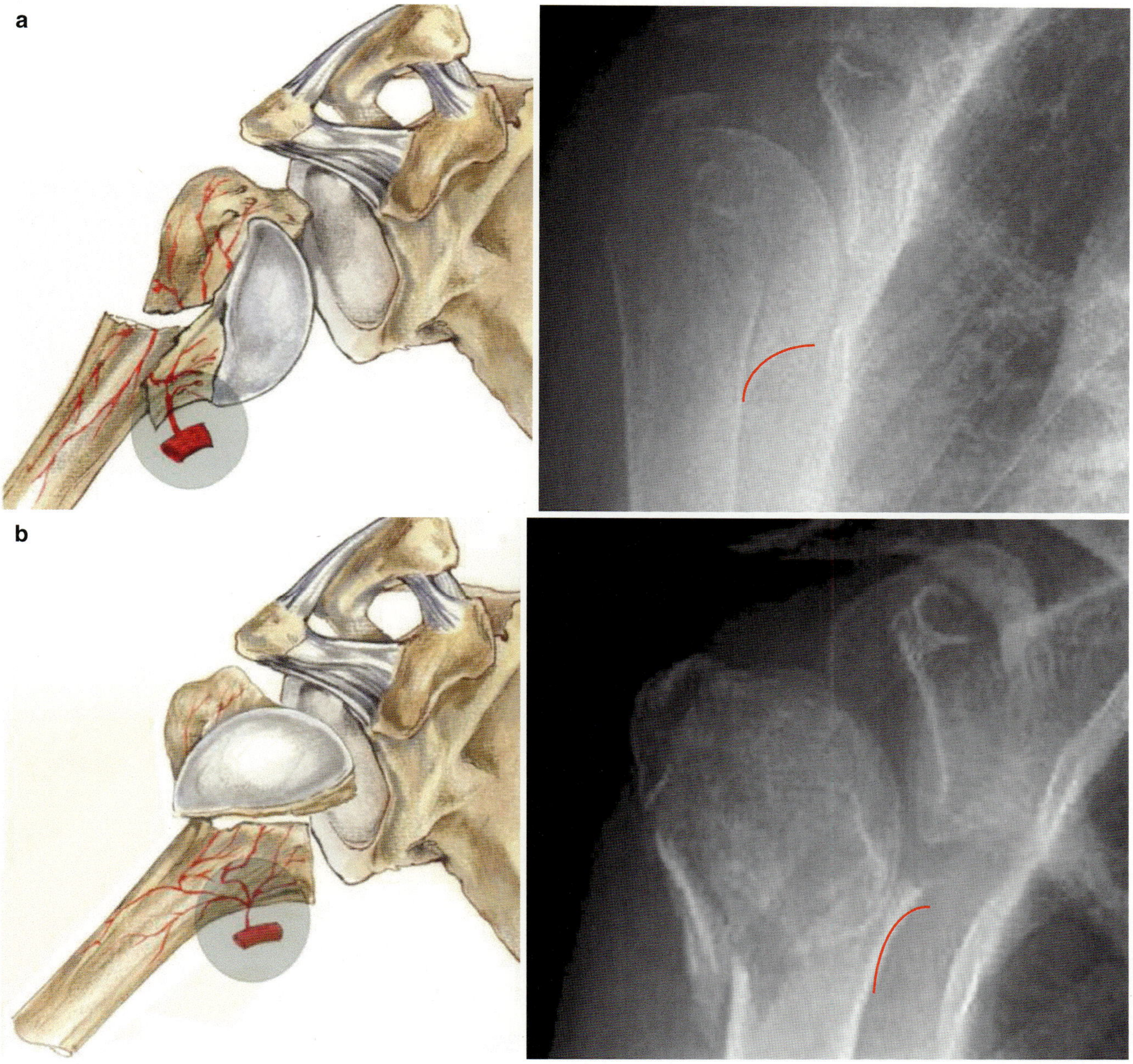

Fig. 1.10 (**a**) Length of the medial metaphyseal head exsension (*red line*), the more likely the head is perfused. (**b**) Integrity of the medial hinge (*red line*) is a predictor of both ischemia and practical feasibility of reduction

Importance intermediate:

- 3–4-part fractures.
- Angular displacement >45°.
- Amount of displacement of the tuberosities over 10 mm.
- Head-split component.
- The mean displacement of the shaft with respect of the head can also be considered a predictor of ischemic head when it is around 13 mm especially if it is medial (Fig. 1.11).

According of Trupka et al., fracture dislocation is not associated with an increased incidence of avascular necrosis of the humeral head (Fig. 1.12) [25].

Perfusion of the head fragment is essential but not the only element for decision-making.

Despite an ischemic head (Fig. 1.13), a head-preserving treatment is an option when revascularization can be expected and/or when a two-staged management protocol is required for local or systemic reasons (first-stage osteosynthesis and second-stage hemiarthroplasty should avascular necrosis not tolerated) (Fig. 1.14).

Generally head-preserving surgery is indicated when the bone quality is good enough to ensure the stable osteosynthesis in order to allow healing (especially of the tuberosities) in an anatomic position.

Anatomical findings [21, 22, 26] and clinical observation [27–30] seem to confirm that perfusion derived from the posterior circumflex vessels alone may be sufficient for head survival.

The most relevant predictors of ischemia, according to Hertel et al. [7], are the length of the dorsomedial metaphyseal extension, the integrity of the medial hinge, and the basic fracture type determined with the binary description system.

Take-Home Message
Gerber et al. [31] stated that in the case of an existing avascular necrosis, it is the deformity rather than necrosis that causes disability. Therefore, the risk of limited blood supply of the articular fragment does not influence our decision-making in terms of treatment.

Like Gerber et al. [31], we believe that the alignment of the tuberosities is very important in cases in which prosthetic replacement might be necessary as a secondary procedure because of head necrosis.

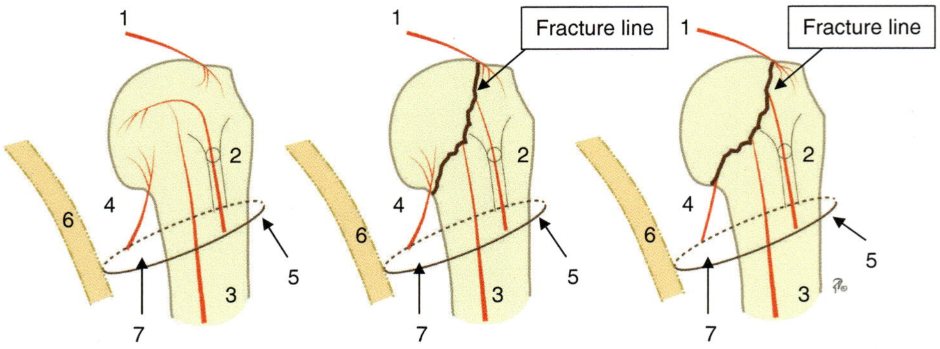

(*1*) Arterial supply of the rotator cuff from the thoracoacromial and suprascapular arteries. (*2*) Ascending branch of the anterior circumflex artery. (*3*) Intraosseous metaphyseal artery. (*4*) Ascending branch of the posterior circumflex artery. (*5*) Anterior circumflex artery. (*6*) Axillary artery. (*7*) Circumflex artery

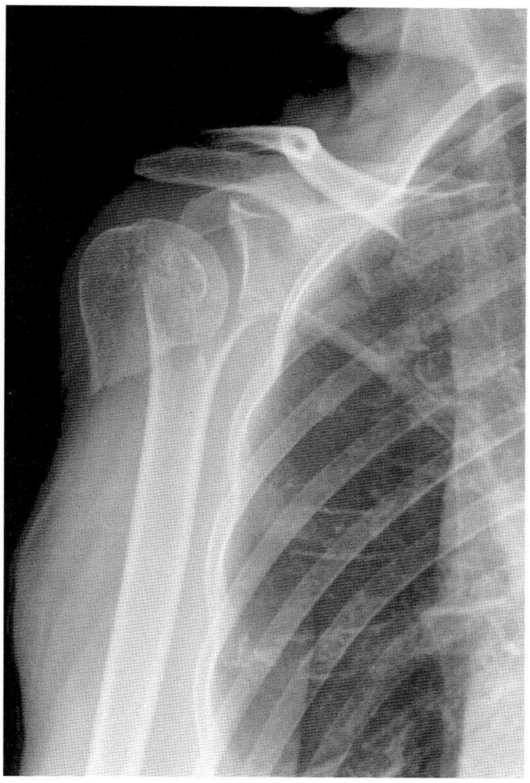

Fig. 1.11 Medial displacement of the shaft

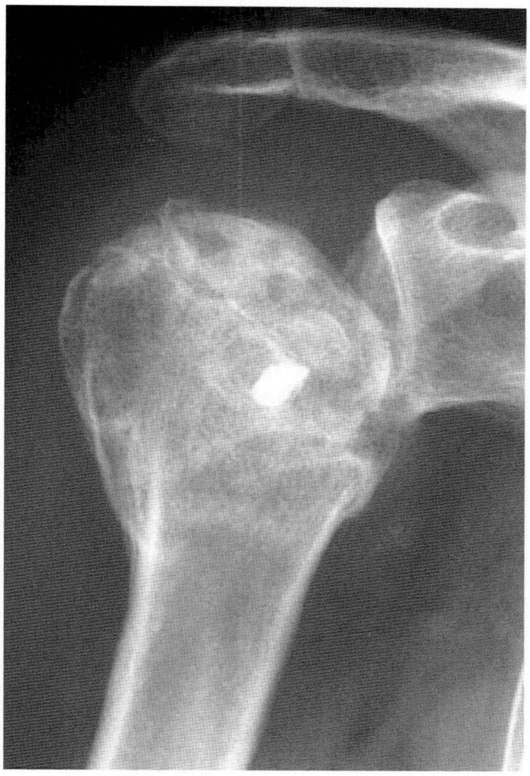

Fig. 1.13 Fracture sequelae of PHF with head avascular necrosis

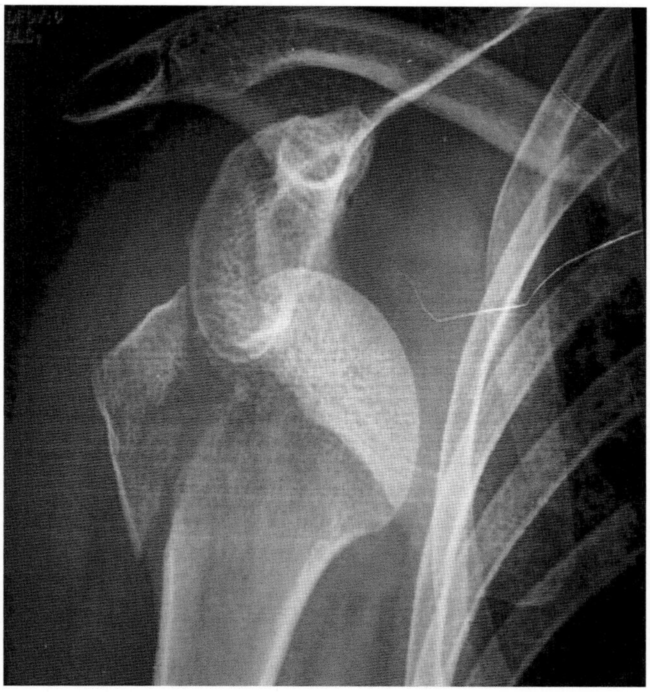

Fig. 1.12 Fracture dislocation

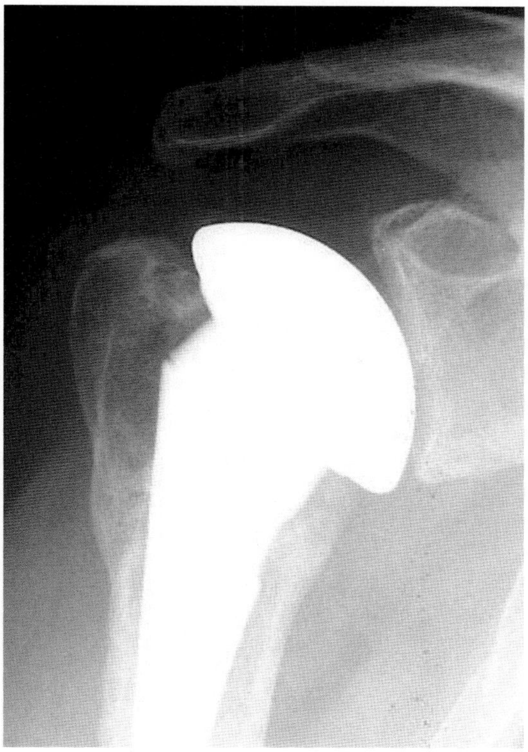

Fig. 1.14 Prosthetic replacement as secondary procedure

1.3 Biomechanics Related to Proximal Humerus Fracture

Different than other pathologies of the shoulder, the third proximal humeral fractures generally occur from a sudden traumatic event, and for this reason, this condition affects the joint from a functional anatomical standpoint.

Therefore after the trauma, only the proximal humeral region is altered from the anatomical and biomechanical point of view.

We assume also that the other joints that make up the shoulder (the acromioclavicular, the sternoclavicular, and particularly the scapulothoracic joints) are functional.

We want, therefore, to focus our attention exclusively to the glenohumeral joint and introduce the concept of biomechanics that, if well understood, will be extremely helpful in making a short or long term: the concept of *fulcrum* and *engine.*

1.3.1 Concept of "Fulcrum" and "Engine"

We define the *fulcrum* as the convex surface of the head of the humerus that rotates inside the concave surface of the glenoid.

The rotation movement is guaranteed by a valid *engine* that is represented by the rotator cuff, its bone insertions (greater and lesser tuberosities), and also by the deltoid.

It is stated that the shoulder can maintain a stable "fulcrum" of motion only when it maintains balance force couples in both the coronal plane (inferior portion of rotator cuff below the center of rotation creates a moment that must balance the deltoid moment) (Fig. 1.15a) and transverse plane (the subscapularis anteriorly is balanced against the infraspinatus and teres major posteriorly) (Fig. 1.15b).

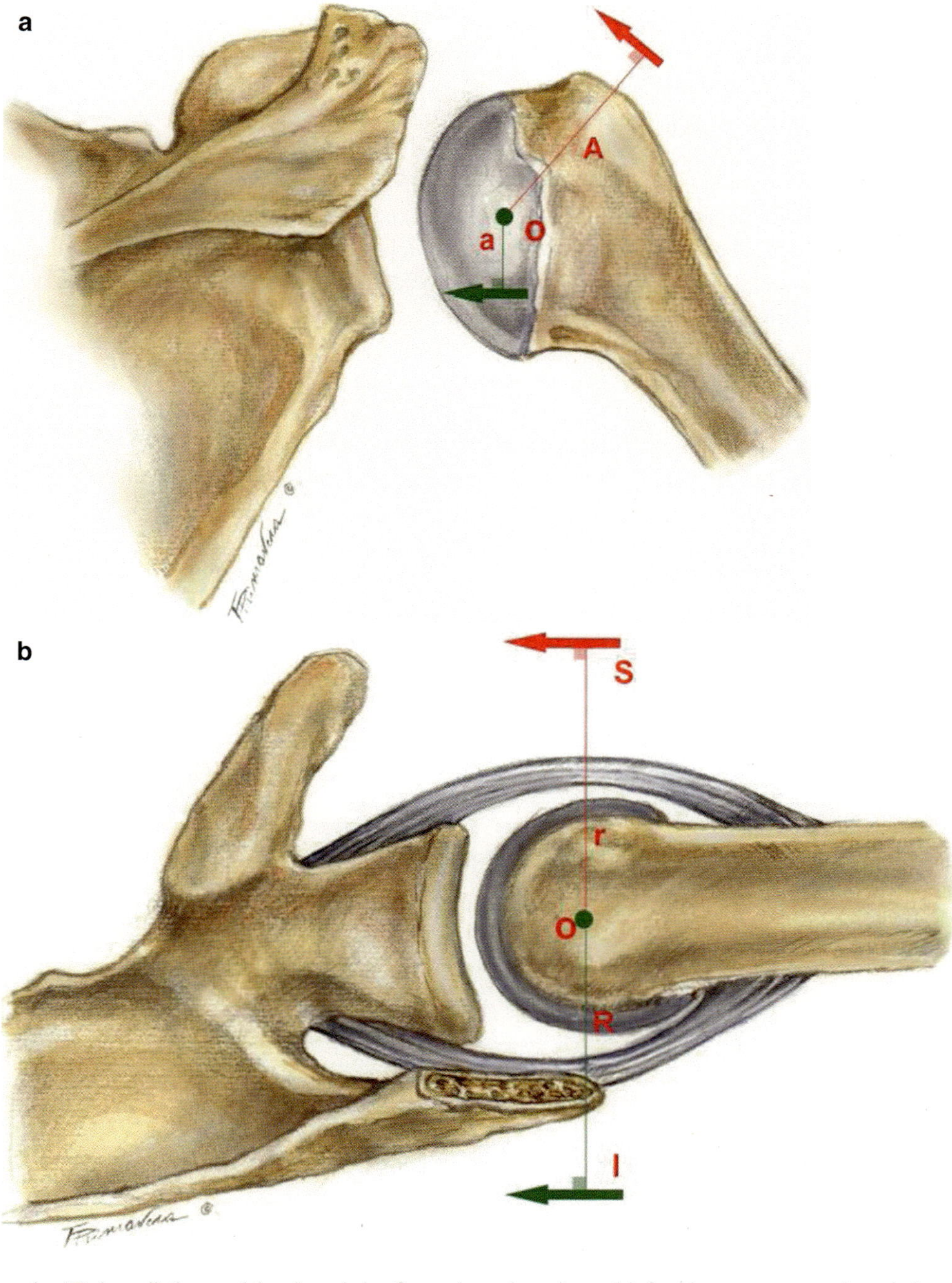

Fig. 1.15 (**a**) Note the "*Fulcrum*" (humeral head) and the Coronal plane force couple ("a" and "A"). "o" correspond to the centre of rotation. (**b**) Transverse plane force couple(S,I). The anatomic and functional integrity of the cuff and of the tuberosities (subscapolaris-lesser tuberosity and infraspinatus- greater tuberosity) represents the glenohumeral "Engine" "b" transverse plane force couple. "o" correspond to the centre of rotation. "R" and "r" corresponds to the ray. "s" and "I" corresponds to the subscapolaris and infraspinatus couple force.

By a rotator cable that works as a stress shielding, a supraspinatus muscle even with a tendon tear can still exert its compressive effect on the shoulder joint by means of its distributed load along the span of the suspension bridge configuration [32].

For this reason, the integrity of the rotator cuff, the infraspinatus and its insertion (greater tuberosity) and the subscapularis and its insertion (lesser tuberosity), represents the "engine."

The anatomical integrity of the *fulcrum* (humeral head) and *engine* (the greater and the lesser tuberosity) are essential to ensure the movement of the glenohumeral joint and therefore of the shoulder.

The functional integrity of the cuff and of the tuberosities (subscapularis, lesser tuberosity, infraspinatus, greater tuberosity) represents the glenohumeral *engine*.

Proximal humeral fractures that affect the head can temporally compromise the "fulcrum," and in case of aseptic necrosis or comminution, it can affect the function of the joint over time (*loss of fulcrum* that can be replaced by a prosthetic element) (Fig. 1.16a, b).

Proximal humeral fractures that affect the insertions of the rotator cuff (lesser tuberosity and greater tuberosity) temporarily compromise the "engine" and, in case of poor healing and bone reabsorption, can affect the function over time (*loss of engine*). It results in a severe damaging event that, from the biomechanical point of view, may be partially replaced by a reverse prosthesis (Fig. 1.17a, b).

We cannot retain valid the functional biomechanics of the shoulder without the following conditions:

- Adequate neuromuscular patterns and proprioception of the scapulothoracic joint
- Integrity of the rotator cuff and of its osseous insertions (integrity of "engine")
- Integrity of the articular surfaces (integrity of "fulcrum": head and glenoid surface)
- Synergistic action between the subscapularis and the infraspinatus which have to guarantee a sufficient balance to stabilize the "fulcrum"
- A well-functioning deltoid muscle that interacts with the cuff during elevation of the arm [33–35]

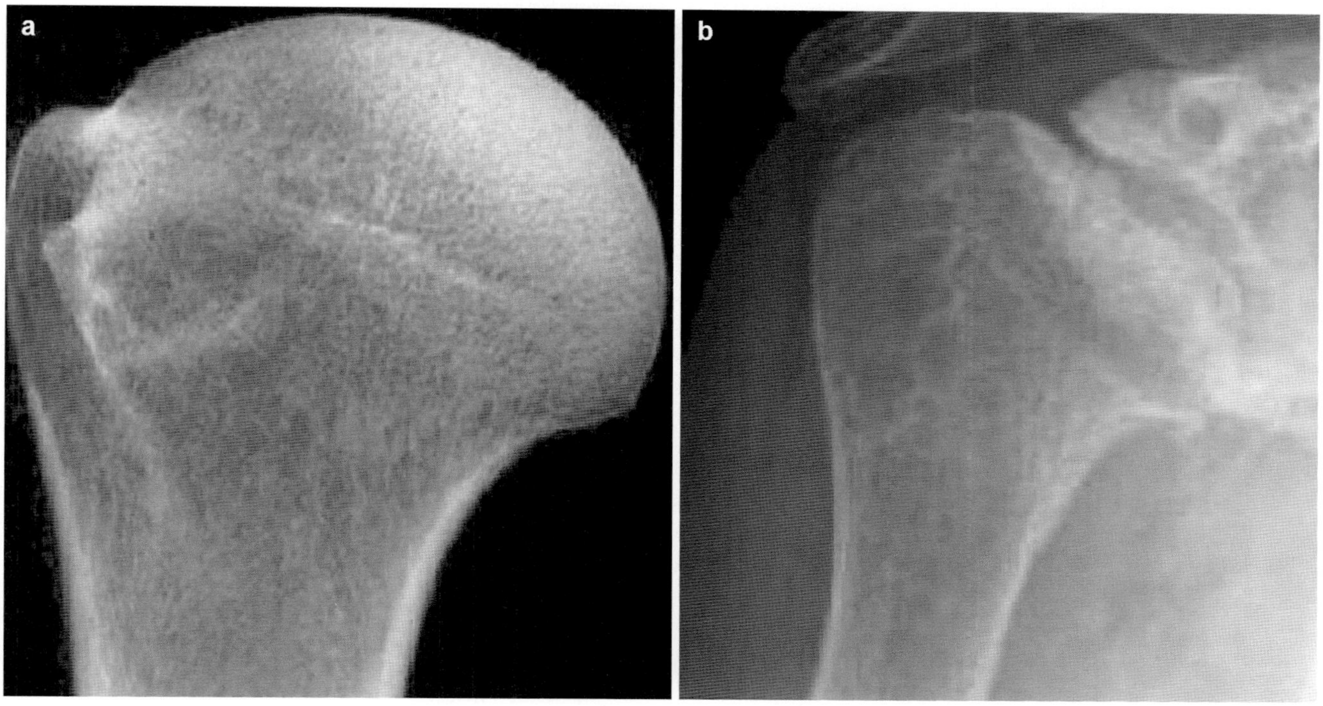

Fig. 1.16 (**a**) Normal humeral head → FULCRUM. (**b**) Aseptic necrosis of the humeral head → LOSS OF FULCRUM

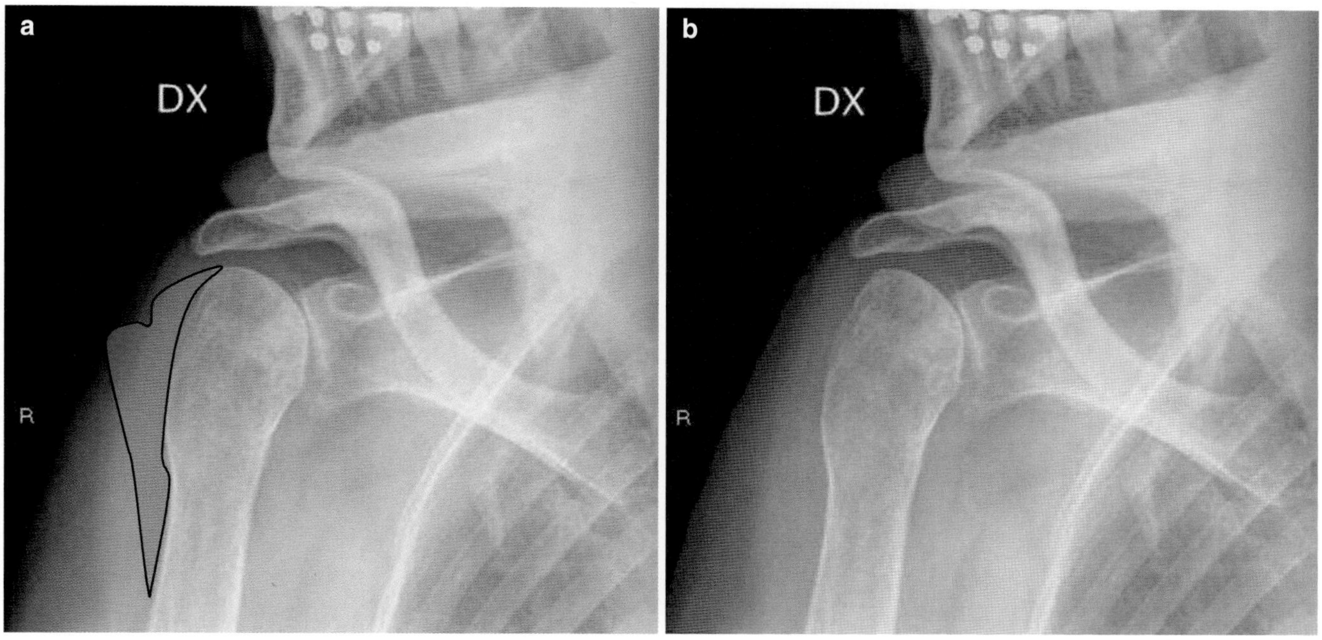

Fig. 1.17 (**a**) Greater tuberosity in *green* → ENGINE dx: right side. (**b**) Reabsorption of greater tuberosity sequelae of PHF → LOSS OF ENGINE

1.4 Conservative Treatment

Nonoperative management is best suited for those fractures that have a high chance of union and will be amenable to an adequate outcome for each specific patient.

These fractures are commonly those in a *stable configuration* and which exhibit *minimal displacement* (<30° varus/valgus angulation of the diaphyseal shaft in relation to the humeral head) (Fig. 1.18).

Conservative management routinely consists of a brief period of immobilization in a sling (from one to three weeks), in order to attain adequate pain control, prior to mobilization under the guidance of physiotherapist (Fig. 1.19).

It is common for a patient to find comfort in resting in the sitting position and this may even extend to times of sleep, particular early on in the fracture healing process.

It should be reiterated to the patient and associated carers alike that prolonged period of immobility is detrimental to the outcome [36].

Shorter periods of immobilization are associated with lower pain scores in the short term; however, at 6 months, there is no difference [37].

More recently, Lefevre-Colau and colleagues found that early mobilization for impact proximal humerus fractures was safe and more effective for performance restoration than a period of immobilization as traditional teaching would suggest [38].

When considering the extent and duration of initial immobilization after fractures, a balance is needed between the advantages of pain relief and avoidance of fracture displacement, as the consequence of immobilization are notably joint stiffness and muscle atrophy.

There is limited evidence that the particular type of bandage used neither influences the time to fracture union nor the functional end result, although an arm sling is found to be generally more comfortable than a body bandage [39].

Patients should be followed with serial radiographs at two weeks (prior to initiation of motion) and then again at 4–6 weeks to ensure fracture stability [40].

Take-Home Message
When conservative treatment is indicated?

- Stable configuration
- Minimal displacement
- No vascular risk

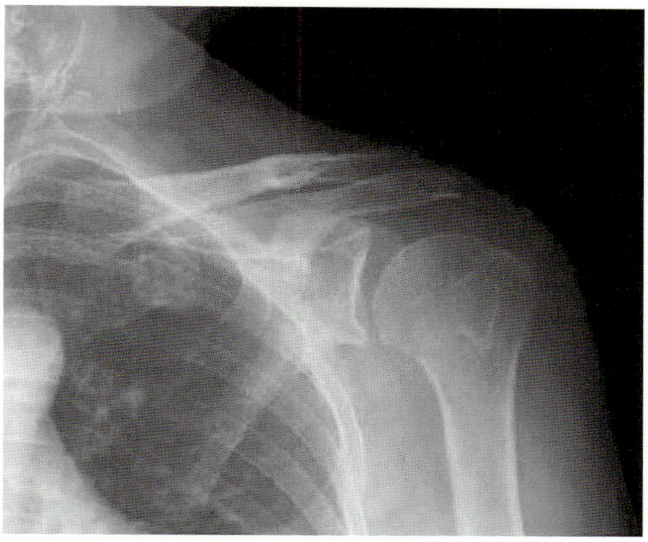

Fig. 1.18 Rx of stable configuration fracture

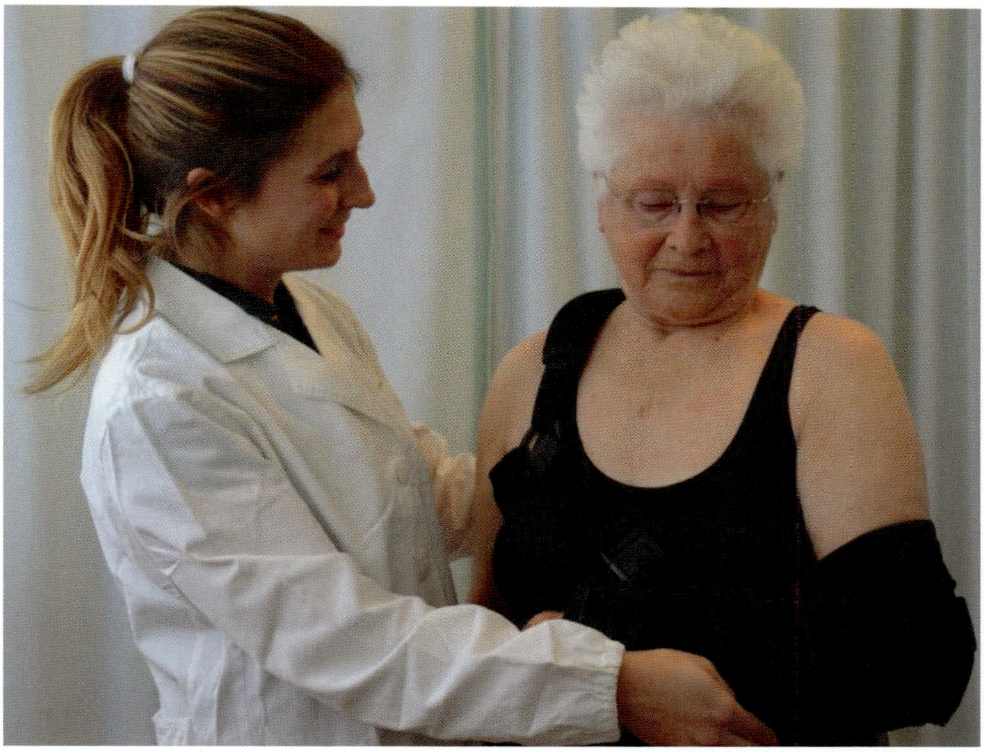

Fig. 1.19 Rest in sling

1.4.1 Rehabilitation in Conservative Treatment

The shoulder is likely the one joint more than any other for which rehabilitation represents a true challenge both with the conservative approach and after surgical ones.

It is universally recognized that non-displaced fractures can be treated conservatively. In these fractures, the surrounding soft tissues are generally intact, and the periosteum, rotator cuff, and joint capsule serve to stabilize the fracture.

Valgus-impacted fractures are also a good indication for conservative treatment.

The conservative treatment of non-displaced or mildly displaced fractures generally yields good results.

Rehabilitation in conservative treatment after PHF is influenced by a variety of factors, in particular the age of the patient.

Consider that in young patients it can be on an accelerated protocol based on maintaining the validity of the different links of the kinetic chain and adding, after healing is completed, the glenohumeral link to the chain as Kibler learns [70].

On the other hand, different is the treatment of the same fracture in the category of patients that are more frequently the victims of this pathology: the peri-/postmenopausal women and men over 70.

In these cases, once a course of rehabilitation is chosen, it is essential to keep in consideration the associated comorbidities, in particular musculoskeletal.

A treatment which is too aggressive could in fact bring out cervical or low back disease, pathological fractures, etc., complicating and stunting recovery.

We want to pay attention to these elements to underline that as well as the correct approach to the specific treatment of the fracture is important, the accuracy of the information gathered from the patient is essential too.

1.4.2 When to Begin Physiotherapy

In literature, when to begin physiotherapy is very controversial; in our experience, besides the patients' age and comorbidities, *the key points are*:

- The stability of the fracture (patterns)
- Quality of the bone
- Compliance of the patient

The following week-based rehabilitation protocol for conservative treatment, ORIF (Open Reduction Internal Fixation), hemiarthroplasty, and reverse shoulder arthroplasty gives a general indication of the time frames involved. The timetable may have to be varied to a greater or lesser extent depending on individual tissue healing times (implant-bone, bone-bone, tendon-bone, etc.) *that must be monitored by imaging techniques and clinical assessment by the surgical team and weighed against the often patient-specific response to rehabilitation.*

Usually we advise to begin *no earlier than one week* immediately after the trauma (*one week off therapy).*

This is important for pain control and also because of the motional patient's adaptation to this new situation, especially in the older one. On the other hand, *we advise not to begin rehab more than three weeks after the trauma* to avoid capsular contracture, muscle atrophy, and loss of the postural control (Table 1.6) [41].

Table 1.6

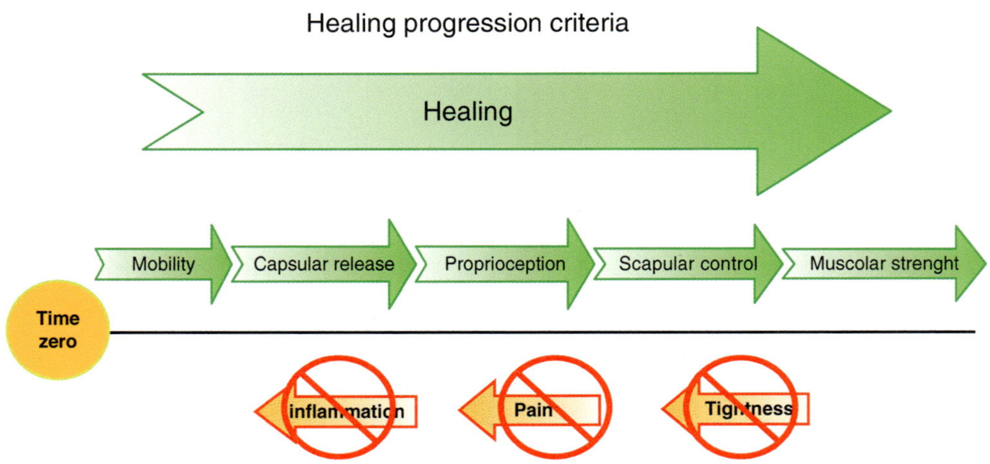

1.4.3 Healing Progression Criteria

According to this, the protocol is divided into *three sections* of work:

1. *Early management (0–4 weeks)* Goal → Pain control and progressive recovery of range of motion (ROM); this phase includes some different steps:
   - *Control pain and inflammation* with immobilization, modalities, analgesics, and nonsteroidal anti-inflammatory drugs.

     Pain, during rehab program, is one of the key points because all the exercises have to be relatively pain-free. It's difficult to progress a painful joint and it is a sign that either the wrong exercise is being done for that time in the recovery process or it is being done improperly.
   - The *education* to prevent inappropriate shoulder movement patterns.
   - *Pain-free passive shoulder flexion on scapular plane exercise* until evidence of fracture healing is present. Early joint mobilization plays an important role in the rehabilitation of the injured shoulder for the return of normal kinematics and shoulder function, avoiding capsular contracture. Prolonged immobilization may predispose patients to muscle atrophy and poor neuromuscular control (Figs. 1.20, 1.21, and 1.22) [71].
   - *Codman's pendulum exercises* (when there is evidence of fracture healing): gravity-assisted pendulum exercises are commonly prescribed after PHF to provide decreased pain, increased flow of nutrients into the joint space, and early joint mobilization [73].

     Shoulder protocols, as well as Codman [72–78] himself, suggest that weight may be added to these pendulum exercises as rehabilitation progresses. In the early management, we suggest to not use weight to avoid compromising the fracture's fragment stabilization.

     The exercise have to follow specific postural conditions: the degree to which the trunk is flexed at the hips have to be, as traditional protocol [72], of *90°* to allow the arm to be in perpendicular line to the ground and not subjected to cutting forces.

     There are different movements that we can ask to the patient: lean over the table, and support body with the uninvolved arm. Let the involved arm hang straight down in a relaxed position; gently swing arm in *circles, clockwise and counterclockwise*, then in a pendulum motion *forward-backward and side to side* (Fig. 1.23a, b).
   - *Scapular control exercises* [70]: after the trauma, we have to pay attention to avoid losing the correct scapular kinematics and to maintain the correct scapular rhythm with exercises that do not necessarily require motion of the shoulder. Restoration of the normal posture and scapular retraction, after the trauma, should be achieved in an upright position with the feet on the ground so as to restore normal physiology and proprioception. All exercises should be initiated with the patient in the "ideal position," with good postural alignment, the pelvis leveled, and the scapular retracted and depressed [74, 75].

     Once the healing process of the fracture has been accomplished, glenohumeral rehabilitation can proceed, with restoration of capsular mobility and rotator cuff activation to restore normal concavity/compression.

     The scapular control is crucial to regain the correct range of motion, being the scapular balance essential to the arms' elevation (proximal stability to distal mobility) (Fig. 1.24).

2. *Intermediate management (4–8 weeks)* Goal → active mobility recovery and to regain complete range of motion.

   It is preferable, in our experience, to have the patient due a little bit frequently rather than overloading muscle tendon units, ligaments, and callus progression. It is more important that patients progress steadily than that they reach landmarks at specific times. The rationale and the quality of the exercise are more important than the quantity being performed.

Exercises have to be done until the muscles fatigue which is when mechanics become abnormal, rather than completing a specified number of sets and repetitions. Progression from submaximal to maximal effort over the course of the program is desirable. The preferred progression in strengthening is isometric to eccentric to concentric training. Closed-chain precedes open-chain exercise. As more exercises are added, the easier ones should be eliminated to prevent boredom on the part of the patient.

This phase includes some steps:

- *Supervised active/assisted shoulder exercise* in the supine position: the regain passive motion is the start point to ask to our patient to begin to make this movement in auto- assisted way. The reason is the importance of the recovery of the functional motion and of the muscle activation. The supine position is preferable to maintain a low activation of upper trapezius during exercises and avoid scapular improper movements. In addition, the patient, especially after the trauma, prefers the lying position to relax the back during the new proposed exercises. In this specific kind of exercise, doing the exercise in lying position helps the patient to regain the range of motion beyond 90°, because we have used gravity on purpose to help the patient to guide the arm to the maximal range of motion out of pain (Figs. 1.25, 1.26, and 1.27) [76–98].
- Light functional exercises without exacerbating pain.
- Use a gentle massage therapy for muscles pain relief (Fig. 1.28) [81, 82, 85].

3. *Late management* (after XR follow-up) Goal is to regain the shoulder functional mobility and strength. This phase includes some steps:
   - Passive stretching of any remaining soft tissue tightness, usually abduction/external rotation and adduction/internal rotation: in this phase we have to regain the last degrees of motion and we can use a more aggressive approach (pain-free) (Figs. 1.20, 1.21, and 1.22).
   - Isometric rotator cuff muscle activation (Fig. 1.29a, b) [79, 80].
   - Progressing to full activity against gravity.
   - Increase focus on isotonic strengthening, restoring upper extremity motion into the kinetic chain.

The perils of nonunion, symptomatic malunion, and avascular necrosis of the humeral head are the main protagonists in preventing a positive outcome.

Table 1.7 Conservative treatment of proximal humeral fractures

Week	Treatment
1st	Gilchrist arm sling, Elbow and hand exercise
2nd–3rd	Pendulum exercises Scapular control exercises
4th–7th	Progressive active assisted physiotherapy
8th	Free mobilization

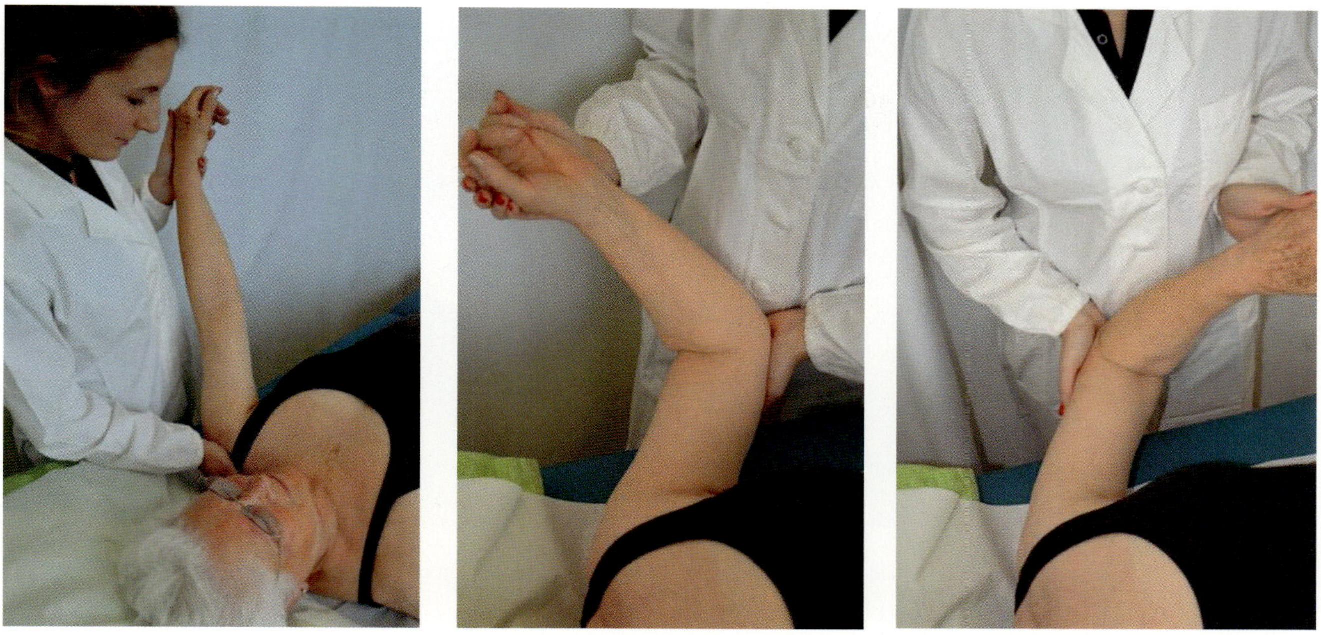

Figs. 1.20, 1.21, and 1.22 Passive shoulder flexion/abduction and external/internal rotation in pain-free stretching

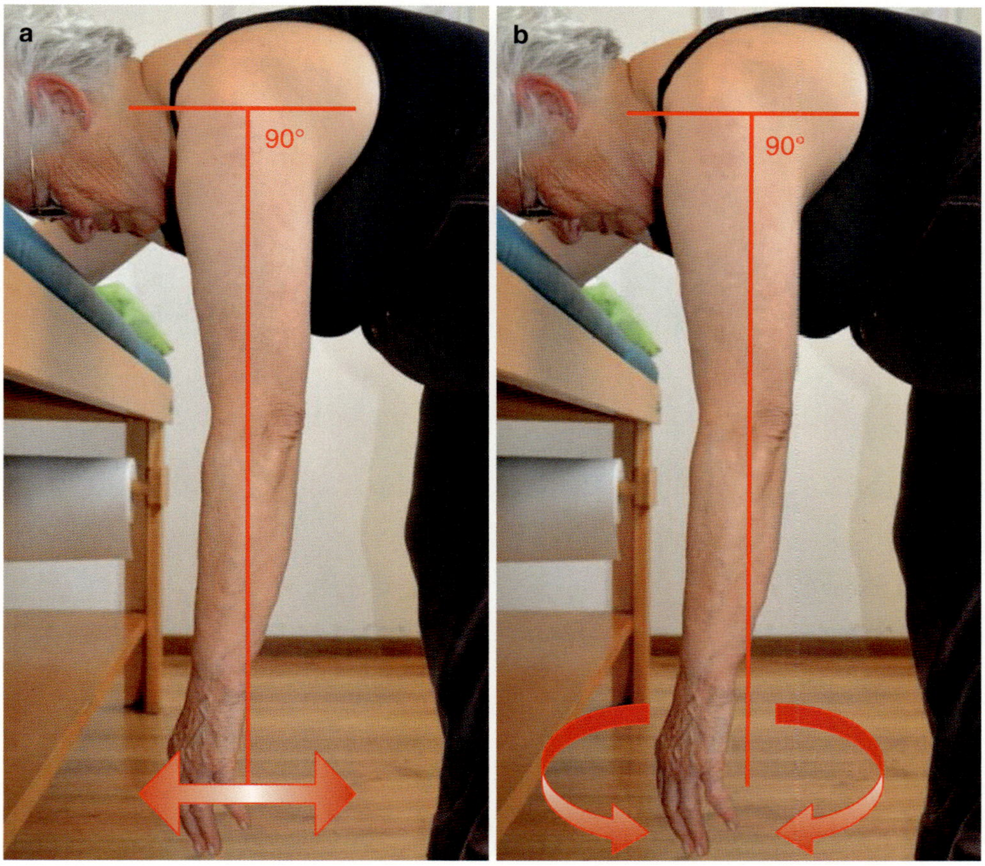

Fig. 1.23 (**a**, **b**) Codman's pendulum exercises → gently swing arm in circles clockwise and counterclockwise, forward- backward and side-to-side

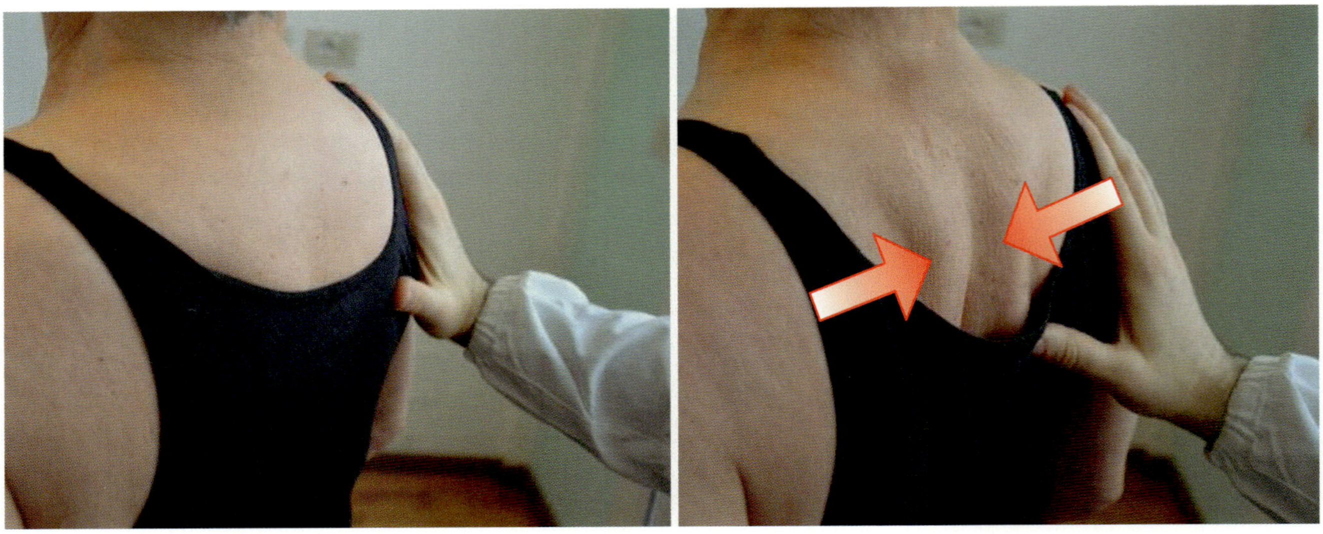

Fig. 1.24 Basic Scapular control exercise → close the scapula emphasizing the lower trapezium contraction

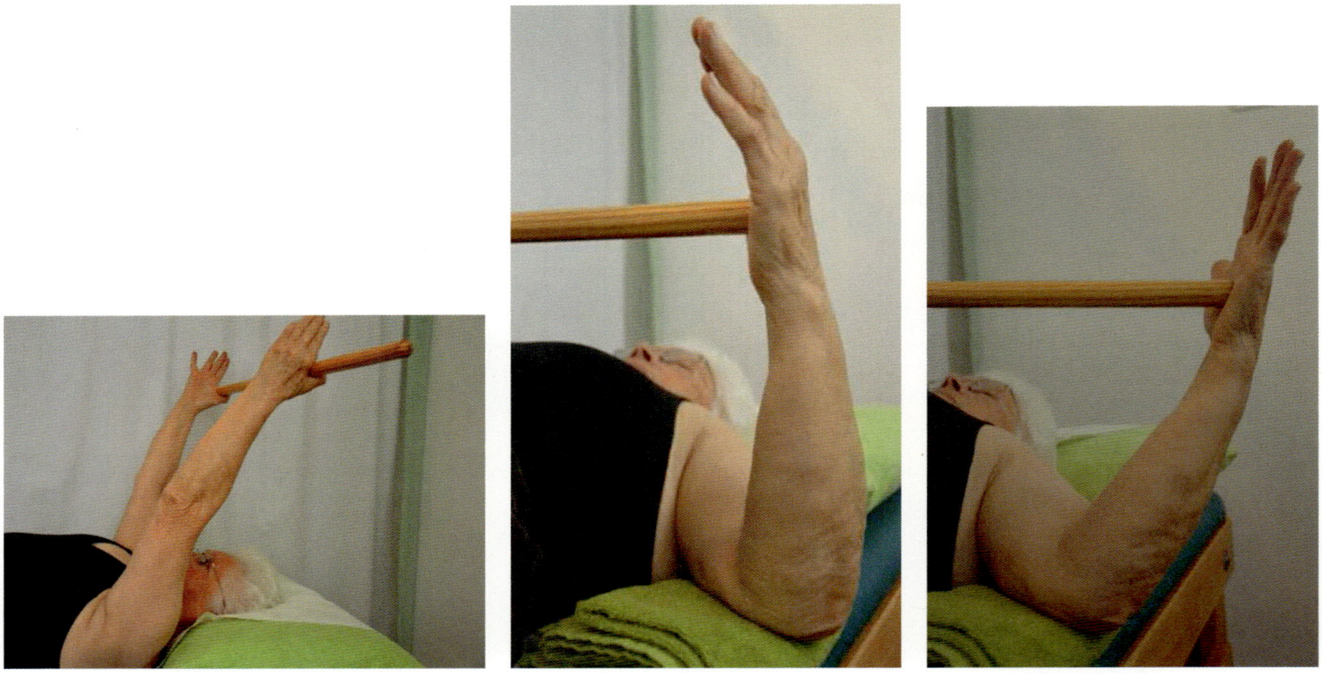

Figs. 1.25, 1.26, and 1.27 Supervised passive and active- assisted exercises in supine position made to increase ROM

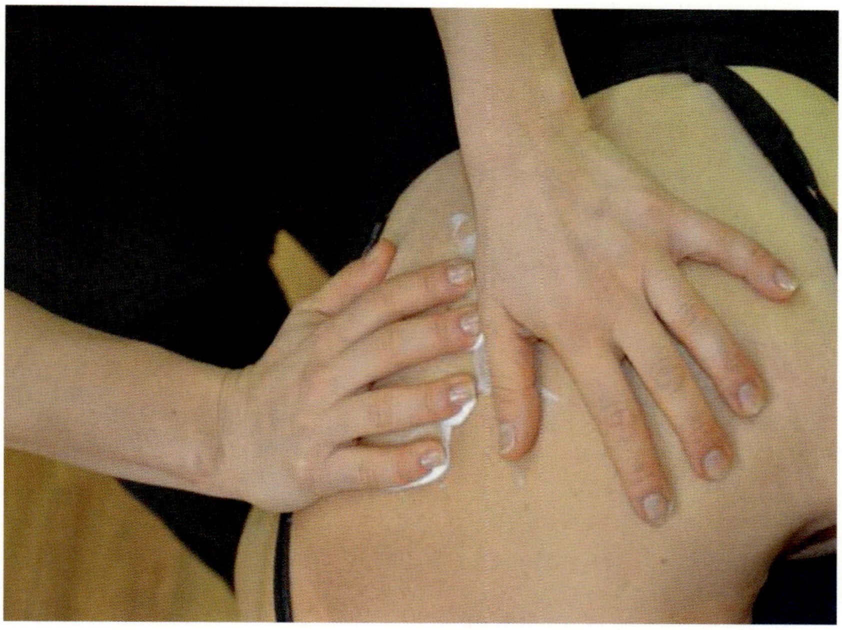

Fig. 1.28 Use a gentle massage therapy for muscle pain relief and to reduce tissue tightness [81, 82, 85]

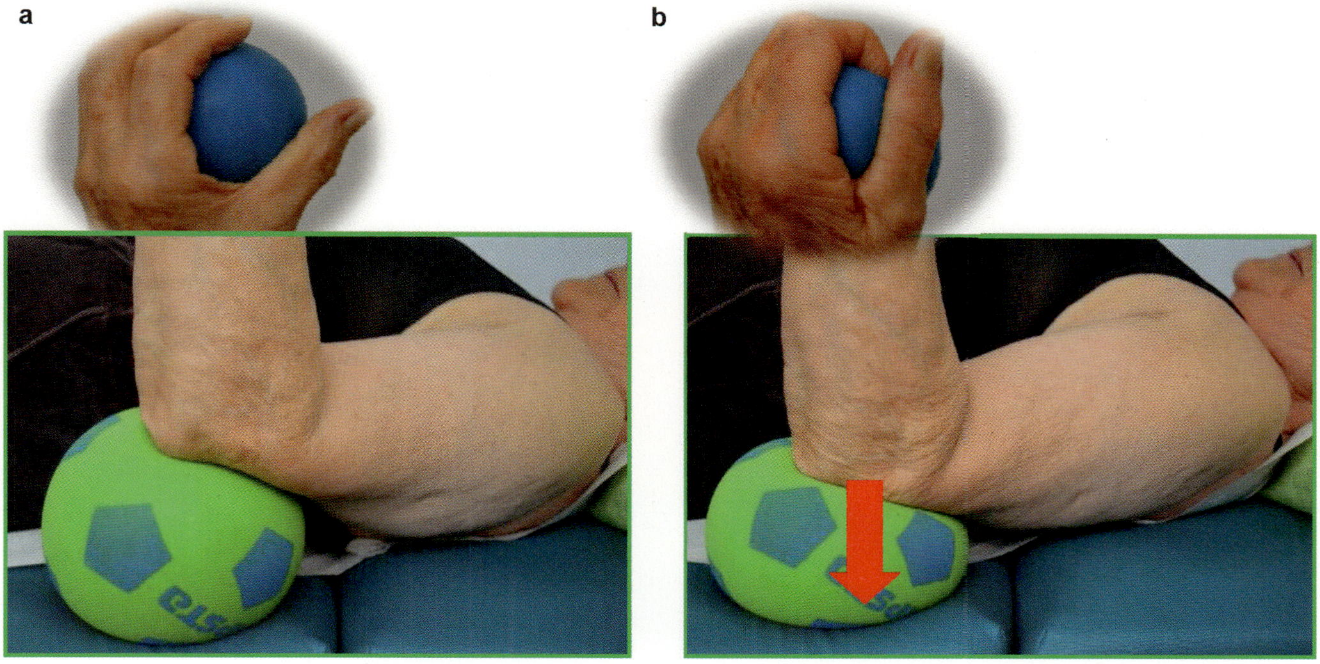

Fig. 1.29 (**a**, **b**) *Double press exercise* → Push the elbow against the ball maintaining the scapula in the correct retracted position and, at the same time, press the ball with the hand. The isometric exercise is important to increase the muscles strength safeguarding the tendon structures [79, 80]

1.5 When to Choose Surgical Treatment?

In *decision-making*, patient expectations are important:

- Young individuals who need to regain preexisting levels of functional requirements
- Elderly patients who wish to resume their activities and their functional autonomy
- Reduction and internal fixation may be indicated in about 20 % of cases comprising both standards under the following condition:
  - Tuberosities are displaced over 10 mm.
  - Risk factors for avascular necrosis (see above vascular patterns).

1.5.1 Surgical Treatments

Ideally the following should be applied:

- The principle reconstruction of the articular fracture.
- The head and tuberosities should be carefully repositioned to avoid weakness due to shortening of musculotendinous units and a decreased moment arm.
- Restoration of the anatomy and stable fixation.
- Stable fixation avoids stiffness to allow immediate passive treatment so that adhesive scarring is limited and recovery of function is possible with minimal muscle atrophy.
- Respect of the soft tissue and the vascular supply.

Surgical approach and the *type of implant* depend on the pattern of the fracture, the quality of the bone encountered (osteoporosis, pathologic fractures), the patient's goals, and the surgeon's familiarity with the techniques.

An adequate surgical technique will minimize complications and an accelerated rehabilitation regime, if possible, will ensure the best possible result [33].

The two main operative approaches are:

- *The deltopectoral approach* (Fig. 1.30a)
- *The lateral trans-deltoid* (AO) (Fig. 1.30b)

Take-Home Message

The influence of the surgical approach, if rightly performed, from the rehabilitation point of view doesn't have a great consequence because the *deltopectoral approach* creates a cleavage between the deltoid and pectoralis major.

The *lateral trans-deltoid* approach, used for isolated tuberosity fractures, creates a cleavage across the deltoid raphe, so it doesn't create any iatrogenic lesion.

Dedicated attention has to be payed to the execution of this approach, concerning the distal extension of the deltoid cleavage that can't be more than 4 cm from the lateral border of the acromion to avoid the axillary nerve that could drastically irreversibly compromise the functional recovery.

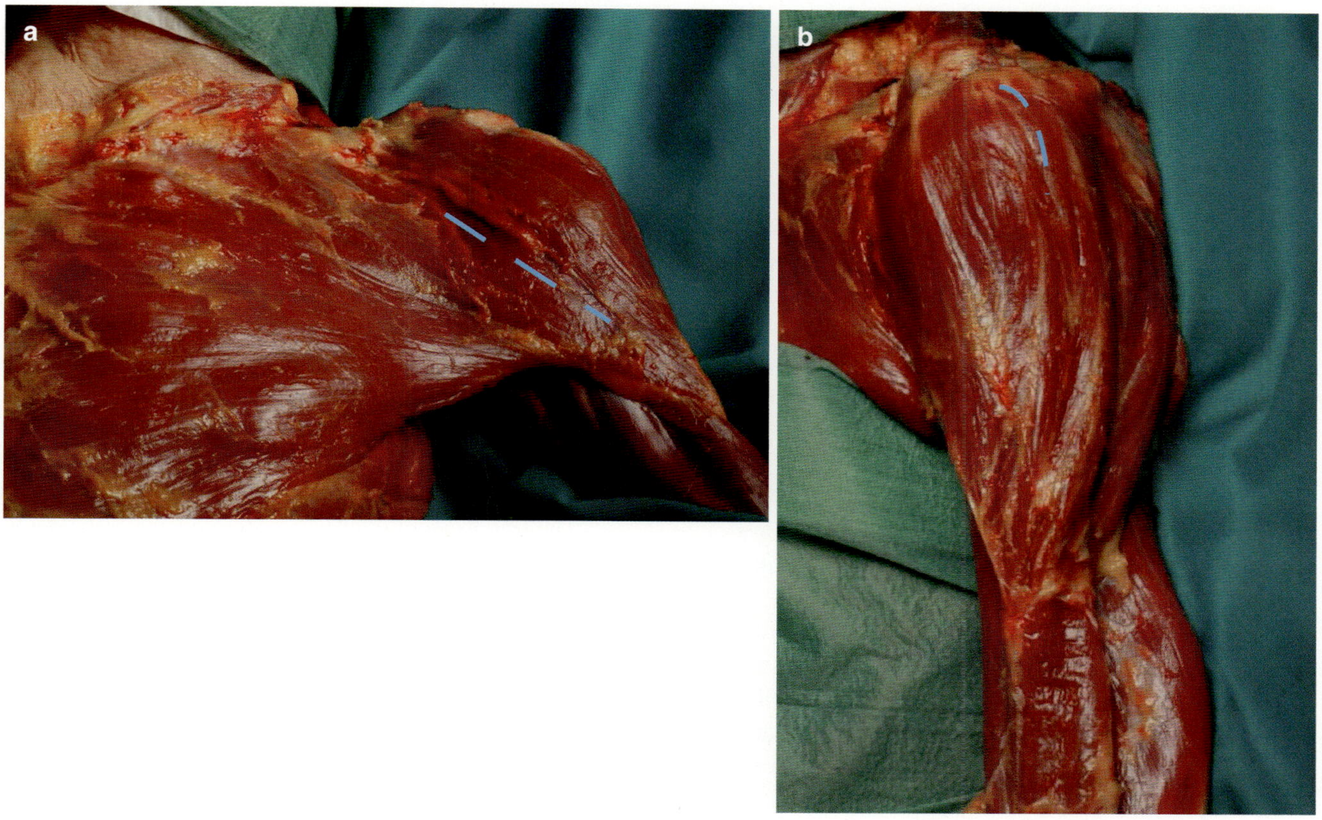

Fig. 1.30 (**a**) Delto-pectoral approach (blue line). (**b**) Lateral trans deltoid approach (blue line)

Reduction and Internal Fixation: Treatment Options

- *Transosseous fixation* → is indicated for two-part greater tuberosity fractures and also when a surgical neck fracture exists [42].

  Nonabsorbable sutures are used to capture rotator cuff tissue fragments anteriorly, laterally, and posteriorly.

  The displaced humeral head or greater tuberosity are reduced and fixated to the shaft through drill holes or suture anchors [43].
- *Closed reduction and percutaneous stabilization* → is a minimally invasive technique with limited indications. Amenable fracture patterns include 2-part proximal humerus fractures, ideally of the surgical neck, and 3- or 4-part fractures with adequate bone stock.

  Theoretically, this technique limits iatrogenic vascular compromise, postoperative pain, operative time, and blood loss while improving aesthetics.
- *Intramedullary fixation* → These devices can be used for fixation of 2-, 3-, and 4- part fractures. Most successful outcomes occur in 2-part fractures. Intramedullary nail fixation with indirect reduction has the benefit of decreased soft tissue stripping. Some surgeons are reticent about intramedullary nailing in the younger patient due to reported rotator cuff damage and persistent shoulder pain. This can be minimized by meticulous placement of the entry point, avoiding the footprint of the supraspinatus tendon. Ensuring the nail is well buried under the bone also helps prevent postoperative discomfort and subsequent need for nail removal.

  Complications of intramedullary nailing include screw penetration, nail impingement, hardware migration, and failure of fixation (Fig. 1.31a–d).

- *Open reduction and internal fixation with locked plate* (Fig. 1.32a–c). Indications have expanded with the introduction of locking plate technology.

Newer designs of implants (*l*ocking *c*ompression *pl*ate) have screwheads which lock into the plate, thus allowing angular stability of the screws in relation to the plate. This type of implant gives improved stability and may therefore speed bony healing and functional recovery.

Initial data on the specific locked fixation devices plate nearly eliminated complications due to hardware failure and subacromial impingement with good functional outcomes if correct surgical technique is employed.

Osteosynthesis is indicated for 2-, 3-, and 4-part fractures in appropriate patients (Fig. 1.33a).

Exceptions include some 4-part fractures, head-splitting fractures, and fracture-dislocations, which are candidates for prosthetic replacement.

The fragments of the fracture must be carefully identified and tagged with stay sutures at the tendon-bone interface using the long head of biceps as a landmark.

Usually it will be possible to reposition the fragment of the head on the metaphysis and to obtain provisional fixation with Kirschner wires.

This is especially true of fractures which are aligned in varus, while in valgus-impacted fractures, if the impaction is extreme, the head may be unimpacted and held in place by an intercalated bone graft.

In this situation, and when using this technique, care must be taken not to disturb the soft tissue attachments of the medial head-neck junction, as reported previously it is in this area that the medial circumflex artery penetrates the humeral head and this tissue may carry the remaining good supply.

The greater and/or lesser tuberosities are also reduced and a contoured T-plate is applied, taking care not to injure the long head of biceps.

Screws are then inserted and the suture bays are either removed or tied into the plate holes or transosseously (Fig. 1.33b).

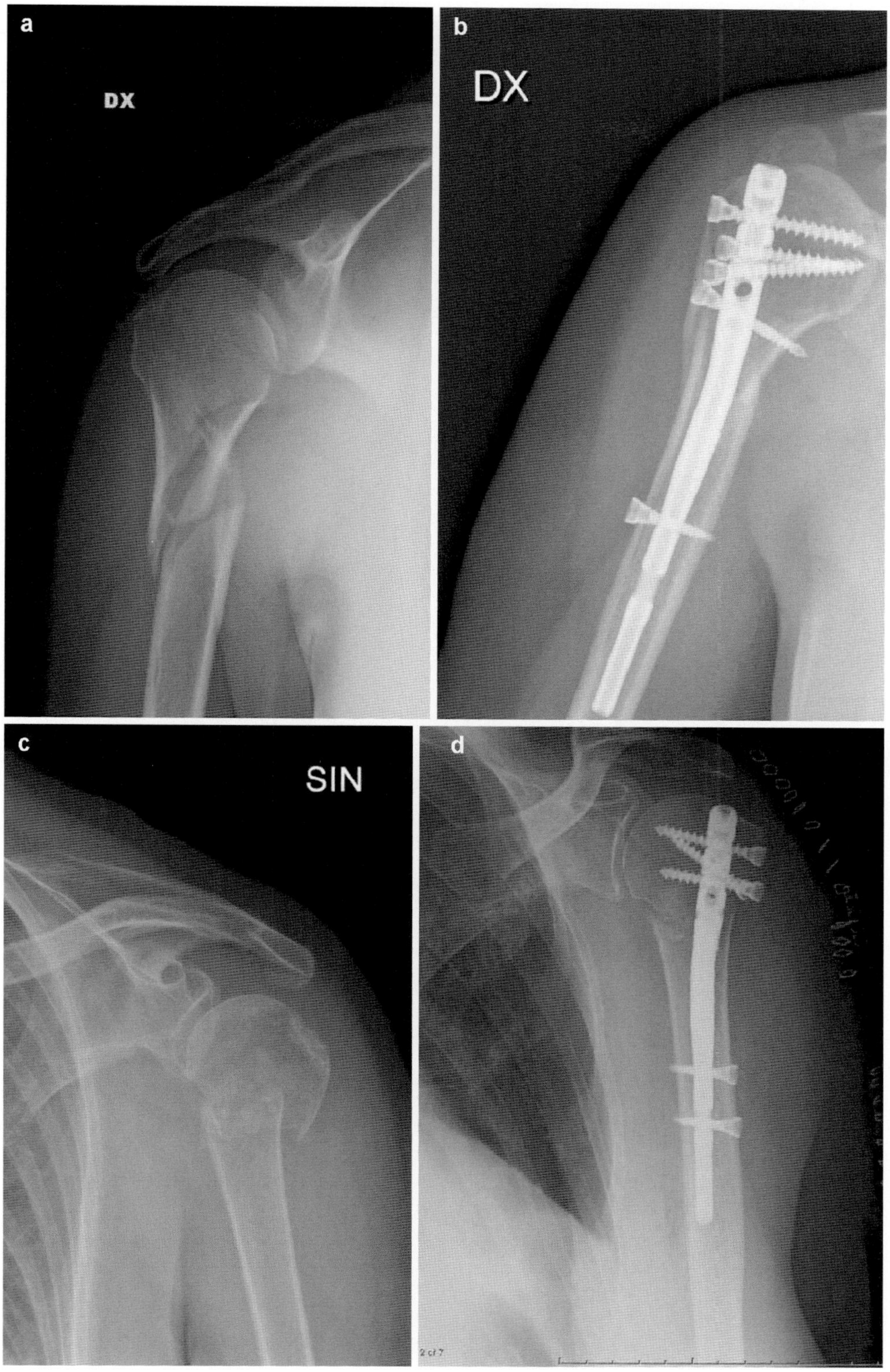

Fig. 1.31 (**a**, **b**) PHF with integrity of the tuberosities and intramedullary fixation. (**c**, **d**) Valgus fracture and intramedullary fixation. dx: right side sx: left side

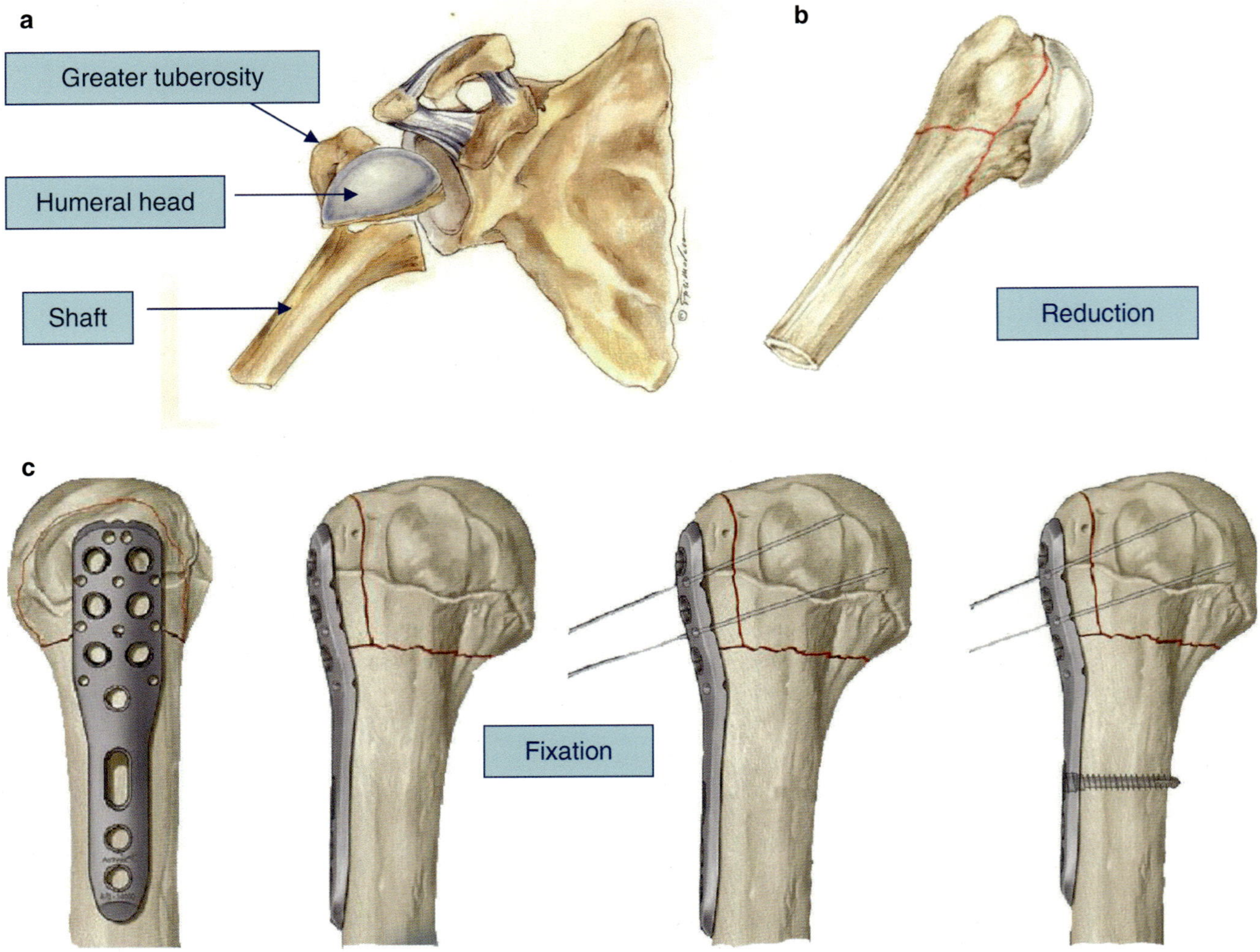

Fig. 1.32 (**a**) PHF. (**b**) Open reduction of the PHF. (**c**) ORIF internal fixation with locked plate

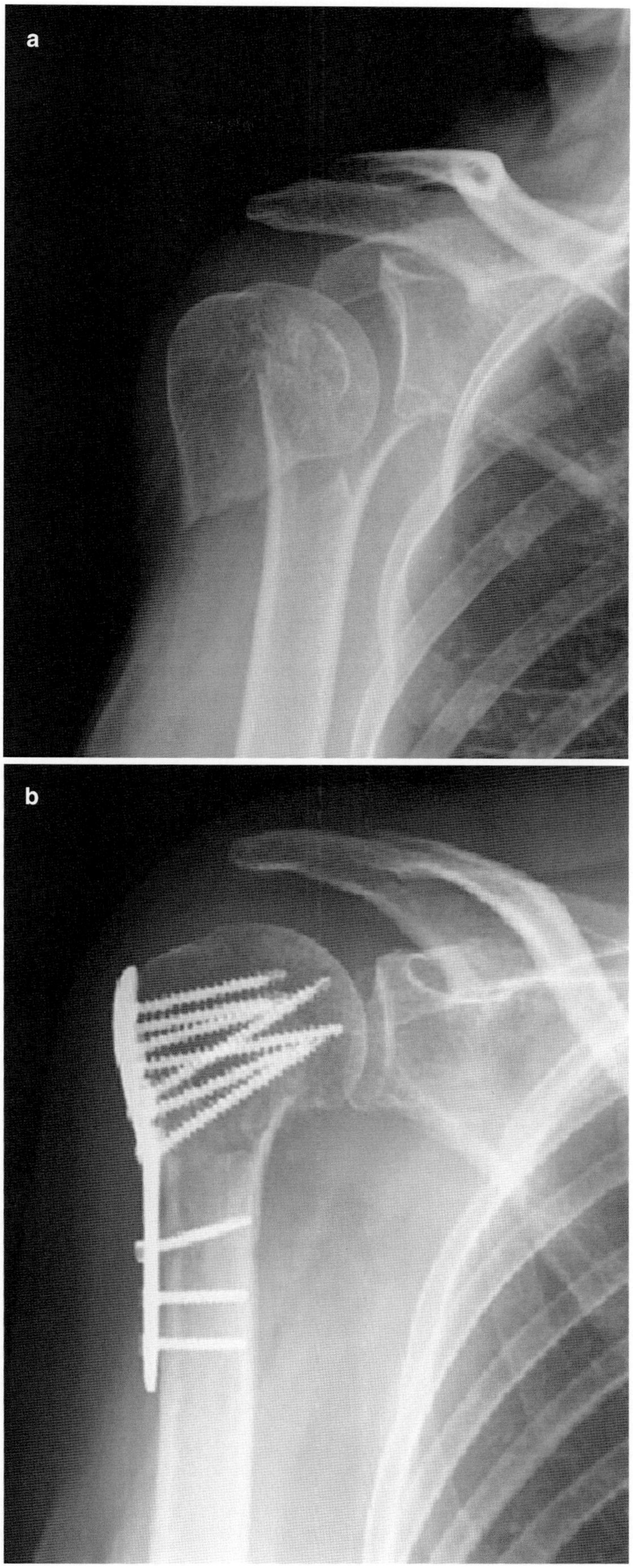

Fig. 1.33 (**a**) PHF with medial displacement of the shaft. (**b**) ORIF with locked plate

Hemiarthroplasty

Hemiarthroplasty for proximal humerus fractures is a good surgical option for low-demand elderly patients or fractures that are not amenable to *ORIF* (*o*pen *r*eduction *i*nternal *f*ixation).

Significant controversy exists as to the best surgical intervention for 3- or 4-part fractures in the elderly osteoporotic patient (Fig. 1.34a, b) [44].

These patients have been shown to have significantly less pain after hemiarthroplasty compared with nonoperative treatment, although range of motion is similar [45].

Patients who present with initial varus angulation greater than 30° are at increased risk for fixation failure, and thus hemiarthroplasty may decrease their need for reoperation [46].

Further, fracture-dislocations may do poorly following osteosynthesis and thus should be treated with arthroplasty, except in the young patients.

It is also important to consider the degree of underlying shoulder pathology, including symptomatic glenohumeral osteoarthritis or rotator cuff arthropathy; if present, these could potentially predispose the patient to poor outcomes following osteosynthesis.

Thus, the presence of osteoarthritis or rotator cuff pathology should influence the surgeon's choice away from ORIF and toward either hemiarthroplasty or reverse total shoulder arthroplasty.

Hemiarthroplasty : the prosthetic element restore the *fulcrum* and the healing of anatomic tuberosity enables a functional rotator cuff (*engine*) and is critical for patient satisfaction and functional outcomes following hemiarthroplasty.

Boileau et al. found that tuberosity malpositioning occurred in half of all patients who underwent hemiarthroplasty for PHF. This was also highly correlated with unsatisfactory results, prosthesis malalignment, decreased range of motion, and residual pain.

Tuberosity healing and outcomes may be improved by use of a fracture-specific humeral component (79 %) compared with those treated by a conventional stem (66 %) [47].

The mean head-to-tuberosity distance (and standard deviation) should be 8 ± 3 mm as shown by Frankle et al. [48] and Mighell et al. [49].

Treatment of PHF with HEMI is a demanding operation, and many variables, including patient factors, surgical technique, and rehabilitation, can influence outcome after this procedure.

To maximize the probability of an optimal outcome, surgeons should play particular attention to two important goals:

- Restoring the tuberosities to an anatomical position (Fig. 1.35a)
- Placing the humeral component in the correct amount of version and height (Fig. 1.35b)

The importance of anatomical restoration of the tuberosities including secure fixation and restoration of humeral length and retroversion cannot be overemphasized.

Ideally, the humeral implant should have a low-profile lateral fin to facilitate proper positioning and suture fixation of the tuberosity (Fig. 1.36a, b).

Malunion, nonunion, or reabsorption of the tuberosities (Fig. 1.36c) is the most common and perhaps most serious complication that can occur after hemiarthroplasty in displaced PHF (*loss of* "*engine*").

Loss of anatomic landmarks makes the restoration of humeral height difficult. Shortening the humerus decreases the lever arm of the deltoid muscle and therefore decreases the motion and power of the muscle in forward elevation. Lengthening may contribute to superior humeral migration and impingement and/or nonunion of the tuberosities.

Most authors recommend 30–40° of retroversion, typically with use of the bicipital groove as the landmark for orientation of the prosthesis [50], although an individualized approach has been proposed in which the contralateral humerus is used for comparison to estimate the proper amount of retroversion for each patient [51].

The tendency is to position the humeral head in excessive retroversion because of imprecise landmarks and the desire to prevent anterior dislocation. Placement of the head in too much retroversion may lead to excessive posterior rotator cuff tension, suture pullout, and malunion or nonunion of the greater tuberosity. Another point to remember is that restoration of the epiphyseal width is critical to reproduce the soft tissue tension of the deltoid and supraspinatus muscle; the opposite shoulder can be used as a template to gauge the epiphyseal width.

Factors that have been shown to be associated with tuberosity malunion include:

- Poor intraoperative positioning of the prosthesis (excessive height and /or retroversion)
- Initial tuberosity position
- Patient age in excess of 75 years
- Female gender [47]

The optimal timing of hemiarthroplasty is also important.

Most recent reports [49–52] have shown that acute treatment is generally preferable to delayed response because acute hemiarthroplasty is technically easier to perform; however, one study found no difference between early or late treatment when a breakpoint of thirty days after injury was used [53].

There is debate in the literature as to hemiarthroplasty versus reverse total shoulder arthroplasty for acute PHF.

Currently indications for a reverse total shoulder arthroplasty in PHF are limited to rotator cuff deficiency and severe tuberosities comminution with intact axillary nerve (Fig. 1.37a, b).

Recently outcomes showing data comparing hemiarthroplasty with reverse for acute PHF showed superior function in a patient who underwent reverse total shoulder arthroplasty [54, 55].

In a patient where there is concern for tuberosities healing due to comminution, as well in patients with glenohumeral arthritis, a reverse shoulder arthroplasty avoids reliance on the rotator cuff and provides the patient with a functional shoulder.

The role of the surgeon, when he matches with PHF, is to correctly interpret the pattern of the fractures to recognize those risk factors previously described that can compromise the healing of the tuberosities and the humeral head.

When surgery is needed and the general clinical condition of the patient is not critical, the tendency, therefore, is to preserve the anatomy (ORIF).

If the fracture is characterized by a significant comminution of the humeral head (*loss of "fulcrum"*), we opt for a hemiarthroplasty.

With a significant damage of the tuberosities and especially of the greater tuberosity (*loss of "engine"*), the only alternative is the inverse prosthesis that represents the *new "fulcrum"* and the deltoid the *new "engine"* (Fig. 1.38a, b).

Treatment algorithm for PHF based on age

Fisiologic age for PHF →

Legend:
RF = Risk Factor

Age	**Young patients <50**	**Middle age 50–70**	**Elderly >70**
2 part	**Conservative** or **ORIF** according to RF	**Conservative** or **ORIF** according to RF	**Conservative** or **ORIF** according to RF
3 part	**Conservative** or **ORIF** according to RF	**Conservative** or **ORIF** according to RF	**Conservative** or **ORIF** according to RF or **HEMI**
4 part	**Conservative** or **ORIF** according to RF	**Conservative** or **ORIF** according to RF	**Conservative** or **ORIF** according to RF or **HEMI**
5 head split	**ORIF**	**ORIF** vs **HEMI**	**HEMI**
6 fracture dislocation	**ORIF**	**ORIF** vs **HEMI**	**HEMI**

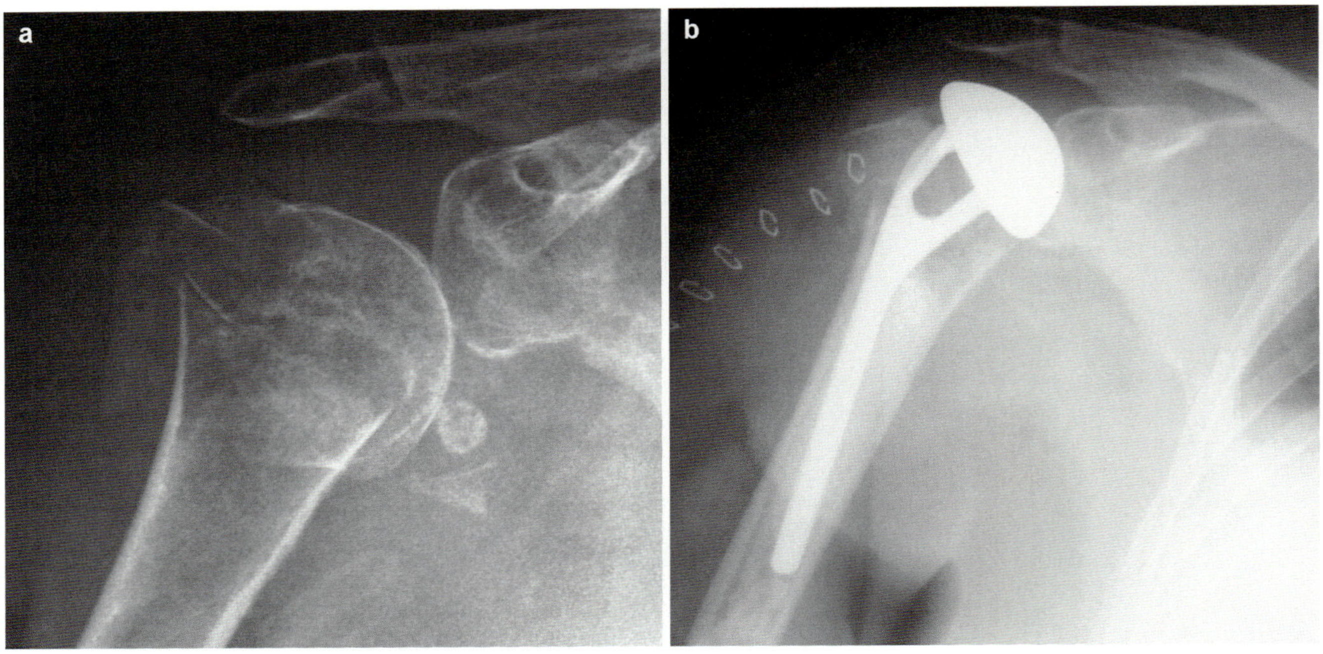

Fig. 1.34 (**a**) PHF in osteoporotic patient. (**b**) Treatment with hemiarthroplasty

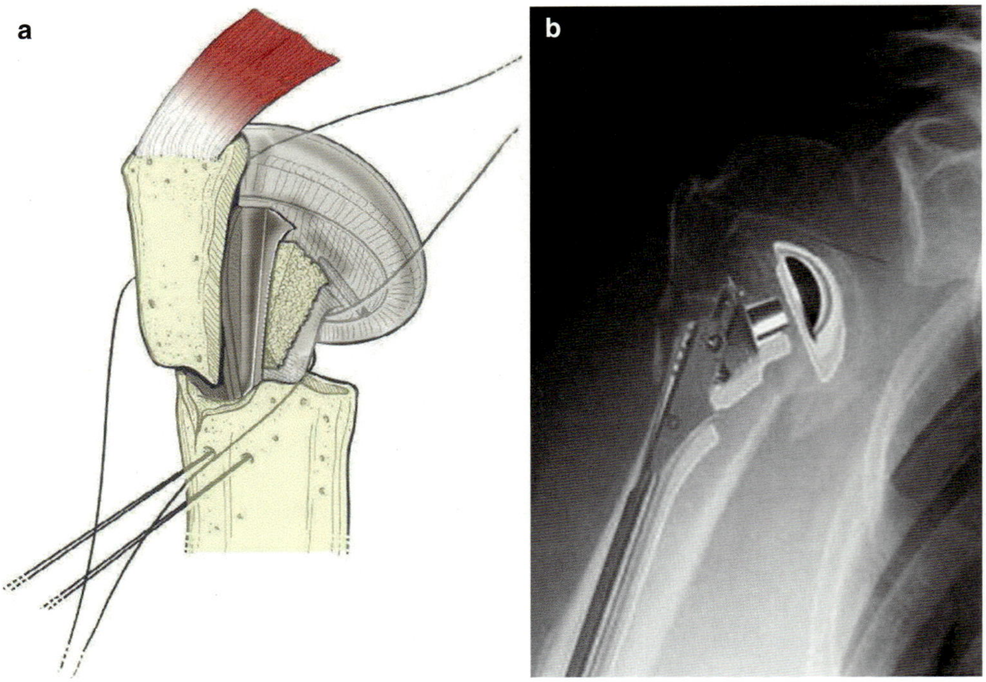

Fig. 1.35 (**a**, **b**) In surgical approach with hemiarthroplasty the healing between the tuberosities and the shaft is crucial to obtain a valid "*engine*" because the "*fulcrum*" is represented by the new prosthetic component

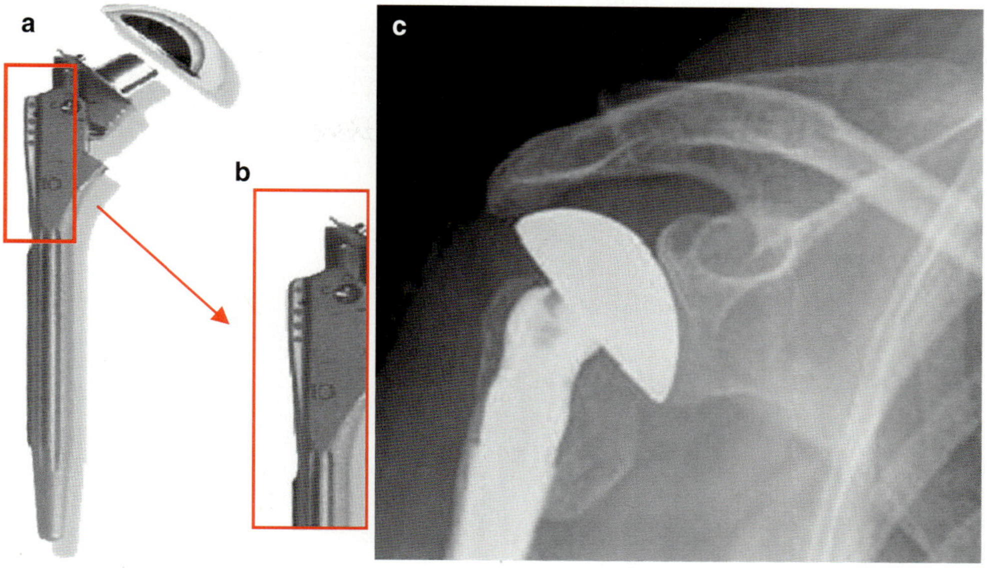

Fig. 1.36 (**a**, **b**) There are some skilled prosthesis that presents anchor points especially designed for the osteosynthesis of the tuberosities. (**c**) PHF sequelae treated by hemiarthroplasty with important tuberosities reabsorption → *loss of "engine"*

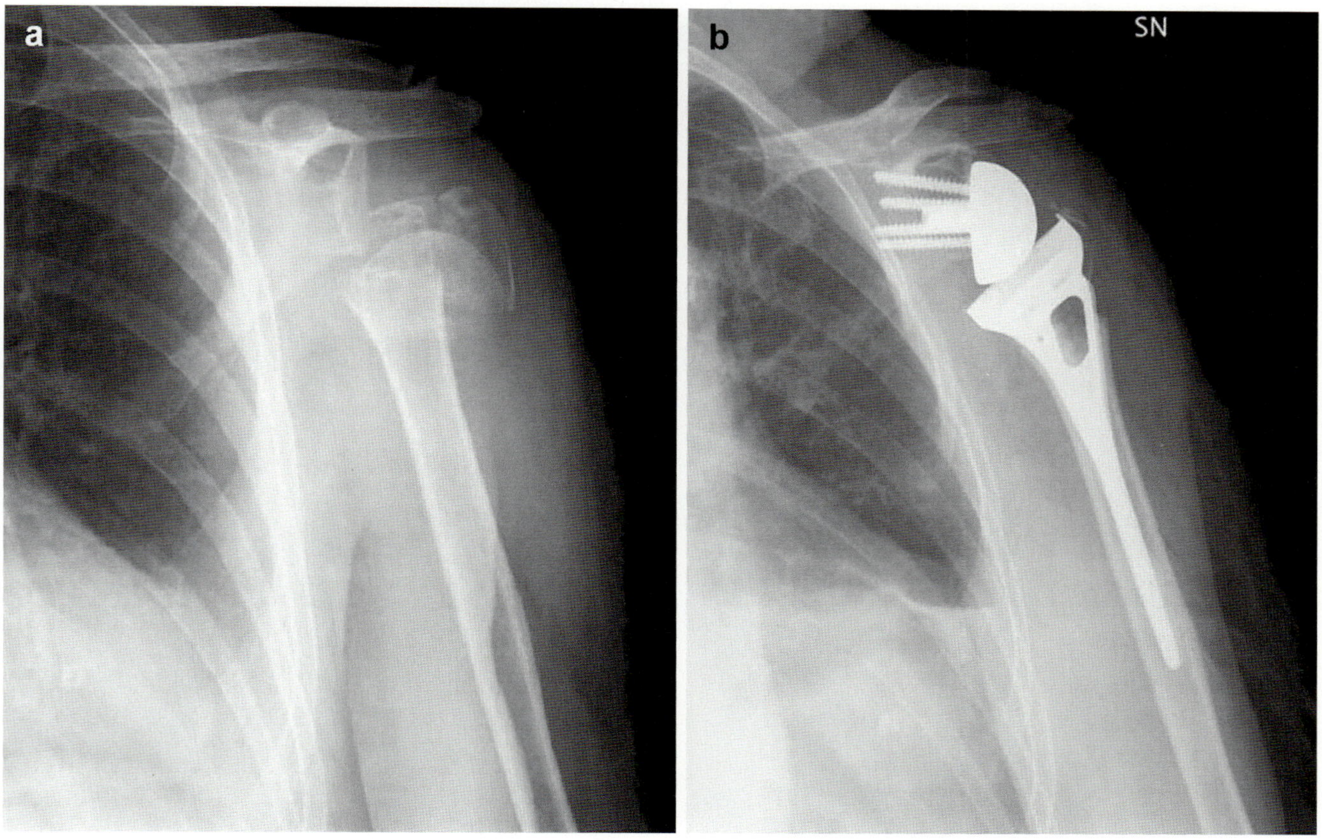

Fig. 1.37 (**a**) PHF with severe tuberosities comminution. (**b**) Reverse prosthesis for fracture **a**. sn: left side

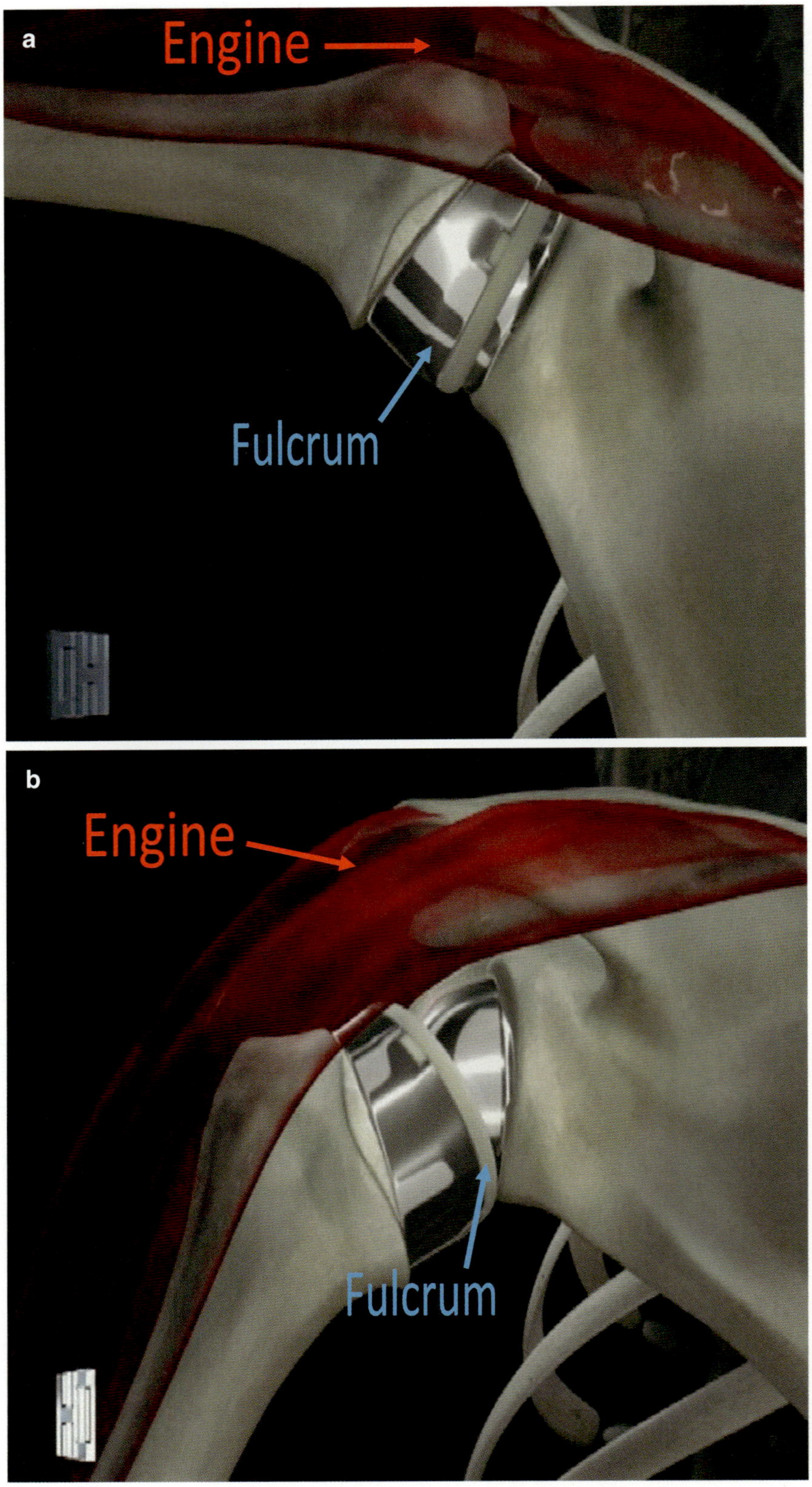

Fig. 1.38 (**a**, **b**) In the reverse prosthesis the "*fulcrum*" is represented by the prosthesis itself (humeral concavity and glenoid convexity), the "*engine*" is represented exclusively by the deltoid

1.5.2 Rehabilitation following Surgical Treatments

Rehabilitation Following ORIF

The rehabilitation after treatment of PHF presents many variables not to be underestimated, even if the choice in surgical treatment allows for early mobilization for the stability of the bone fragments obtained by the synthesis.

We need to take in to consideration the fact that if the surgeon opted for the surgical treatment, evidently the pattern of the fracture was at risk for biomechanics (displaced fractures) and biology (reabsorption of the humeral head and of the tuberosities) or the patient presented with comorbidities which rendered him or her at risk candidate for conservative treatment.

For this reasons, in the postsurgically rehabilitative approach, the physical therapist must monitor diligently the progression of the rehabilitation in a way to readily identify the patients that warrant a reexamination from the surgical team.

In the postsurgical patient treated with ORIF, the pain management and the progression criteria of the rehabilitation protocol overlap with the rational that we underlined in the conservative treatment chapter.

Sling Use

In the postsurgical treatment, to relieve pain and as a protective mechanism, we advise the use of an arm sling (neutral rotation to avoid stress on greater or lesser tuberosity (Fig. 1.39a)) for 7–10 days during which, however, the arm sling can and should be removed temporally for flexion and extension of the elbow. In the case of elderly osteoporotic patients, another 3 weeks of sling to protect the fracture healing could be (Fig. 1.39).

1° day → In the immediate postoperative period, control of pain is a primary concern. Patients should benefit from scalene block performed immediately before operation [33], and if possible, the catheter should be left in place and the pain controlled by PCA (patient-controlled anesthesia) computerized pump.

Pain in the initial post-op period is due to the iatrogenic injury made necessary by the surgical procedure and to muscles that have become shortened and contracted, giving rise to defensive antalgic posture. Although NSAID administration will help relieve pain, the physiotherapist is key to pain management in the preliminary rehabilitation phase.

Conditions can delay the beginning of passive range of motion:

- Poor screw adhesion in osteoporotic bone
- Problems relative to healing of the soft tissue (tendon or ligamentous)
- Other particular conditions (as in closed reduction and percutaneous stabilization)

2–9°day → Even if the international literature reports aggressive treatment protocols advising to begin passive exercises from the second postsurgical day [76], on the other hand, according to our experience, in older patients we prefer to wear a brace in neutral position for 7–10 days after the surgery to adapt to this new physical and emotional situation; after that we begin the rehab protocol. Anyway in younger patients with stability of the fracture and good quality of the bone and of the soft tissue, we also follow an accelerated protocol.

The rehabilitation protocol should be rolled out in line with each individual patient's progress, which in turn is closely linked to compliance and tissue healing times.

The following protocol must therefore be modulated not only in terms of the specific exercise to be chosen for a specific purpose but also when to introduce an exercise, a decision that should be taken in agreement with the surgeon.

Although goal achievement rates will closely depend on team experience, patient progression can be based on the following *three-phase* strategy:

- *Phase 1*

  10° days to 6 weeks → on removal of stitches (12 days) (Fig. 1.39b): rehabilitation protocol starts. What are the goals?

  Confidence: Create a sound patient-therapist relationship based on trust and empathy.

  Pain Control: The sling may cause the patient to adopt defensive antalgic posture (anterior scapula tilting) with consequent contraction of the peri-scapular muscles and shortening of the anterior muscles (pectoralis minor). The physiotherapist can help in this with:

  - Gentle massage of the peri-scapular muscles to avoid or eliminate antalgic contracture
  - Stretching

  PROM: We start passive range of motion on the scapular plane in relation to pain. The physical therapist's role is crucial (Fig. 1.40a, b). The main aim in this phase is to regain passive ROM; therefore the rehabilitation program must be tailored to patient compliance and expectations as well as to the quality and stability of the reconstruction. Is advised. in this phase, to propose the PROM and the auto-assisted exercises in supine position to mantain a low activation of upper trapezius during the shoulder movement and avoid to activate scapulars' imballances. [76–98]

  Active Assisted: Once the patient has achieved 90° *pain-free* passive range of motion with *stable, X-ray documented, osteosynthesis*, active/assisted kinesis in the scapular plane can be started. Care should, however, be taken with external rotation if there are any concerns about the lesser tuberosity and with internal rotation if the stability of the greater tuberosity is in doubt.

Proprioception Exercises: Proprioceptive control (the ability to identify, control, and coordinate the different body segments in relation to each other, with or without visual afference) is crucial for functional recovery. Neuromuscular exercises develop the basic stability that must underpin range of motion recovery.

Scapulothoracic: Proprioception exercises can be combined with scapulothoracic exercises extending to less than 90° so as to ensure gradual, gentle recovery; these exercises aim to maintain peri-scapular neuromuscular control so as to allow progression to the next rehabilitation phase.

Take-Home Message

We suggest in the first postoperative weeks repeated clinical controls to identify those patients who for varying reasons are predisposed to postsurgical capsular retraction. If these patients who present with this individual predisposition are identified early, an accelerated treatment plan (if allowed to stability of the fracture) and *hydrotherapy is a valuable adjunct.*

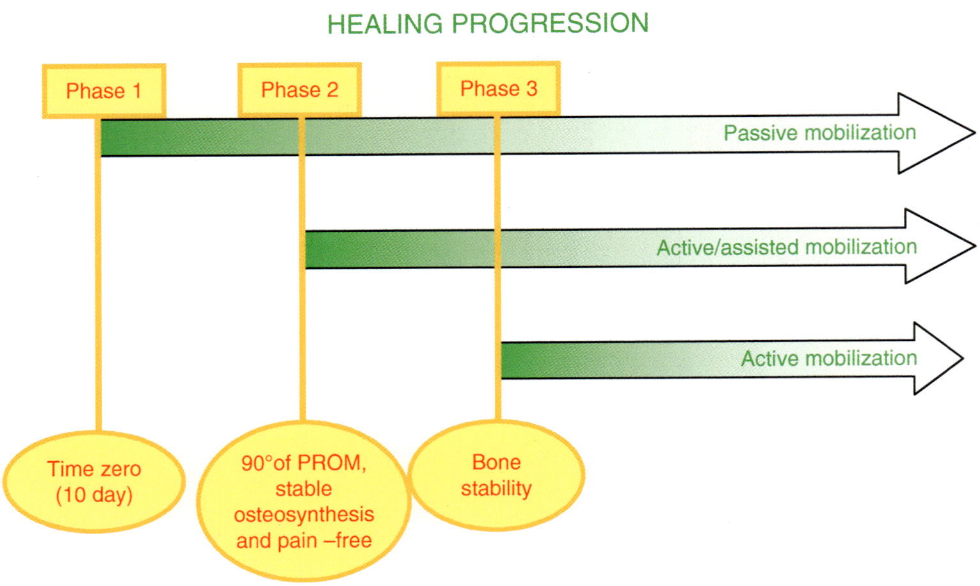

- *Phase 2*

  6–10 weeks: Goals → To achieve satisfactory passive ROM, approximately 80/90 % of the contralateral arm. This part of the rehab program aims to improve activation of the rotator cuff and scapulothoracic muscles to regain kinetic chain shoulder function once there is documented evidence of tuberosity healing. Exercise progression criteria are the following:

  Passive and Active Assisted Mobilization: passive mobilization in this phase aims to achieve 90 % ROM while the assisted active exercises started in Phase 1 are progressively increased with a view to regaining active mobility in Phase 3.

  Advanced Scapulothoracic Exercises: while always taking into account patient ability and compliance, advanced scapulothoracic exercises extending beyond 90° aim to increasingly recruit and strengthen the scapular muscles and improve the dynamic stability of the shoulder joint (Fig. 1.41a–c).

  Isometric Exercises: isometric exercises actively recruit the rotator cuff and deltoid muscles, the latter being the "engine" of the system. They pave the way for the full active functional recovery to be obtained in the subsequent phase (Fig. 1.41d, e).

- *Phase 3*

  10–12 weeks: Goals → Once PROM is 90–100 % of the contralateral arm and there is X-ray evidence of healing, the goal of rehabilitation becomes regaining full correct functional capacity. This phase will proceed with:

  Active Exercises: Progressive strengthening exercises are added to the regime at this point.

  Gradually the patient is taught to use operative arm more and withdraw assistance from the contralateral arm during therapy.

  – Patients are allowed and encouraged to perform activities of daily living.
  – *Theraband resistance* (Fig. 1.42a–c) exercises and *light weight* (Fig. 1.43a–e) are begun when the patient is pain-free and has achieved almost complete motion.
  – *Balance stabilization exercise's* (Fig. 1.44a, b) purpose is for muscle and strength activation.

→ *If at this point the passive ROM is under 80 % with respect to the contralateral, we advise for a clinical and radiographic evaluation to rule out unstable fixation*:

- Unstable fixation →specific orthopedic treatment
- Stable fixation with good healing →emphasize stretching program

Usually the shoulder takes about a year to achieve optimum function, but this may still improve for a further 12 months.

What must I know?	Symptoms	Solutions
Postsurgical phase	*Unrelenting pain that lasts in postsurgical days,* specifically resistant to medical treatment → must be a sign of alarm *Rigidity in internal and /or external rotation during the first phase of the rehabilitation → can be a sign of capsular retraction.* *Alterations in sensation, accompanied by a severe pain, can mean* → movements of the plate or fragments migration → advise to examine radiographically	Seek assistance from the referring surgeon
Since surgery to 10 weeks	Pain that extends down the arm and into the hand in the first postsurgical weeks → can be a sign of algo-neuro-dystrophy reflected or incipient or can be a sign of unmask of a cervical-brachial pain	Seek assistance from the referring surgeon
Since 10 weeks to 1 year	If the active range of motion is limited but passive is normal → one may assume reabsorption of the tuberosity (*loss of engine*) Progressive degradation of the articular range of motion, also after a year, can have significant → avascular necrosis of the head of the humerus (*loss of fulcrum*)	Seek assistance from the referring surgeon. Advise radiographic consultation and eventually CT scan

Take-Home Message

- *The final objective is to regain functionally and strength.*

  The worse the initial fracture is and the older patient, the more the possibility exists of left over rigidity of the joint.
- Fundamentally in the rehabilitation post- surgical timing is the balance between the need of biological healing of bone tissue, that doesn't have to be stressed too much, and the need to mobilize the joint in order to avoid a capsular stiffness that can be complication of this type of fracture.

  In a *young patient* with a good bone quality and stable plate, we can opt for a relatively aggressive functional rehabilitation.

In *patients in their 70s and 80s* with osteoporotic bone, the post-surgically management is extremely delicate and must be managed with a clear and precise communication between the surgeon and the rehabilitation team.

The surgeon must inform the phisioterapist about the quality of the bone, about the bone-plate stability complex and on the evolution of the callous formation monitoring with periodic x-ray exams. The therapist, on the other hand, correctly informed by the surgeon, mobilizes the shoulder joint according to the parameters given by the surgical staff, representing fundamental feedback for the surgeon on how the patient is responding to treatment.

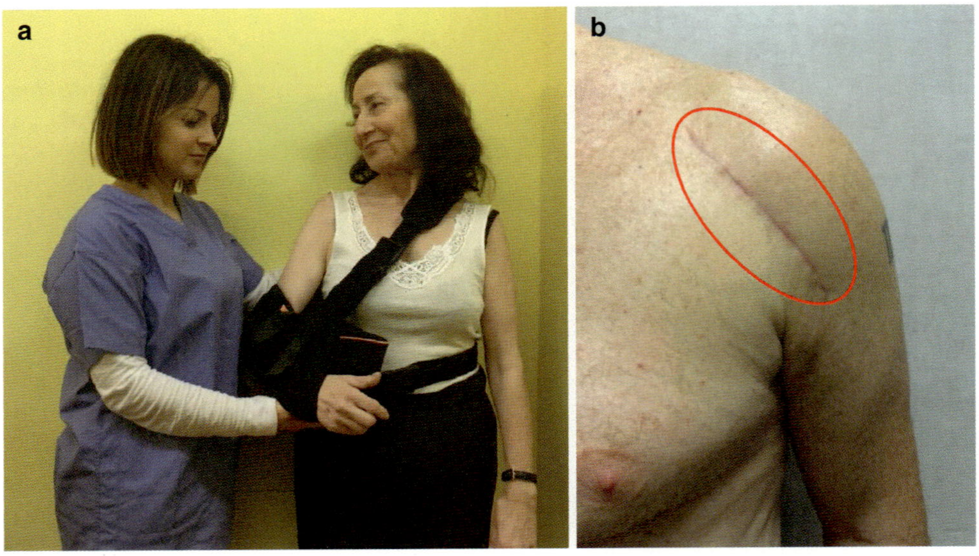

Fig. 1.39 (**a**) Rest in sling in netural position. (**b**) Delto-pectoral approach

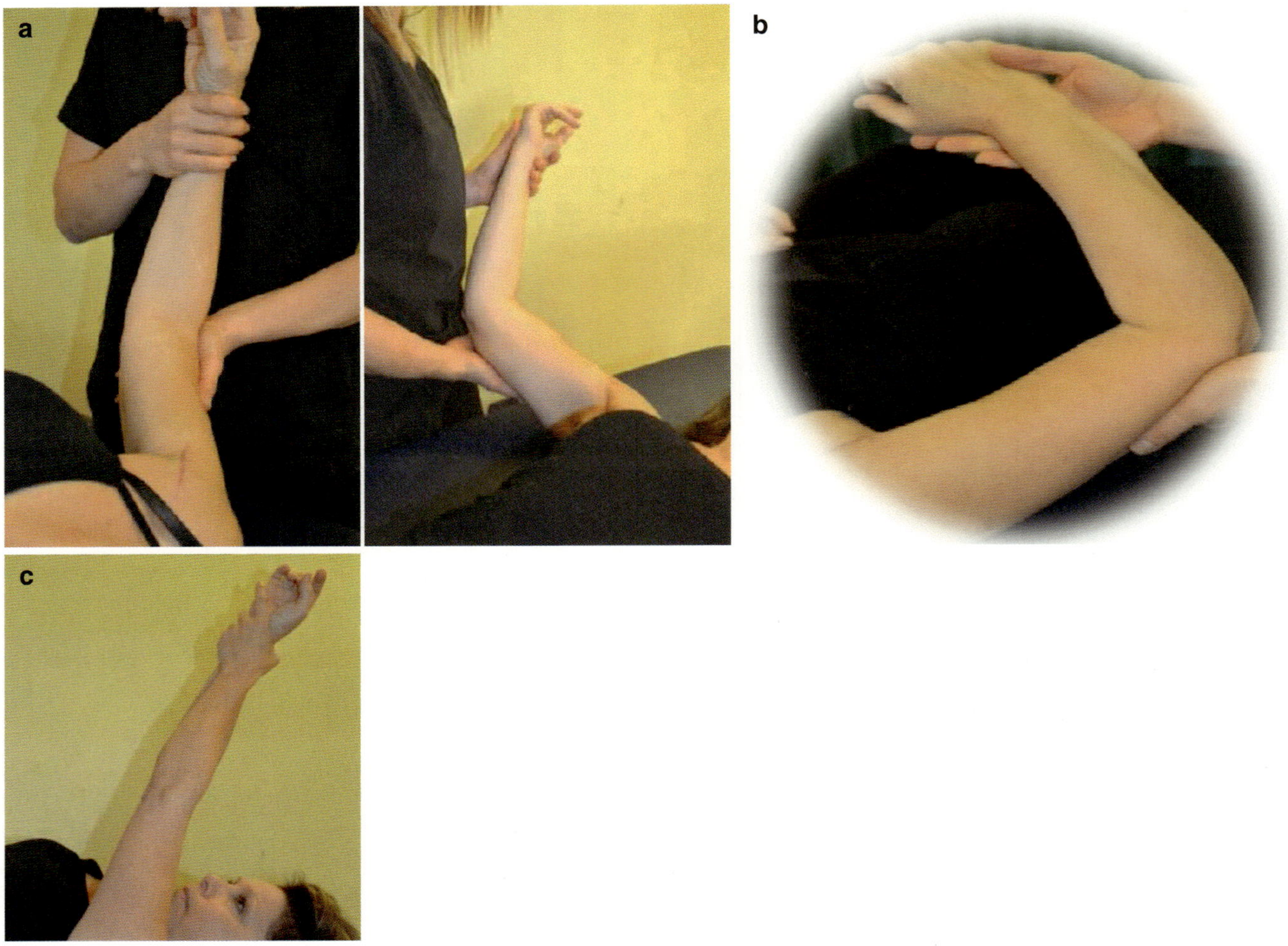

Fig. 1.40 (**a**, **b**) Passive stretching playing attention to the internal and external rotation in relation to the healing of the tuberosities. (**c**) Active assisted exercises

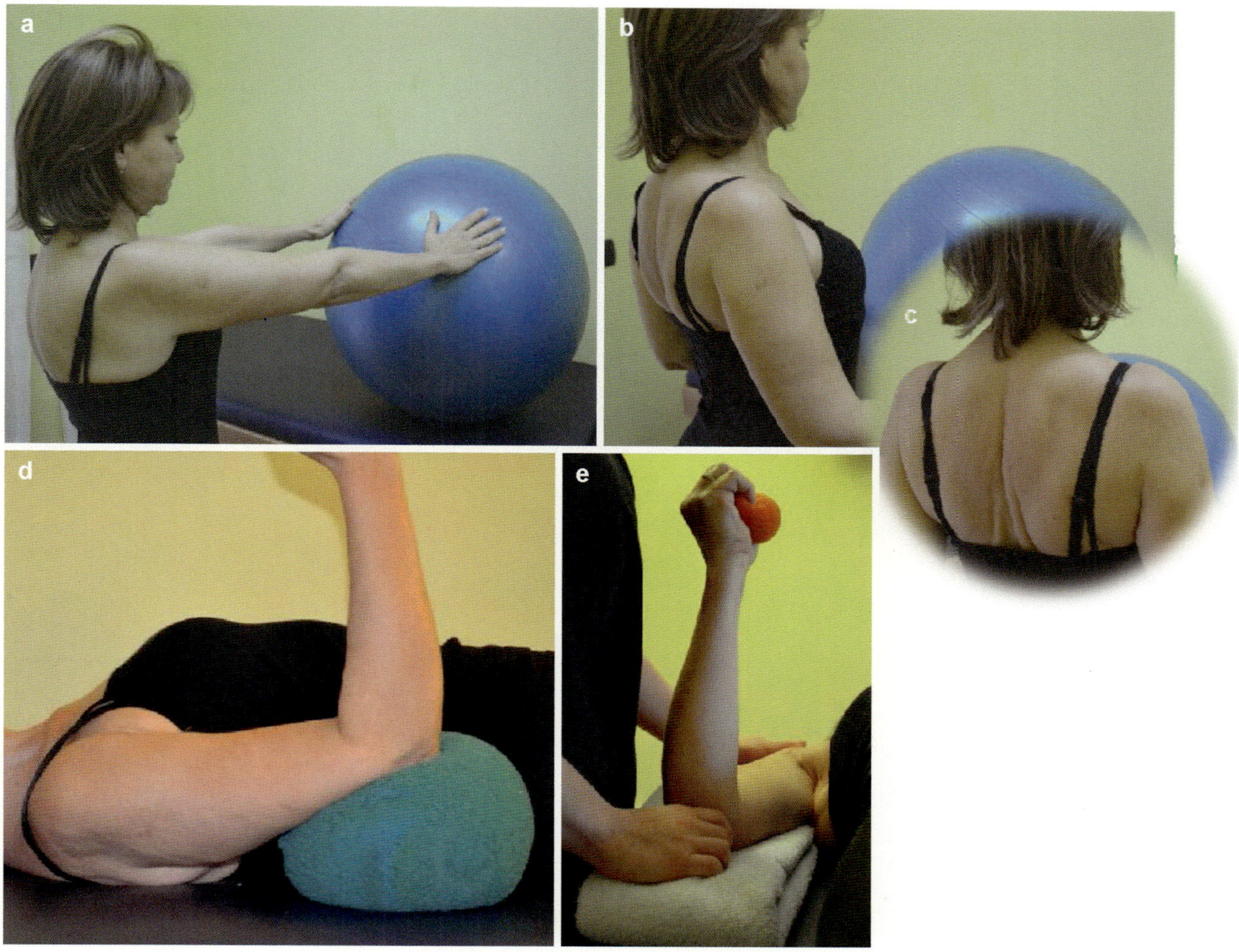

Fig. 1.41 (**a-c**) *Slide ball exercise* → Push forward the ball sliding it and come back pushing the scapula in the correct retracted position [70]. (**d**, **e**) Isometric exercises

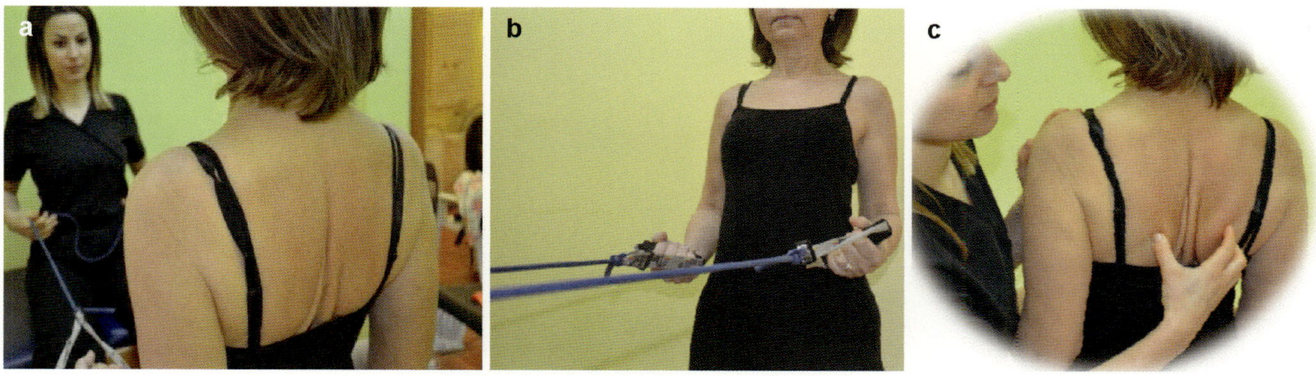

Fig. 1.42 (**a–c**) *Scapular control exercises using tube* with the PT assistance paying attention to the scapular retraction. We have to put in back the scapula in the kinetic chain → for this reason we must to emphasize the trunk and the hip stabilization [70]

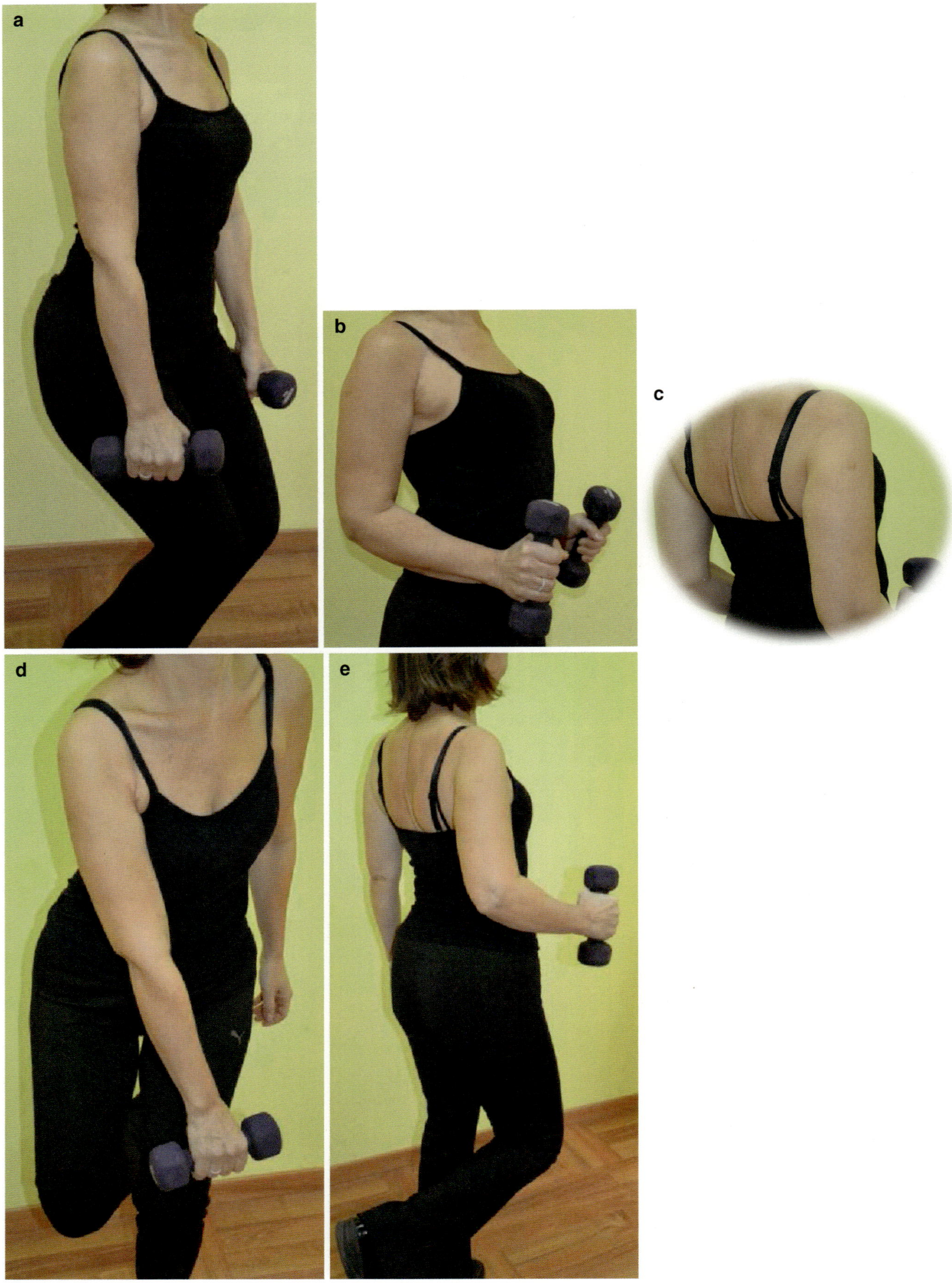

Fig. 1.43 (**a–e**) Scapular control exercises using light weights. After 10 weeks we can use the weights to emphasize the scapular retraction with the PT assistance [70]

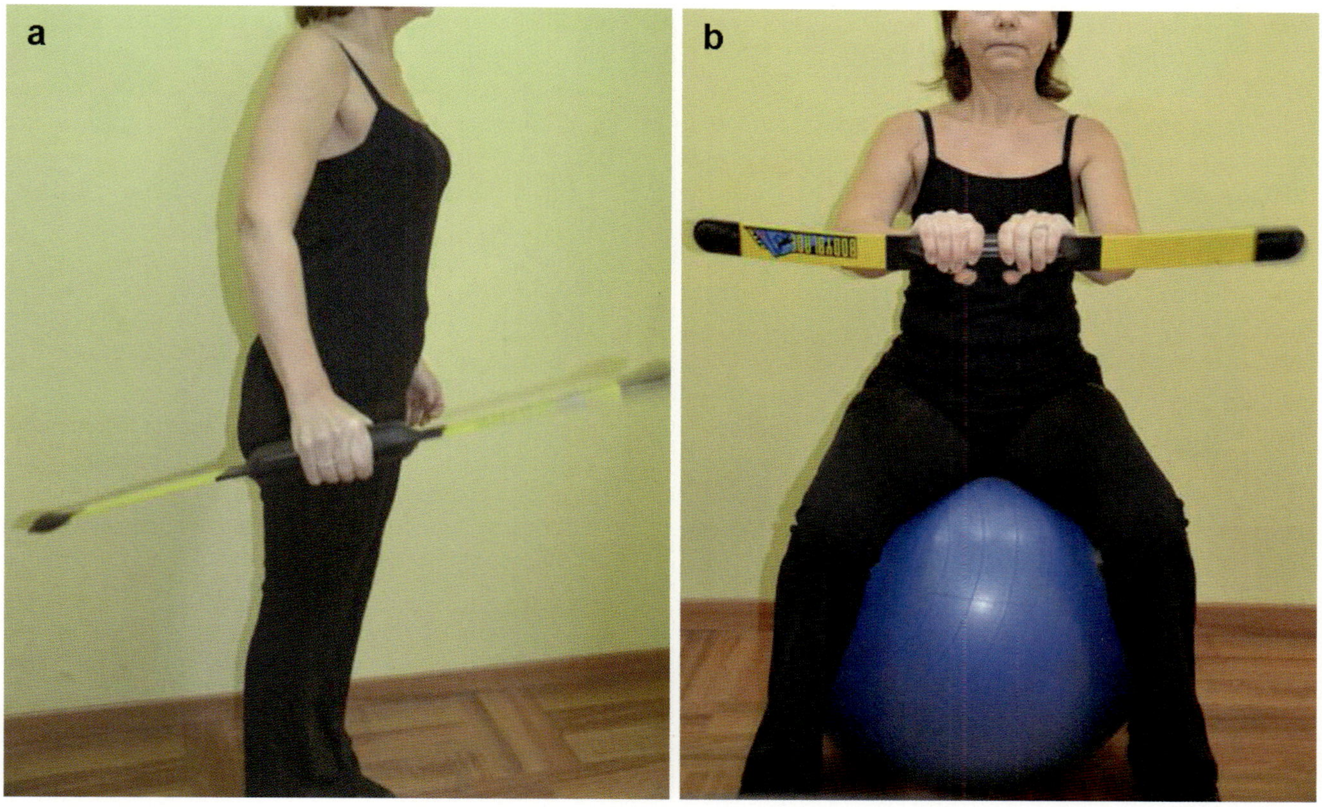

Fig. 1.44 (**a**, **b**) *Body Blade stabilization* → This exercise is helpful to improve the muscle balance and the stability of the shoulder in the final phases of the physical therapy [83, 84]

1.6 Rehabilitation following Hemiarthroplasty

While hemiarthroplasty after proximal humeral fractures has been shown to provide good pain relief, the achievement of excellent range of motion with this method has been less predictable.

Rehabilitation, particularly passive range of motion in the early stage and long-term active range of motion and strengthening, is considered essential to the achieving an optimal outcome after shoulder hemiarthroplasty [51, 53, 56].

Immediately after surgery, the affected extremity is placed in a sling in a slight external or neutral rotation to relieve stress on the greater tuberosity.

The following week-based timetable is only a general postsurgical rehabilitation program since work will be conditioned by individual tissue healing times (implant-bone, bone-bone, tendon-bone, etc.) *that must be monitored by imaging techniques and clinical assessment by the surgical team and weighed against the often patient-specific response to rehabilitation.*

In general, rehabilitation begins within the first week.

- 1/6 week → The decision to initiate passive ROM exercise should be individualized to the patient and it depends on the surgeon's confidence in the strength of tuberosity fixation.

  Passive ROM exercises to 90° of forward elevation on the scapular plane, *very gentle external rotation*, and *paying attention to internal rotation* to avoid stress on the greater tuberosity are performed with the patient supine (Fig. 1.45a, b and 1.46) [99].

  With tenuous tuberosity fixation, ROM exercise can be delayed for 2–3 weeks to minimize stress on the repair, and if repair of the lesser tuberosity was performed, avoid early external rotation.

  Gentle active motion of the wrist and elbow is encouraged immediately postoperatively to avoid stiffness and pain due to immobilization.

  Pendulum exercises are allowed to the patient, as we explain in previous rehabilitation paragraph, if pain-free.
- 6/8 WEEK → Active/assisted forward elevation and external rotation exercises are delayed until radiographic evidence of tuberosity healing is present (Fig. 1.47).

  Once tuberosities healing is confirmed radiographically, gentle isometric rotator cuff and scapular strengthening can begin, typically at 6–8 weeks following surgery (Figs. 1.48 and 1.49).

  The rehabilitation program have to obtain the regain of the functional utilize of the arm and improve the articular range of motion as well as possible emphasizing the scapular control to restore the correct kinematic and validity of the kinetic chain in relation to the real general condition and comorbidities of our patient (Fig. 1.50).

  The estimated maximum level of improvement can be achieved 9 to 12 months postoperatively.

Take-Home Message

The rehabilitation time in hemiarthroplasty as well as in the case of ORIF of the PHF, are given by a biological healing time bone to bone. In the prosthetic the two bone components that must necessarily heal are the greater TUBEROSITY and the DIAPHYSIS (Fig. 1.32a).

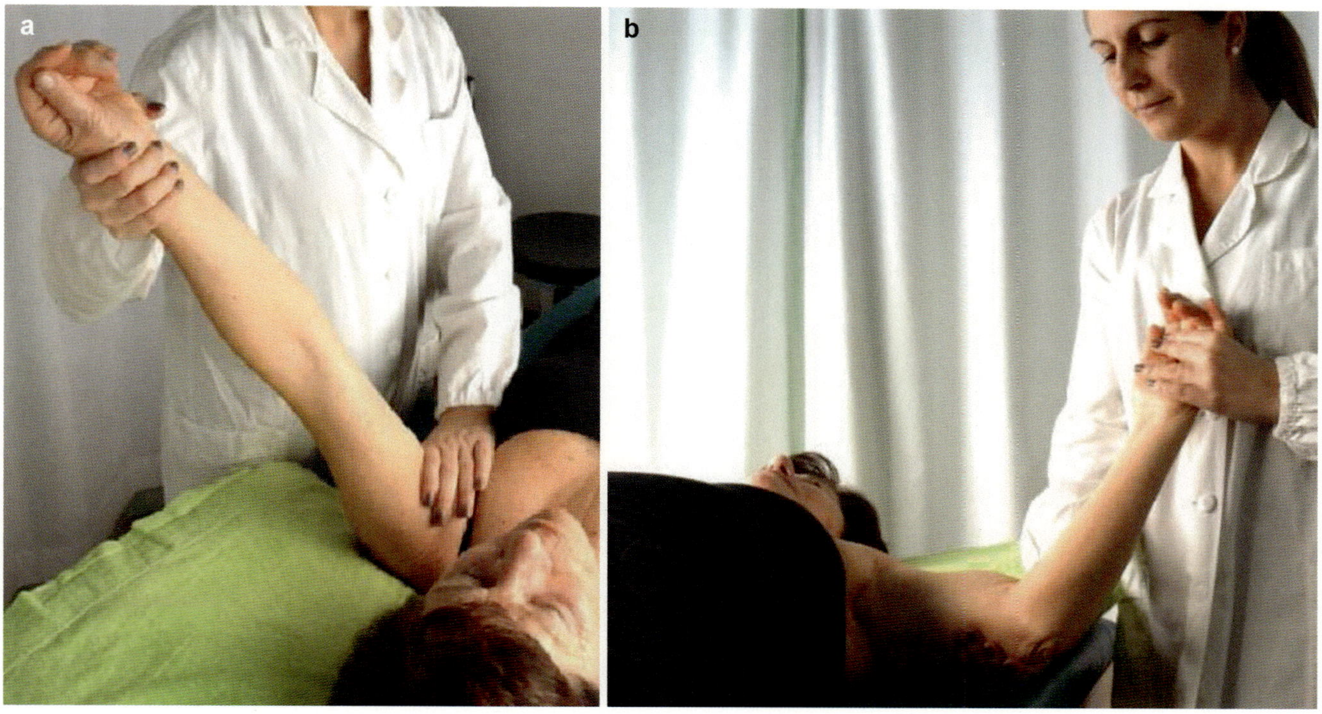

Fig. 1.45 (**a**, **b**) Passive ROM exercises on scapular plane and gentle external rotation

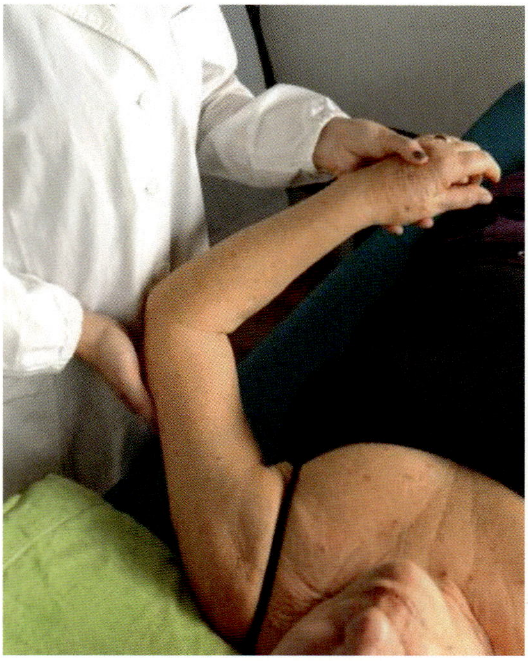

Fig. 1.46 Pay attention to internal rotation

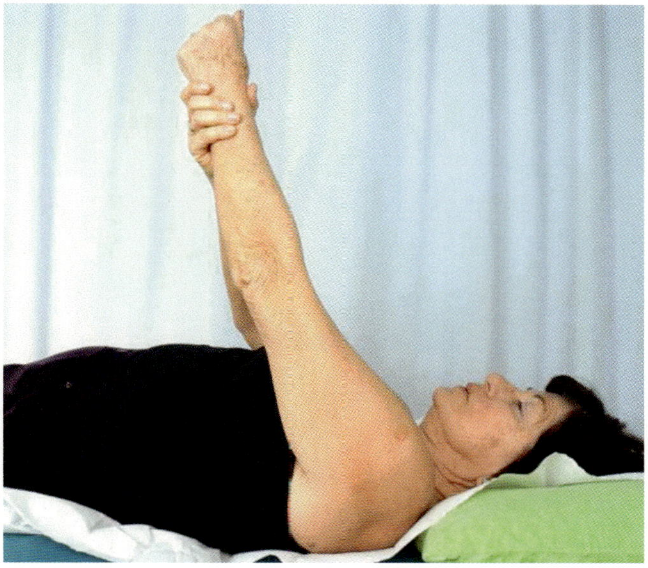

Fig. 1.47 Active/assisted forward activation

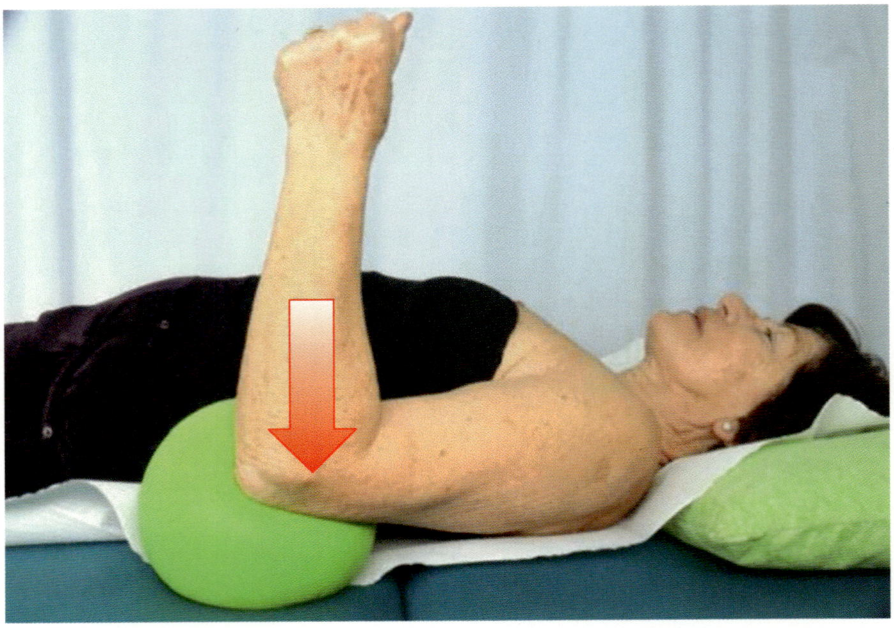

Fig. 1.48 Isometric exercises

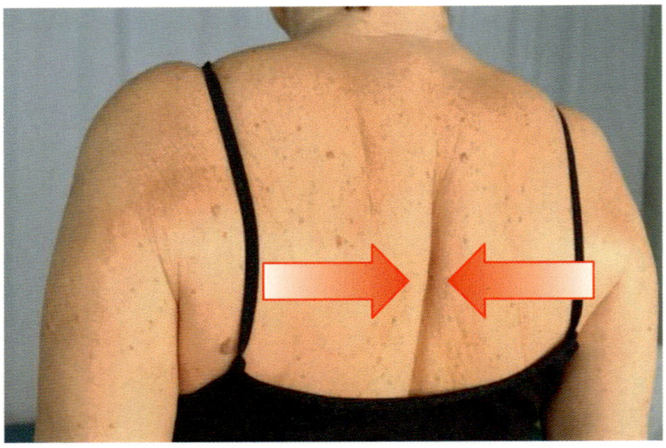

Fig. 1.49 Scapular control exercises

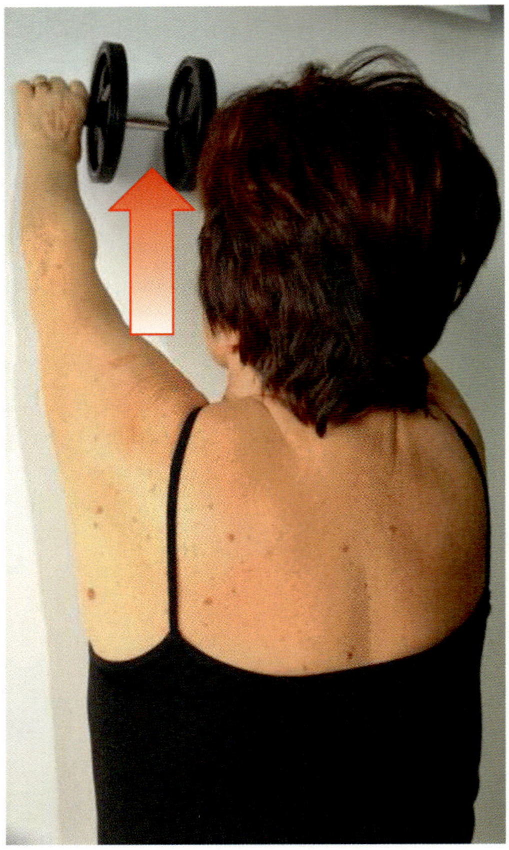

Fig. 1.50 Arm stretching elevation

1.7 Complications

1.7.1 Neuroanatomical and Neuromechanical Aspects of the Shoulder following Proximal Humeral Fractures

Mechanical stresses and loads potentially can injure specialized connective tissues of the shoulder.

The pain felt at the shoulder as a result of mechanical stresses after a proximal humeral fracture is often also due to the physical distortion of nociceptors that lie within these tissues or is a consequence of chemical activation of the resident nociceptive free nerve endings that are depolarized as a result of damage to the cell walls of the tissues (DEAFFERENTATION).

Nociceptors are the biological transducers that convert physical and chemical energy stimuli into action potentials.

When muscles, tendons capsuloligamentous structures are damaged partial deafferentation leads to proprioceptive deficit.

In addiction to injury to the specialized connective tissue or damage to the muscolotendinous tissues, pain felt within the shoulder after a trauma that lead to a PHF may be caused by several other neuroanatomical or neurophysiological factors.

The *axillary nerve* is the most frequently injured nerve in proximal humerus fractures, and the suprascapular nerve is the second most commonly injured [94].

The axillary nerve enters the quadrangular space along with the PCHA at an average distance of 1.7 cm from the surgical neck [95].

In the quadrangular space, the nerve divides into anterior and posterior branches, the latter of which provides motor input to the posterior and middle heads of the deltoid before terminating as the superior lateral brachial cutaneous nerve [95].

The anterior branch of the axillary nerve continues along the undersurface of the deltoid, crosses the anterior deltoid raphe, the avascular region separating the anterior and middle heads of the deltoid, at an average of 3.5 cm from the lateral prominence of the greater tuberosity and 6.3 cm from the anterolateral border of the acromion [96].

Gardner and colleagues showed that this nerve can be reliably palpated as a cord-like structure at this location.

The proximity of the axillary nerve makes it particularly vulnerable to both traumatic and iatrogenic injury [97].

The suprascapular nerve runs posteroinferiorly through the suprascapular notch to supply the supraspinatus and infraspinatus muscles, the motor branch of the nerve arises about 1 cm from the base of the scapula spine and courses 2 mm posterior to the glenoid rim [95].

The nerve is particularly vulnerable to traction injury at two distinct locations: its branch-point from the upper trunk and at the suprascapular notch where it runs deep to the transverse scapular ligament.

1.7.2 Complications Following ORIF

A favorable outcome is generally achieved if some complications can be avoided: AVN (Avascular Necrosis), non-union and tuberosities mal- union, post-operative infections.

These can be sequelae of either the original injury of subsequent management:

1. *AVN* is more commonplace in comminuted fractures, although associated dislocation also increases the risk of impairment of vascular supply to the humeral head. As previously mentioned, the infero-medial portion of the head is believed to be a critical area with regards to maintaining adequate blood supply. Pain and loss of function are commonly seen in those patients who develop AVN.
   How to search?
   - Plain radiographs may show changes somewhere on a spectrum between sclerotic patches to collapse and resorption of the affected bone.
   - MRI is commonly used to further evaluate the extent of damage.

   What to do?
   - Core decompression has been advocate in early disease, however most require humeral head replacement [31, 57].
2. *NON UNION OR MAL UNION* :The normal contributory factors for non- union apply to PHF as well such as infection are poor physiological reserve, smoking, diabetes, inadequate fracture stabilization and excessive soft tissue stripping [58, 59]. Mal- union is common after these fractures. The elderly population tend to cope well, undoubtedly due to lower expectation demands. Younger patients would notice a decrease in function particularly when the tuberosities and their adjoining cuff insertions are involved.

   Though some amount of stiffness is expected after these fractures, other significant limitation should be investigated and treated.

Capsular tightness, tuberosities mal-union or reabsorption, (Fig. 1.51) impingement secondary to plate misplacement, screw protrusion (Fig. 1.52a–c) and cuff dysfunction can all contribute to a stiff shoulder.

How to search?

- Radiographs may show the non-union, but a CT scan may be required for confirmation and also provides useful information for pre-operative planning.

What to do?

- If a non-union is present either shoulder hemiarthroplasty or ORIF with bone grafting is usually required.

3. *POSTOPERATIVE INFECTION* is always a possibility and must be kept in mind at all times. The signs and symptoms may be minor, such as loss of GO joint space accompanied by persistent pain and discomfort. These symptoms could be the first indication of infection.

How to search?

- Radiological evidence
- Biological evidence with intra-articular aspiration that could show if the infection is acute (<3 weeks), intermediate (between 3 and 8 weeks) or chronic (>8 weeks).

What to do?

In this situation an intravenous antibiotic regime must to be started preferably under the guidance of an infectious diseases' specialist.

- *Acute infections* → The implant may be left in place if it contributes to stability
- *Intermediate infections* → in this situation a secondary intervention may be contemplated, such as a fusion or reimplantation of the prostheses.
- *Chronic infections* → Removal of the implants is *mandatory.*

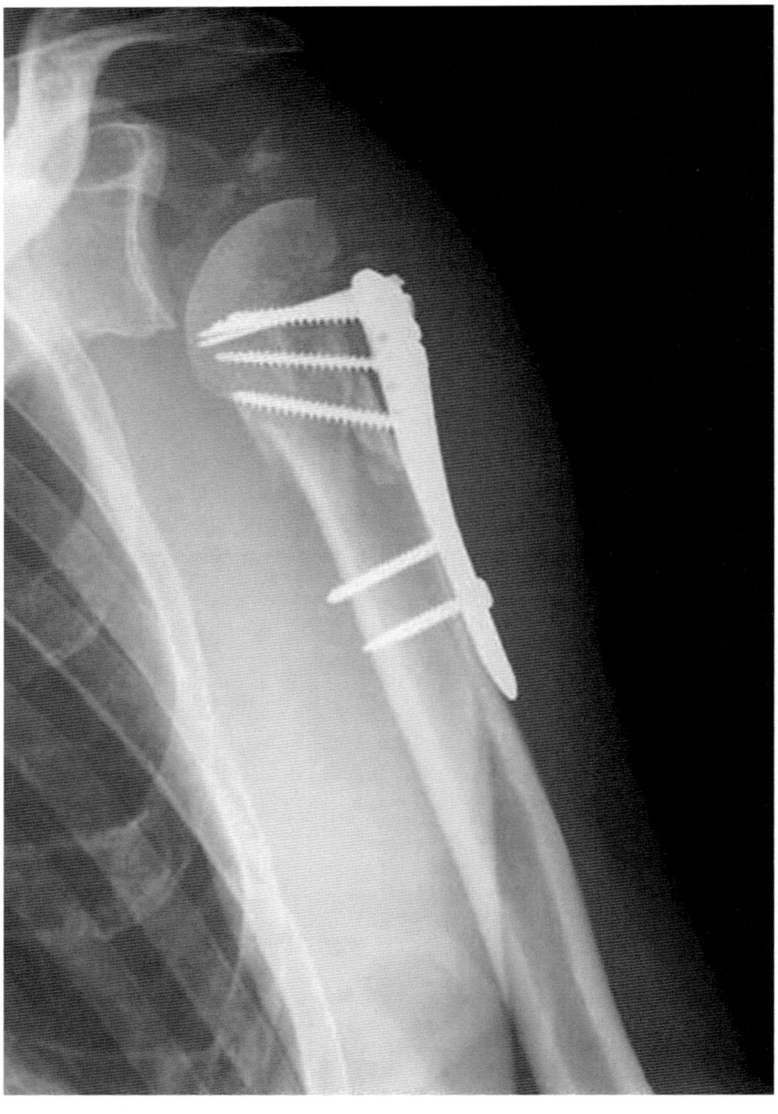

Fig. 1.51 Tuberosity mal union and reabsorption

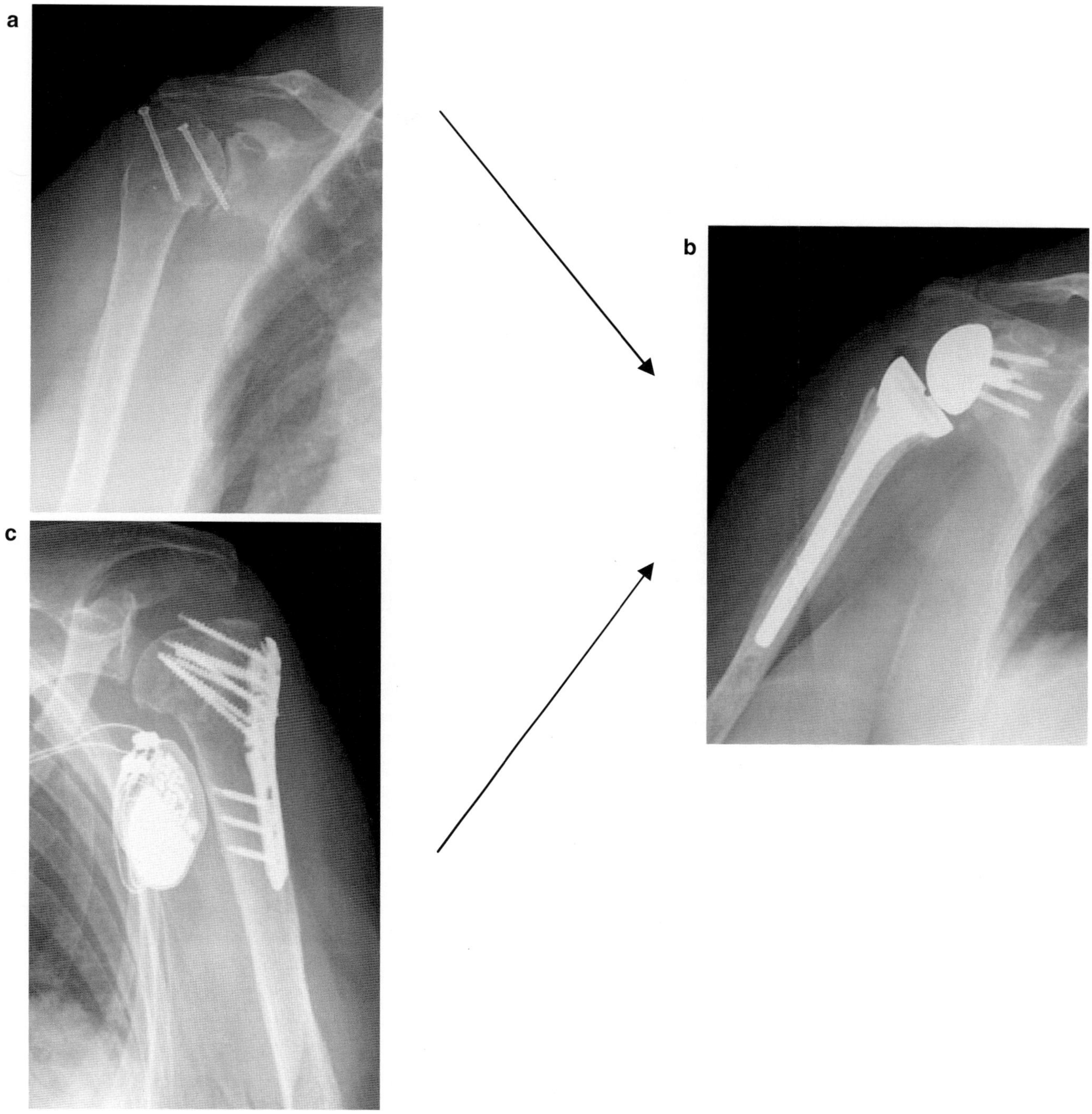

Fig. 1.52 (**a**) Screws protrusion. (**b**) Solution

1.7.3 Complications following Hemiarthroplasty

The literature describes some different complications that can occur after hemiarthroplasty.

Bigliani et al. [60] identified tuberosities non-union as the most common cause of failure in a series of 29 failed shoulders in which hemiarthroplasties were performed to manage acutely displaced PHF.

In a meta-analysis of 810 failed shoulders hemiarthroplasties, complications included superficial and deep infection, heterotopic ossification (8.8 %), and proximal migration of the humeral head (6.8 %) (Fig. 1.53) [61].

In general the most common complications that we can manage are just two: *Tuberosity non-union and the infection of the implant.*

1. *TUBEROSITY NON-UNION* : is the most common and devastating cause of poor outcomes following for displaced 3–4 part PHF treated with Hemiarthroplasty.

   Boileau et al. found that [47] tuberosity malpositioning occurred in half of patients who underwent hemiarthroplasty for PHF, and this was also correlated with unsatisfactory results. Prosthesis malalignment decreases range of motion and residual pain.

   How to search?
   - Radiographs control and CT scan

   What to do?
   - Reverse total shoulder arthroplasty
2. *Infection*: The risk of periprosthetic shoulder infection increases when the operation is performed for fractures, cuff arthroplasty, or radiation induced osteonecrosis. These infections are specifically influence by:
   - Obesity
   - Malnutrition
   - Systemic steroids
   - Malignancy
   - Chemotherapy
   - Diabetes mellitus
   - Synchronous infection
   - Postoperative hematoma formation
   - Revision surgery

The most common species of isolated organisms from the cultures of postoperative shoulder infections are: Staphylococcus Aureus, S Epidermitis, Propinobacterium acnes, and Corynebacterium [62, 63].

In general antibiotic prophylaxis has been shown to reduce the incidence of hemiarthroplasty shoulder infections and to be cost effective.

Surgical side preparation with an antiseptic prophylaxis antibiotic administration before the start of procedure will predictably eradicate the offending organism.

Shaving and draping the axilla have been proposed as additional means of reducing the incidence of surgical site infections, but the efficacy of this intervention has not be proved [64, 65].

Symptoms: Symptoms usually develops within a few days after surgery and are characterized by localized wound erythema and skin sensitivity.

Deep infections are more difficult to recognize and may present in an early or delayed manner.

Increased pain and stiffness are the most common symptoms associated with deep soft tissue [63, 66, 67, 69].

Systemic symptoms (fever and chills) are less common.

Diagnosis:

- *Radiological evidence*: with early pyogenic infection, radiographic findings are typically normal. In contrast, radiographs in sub-acute and delayed case may show osteopenia, lucencies around a prosthetic component and pseudo-subluxation of a prosthetic humeral head [68].
- *Biological evidence*: aspiration of the GO joint with a synovial fluid analysis should be considered in all cases of suspected deep infection. White cell blood count >50,000 cells/mm with more than 75 % polymorphonuclear cells are highly suggestive of infection.

  The peripheral blood leukocyte count in a deep infection is rarely abnormal whereas the erythrocyte sedimentation rate (ESR) and C- reactive protein (CPR) level are frequently elevated [62, 63, 66, 67].

Treatment:

- *Systemic approach*: antibiotic suppression
- *Local approach*: debridement with retention of the prosthesis, resection arthroplasty, arthrodesis, direct prosthesis exchange with temporary placement of antibiotic spacer.

  The varied management approaches, absence of uniform protocols and the use of multiple outcomes measures make it difficult to draw definitive conclusions regarding treatment of infected shoulder arthroplasties.

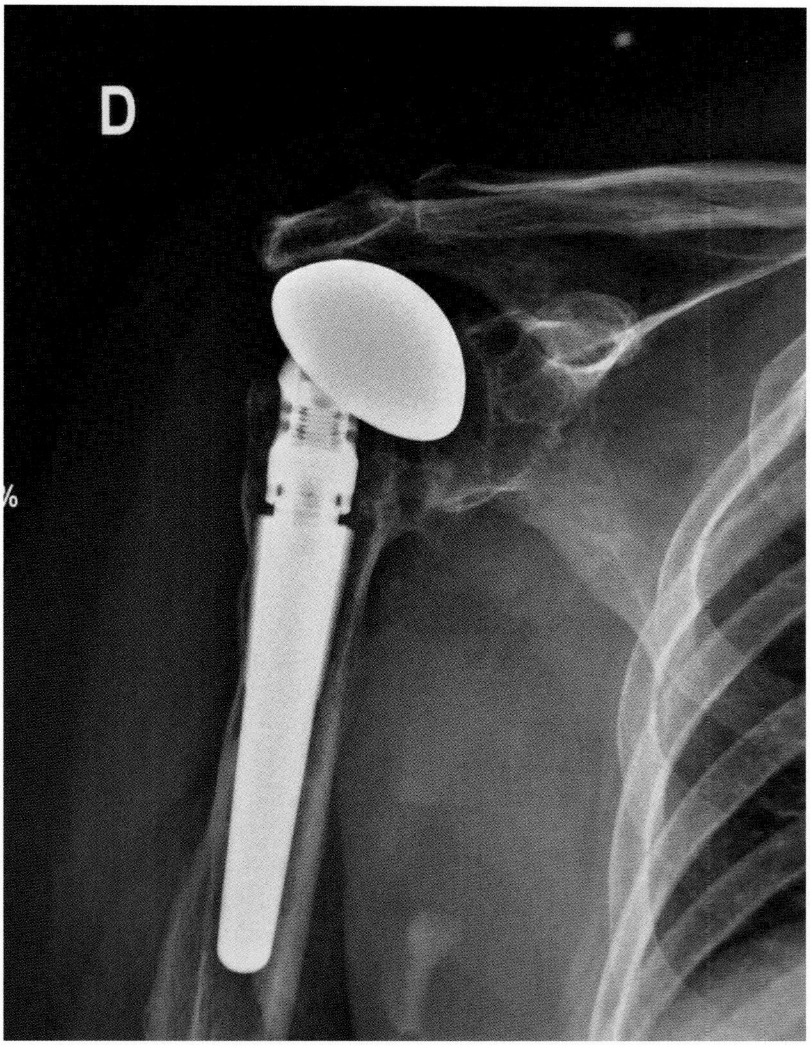

Fig. 1.53 Proximal migration of humeral head in HEMI for PHF treatment

1.8 Sequelae of Proximal Humeral Fractures

The treatment of complex humeral fractures or fracture dislocations presents several challenges. Late complications such us mal-union, avascular necrosis or non-union are frequent and often lead to articular incongruence.

Patient can be severely handicapped, presenting with considerable pain, stiffness, and important functional impairment.

Stiff shoulders with distorted proximal humerus, soft tissue damage, a scarred deltoid and rotator cuff tears make shoulder arthroplasty a challenging procedure often with unpredictable results and a high risk of complications.

The overall results of patients with old trauma are inferior to the results currently obtained in patients with primary osteoarthritis or with recent 4-part fractures who are treated initially with humeral head replacement. In symptomatic fracture sequelae there are different surgical approaches that we are going to discuss.

Among these fracture sequelae, some cases of avascular necrosis with subchondral bone collapse, certain locked dislocations and fracture- dislocations, some non-unions of the surgical neck with a small osteoporotic head fragment, and some mal-unions of the tuberosities with incongruity of the humeral articular surface may be indications for the insertion of a shoulder prosthesis [86–89].

From a surgical point of view, fracture sequelae can be distinguished whose natural history, functional outcomes, and prognosis are very different [92].

The sequelae of PHF can be divided into moderate and major, depending on the impaction/disimpaction of the humeral head and the connection/disconnection of the tuberosities especially of the greater tuberosity. The disimpaction of the humeral head and the disconnection of the greater tuberosity from the shaft are more frequent in case of extracapsular fractures of the proximal humerus as Boileau observed [86].

Boileau et co-authors have also classified sequelae of PHF in *two categories* and *four types*:

Category 1:

- *Intracapsular impacted fracture sequelae*: in which an osteotomy of greater tuberosity *is not required.*
  - *Type one → Cephalic collapse and/or necrosis* (Fig. 1.54a, b): integrity of *engine* (greater and the lesser tuberosity), we have only to change the *fulcrum* (humeral head) → *HEMI*
  - *Type two → Locked dislocations or fracture dislocations* (Fig. 1.55a, b): integrity of *engine*, we have only to change the *fulcrum → HEMI*

Category 2:

- *Extracapsular disimpacted fracture sequelae*: in which a humeral implant cannot be inserted *without osteotomy and repositioning of the greater tuberosity.*
  - *Type three→ Non-union of the surgical neck* (Fig. 1.56a, b): conservative surgical treatment is possible→ *PEG BONE GRAFT* (Fig. 1.61b)+*ORIF or INTRAMEDULLARY FIXATION (with or without osteotomy)*
  - *Type four→ Severe tuberosity mal-union* (Fig. 1.57): loss of *fulcrum and engine→ REVERSE*

Cephalic collapse and/or necrosis and chronic fracture dislocations (Category 1) are usually associated with impacted intracapsular fracture sequelae, in which to perform an arthroplasty osteotomy of the greater tuberosity is not required.

On the other side, non-unions of the surgical neck and severe mal-union of the tuberosities (Category 2) are associated with disimpacted extracapsular fracture sequelae in which a humeral implant cannot be inserted without osteotomy and repositioning of the greater tuberosity.

Take-Home Message

Reverse prosthesis is advised in cases of fracture sequelae in which distortion of the proximal humeral anatomy around the cuff insertion result in the functional unless cuff.

Category and type	Possible sequelae	Biomechanic implications	Solution
Category 1 Type 1 (Fig. 1.58a, b)	Cephalic collapse or necrosis	Integrity of ENGINE →change the FULCRUM	HEMI
Category 1 Type 2 (Fig. 1.59a–c)	Locked dislocations and fracture dislocations	Integrity of ENGINE →change the FULCRUM	HEMI
Category 2 Type 3 (Figs. 1.60a, b and 1.61a, b).	Non-union or mal-union of the surgical neck	conservative surgical treatment is possible	PEG BONE GRAFT + ORIF or INTRAMEDULLARY FIXATION
Category 2 Type 4 (Fig. 1.62a, b)	Severe tuberosity mal-union	Loss of FULCRUM and ENGINE	REVERSE

The results of shoulder hemi/non-constrained arthroplasties (NCA) for old trauma are much less favorable than those of primary osteoarthritis or HEMI performed for acute fractures. On the basis of a literature review [90], satisfactory results may be expected in 15–72 % of the cases, with pain relief in more than 85 %.

Motion is usually limited with an active anterior elevation around 110° and an active external rotation around 20°. The complication rate is usually higher than that for other etiologies.

The percentage of complications varies from 20 to 48 % depending on the series. The revision rate varies from 3.5 to 35 %.

Several factors seem to influence the final results [93] (NCA):

1. The role of the initial fracture treatment (initial conservative treatment with better outcome when compared to initial surgical treatment).
2. The type of sequelae with better results are reported after post-traumatic arthritis without any distortion of the tuberosities, as the best outcomes occurred in cases of isolated necrosis of the humeral head.
3. Outcomes is also good and predictable in patients with valgus deformity. In contrast, the outcomes in patients with varus malunion is significantly poorer than those in patients with valgus malunion Two hypotheses could explain this difference. It is technically more difficult to implant a humeral head prosthesis in a patient with substantial varus deformity because of the risk of greater tuberosity or diaphyseal fracture. In addition, the humeral medialization resulting from the varus deformity leads to circumferential tightening of the soft tissues and a severely stiff shoulder. The presence of fatty infiltration of the rotator cuff muscles is also associated with significantly poorer clinical outcomes. On the basis of the results of the present study, different authors [91] consider patients with type-1 fracture sequelae with varus malunion and/or fatty infiltration of the rotator cuff muscles to be poor candidates for an anatomic prosthesis. In these situations, reverse shoulder arthroplasty may be preferable, especially if the patient is elderly.

The most significant factor affecting functional outcomes is greater tuberosity osteotomy.

All of the excellent and good post operative Constance scores are obtained in Type 1 and Type 2 sequelae in which osteotomy of the greater tuberosity is not required.

Patients in Type 3 and Type 4 who require a greater tuberosity osteotomy, have either fair or poor results and do not regain active elevation above 90°. It is general consensus that shoulder arthroplasty for the treatment of the sequelae of proximal humerus fractures should be performed without an osteotomy of the greater tuberosity. If prosthetic replacement is possible without an ostectomy, surgeons should accept the distorted anatomy of the proximal humerus and adapt the prosthesis and their technique to the modified anatomy.

In 2008 Boileau at al [93].compared the results of non-constrained arthroplasty (NCA) to reverse shoulder arthroplasty (RSA) in the treatment of fracture sequelae:

- *In Type 1* the result of RSA were equivalent to those observed with NCA except for external rotation which was lower. Therefore it's recommended preferring NCA prosthesis in this cases in order to restore bought active elevation and external rotation; only patient with muscle atrophy or rotator massive cuff tear may benefit from Reverse (Fig. 1.58a, b).
- *In Type 2* bought Anatomical (NCA) and Reverse (RSA) can be indicated although a NCA may be preferred for posterior dislocation, a RSA must be preferred in case of chronic anterior dislocation in which anterior stability may be a problem with NCA (Fig. 1.59a–c).
- *In Type 3* RSA produced unexpected poor functional result. Therefore patients with isolated surgical neck non-union should be considered as a group at risk for Anatomic and Reverse arthroplasty. The most adapted procedure is fixation of the non –union with bone PEG graft and internal fixation (Fig. 1.60a, b and 1.61a, b). In cases where surgical neck non- union is associated with tuberosity non-union, severe humeral head cavitation or osteoarthritis, other option such us humeral head replacement and tuberosity fixation with bone graft should be considered.
- *In Type 4* NCA demonstrated that prosthetic implantation required greater tuberosity osteotomy. This option has clearly been identified as pejorative on the final outcome. RSA provided better early results than those achieve with NCA with acceptable results despite non-union or malunion of the greater tuberosity (Fig. 1.62a, b).

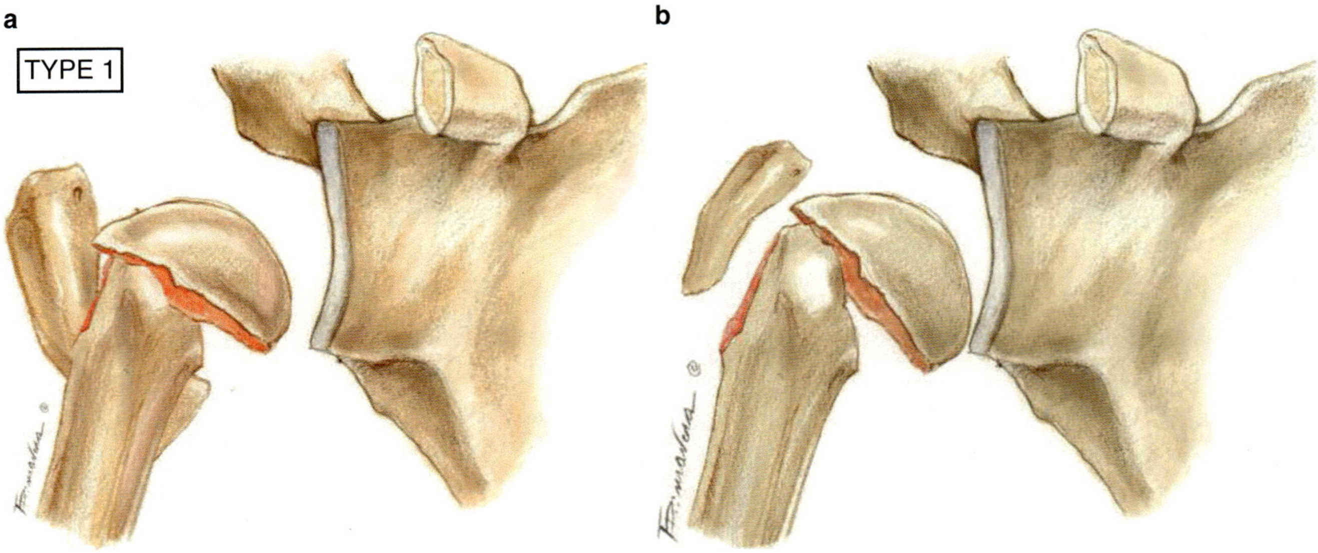

Fig. 1.54 (**a**, **b**) Cephalic collapse or necrosis

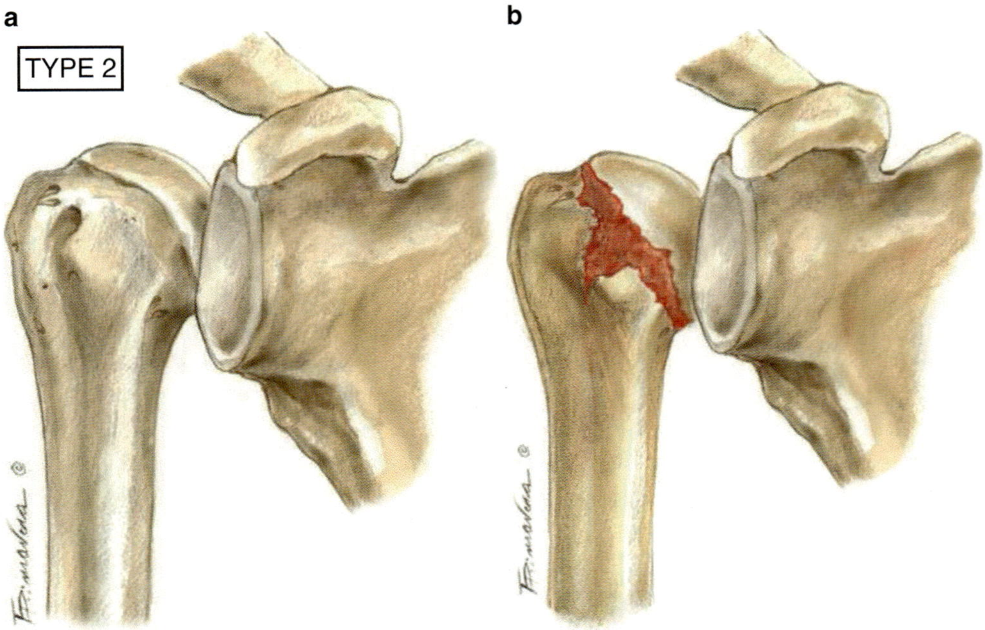

Fig. 1.55 (**a**, **b**) Locked dislocation and/or fracture dislocation

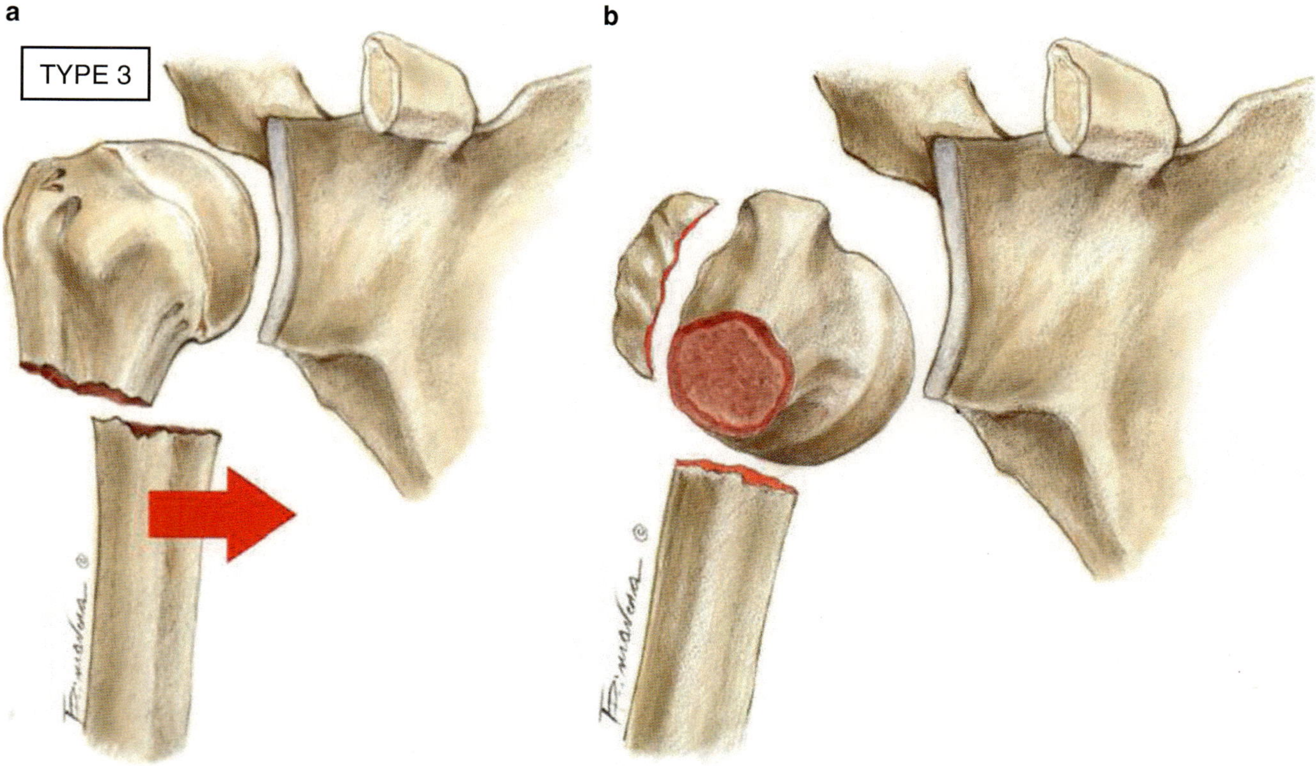

Fig. 1.56 (**a**, **b**) Surgical neck non-union

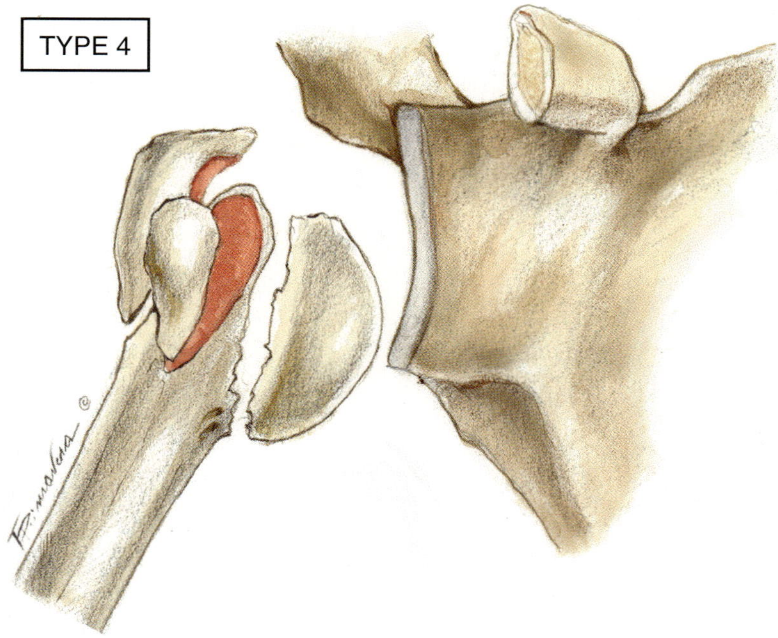

Fig. 1.57 Fracture dislocation

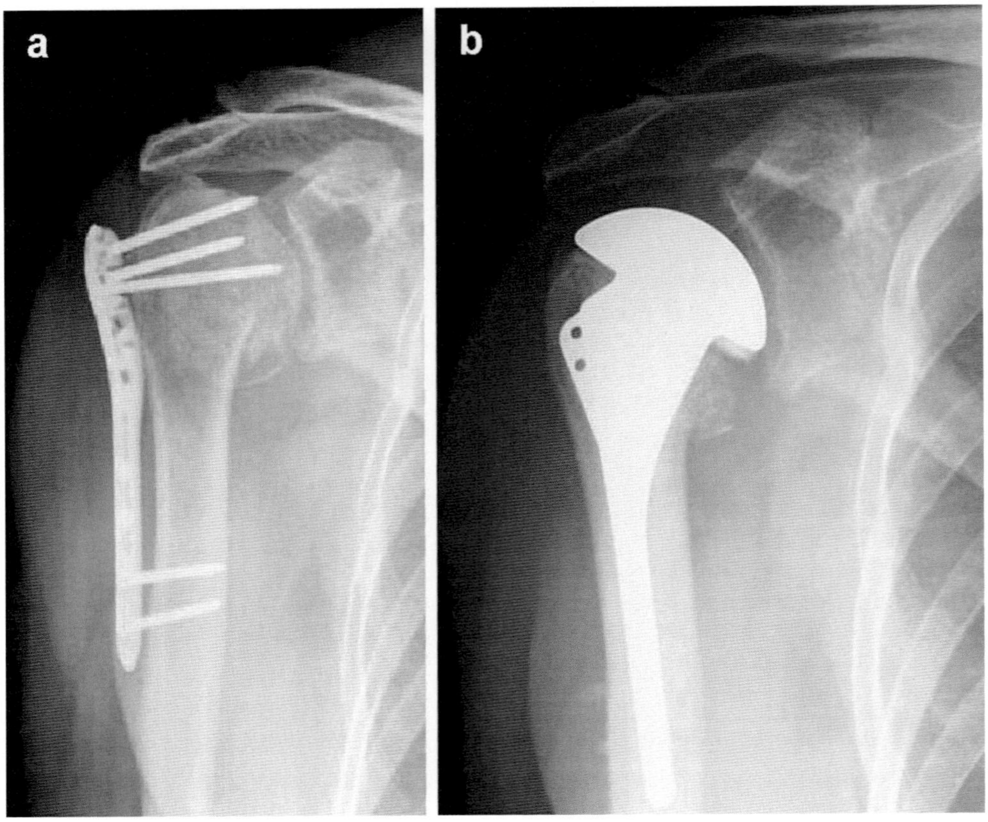

Fig. 1.58 (**a**) *Type 1*-Fracture sequelae. (**b**) Surgical solution with HEMI

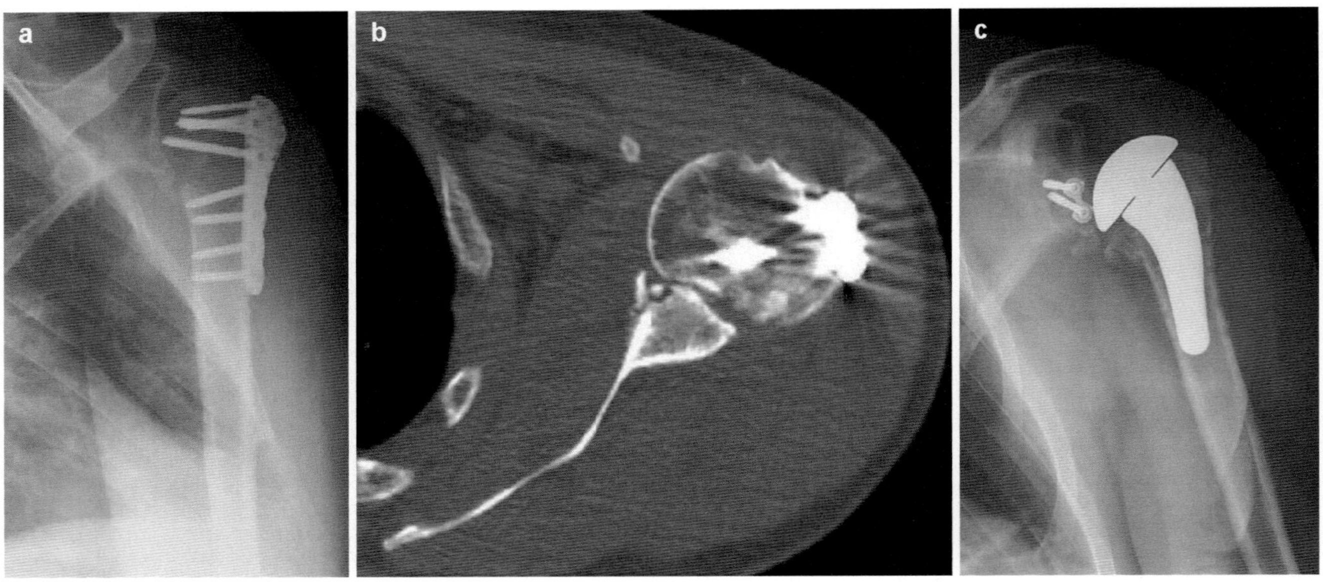

Fig. 1.59 (**a**) *Type 2*- Fracture sequelae. (**b**) Locked fracture dislocation. (**c**) Because the integrity of *Engine* (tuberosities), we performed HEMI to regain the *Fulcrum* and bone graft on the glenoid (Latarjet) to restore the *Glenoid track*

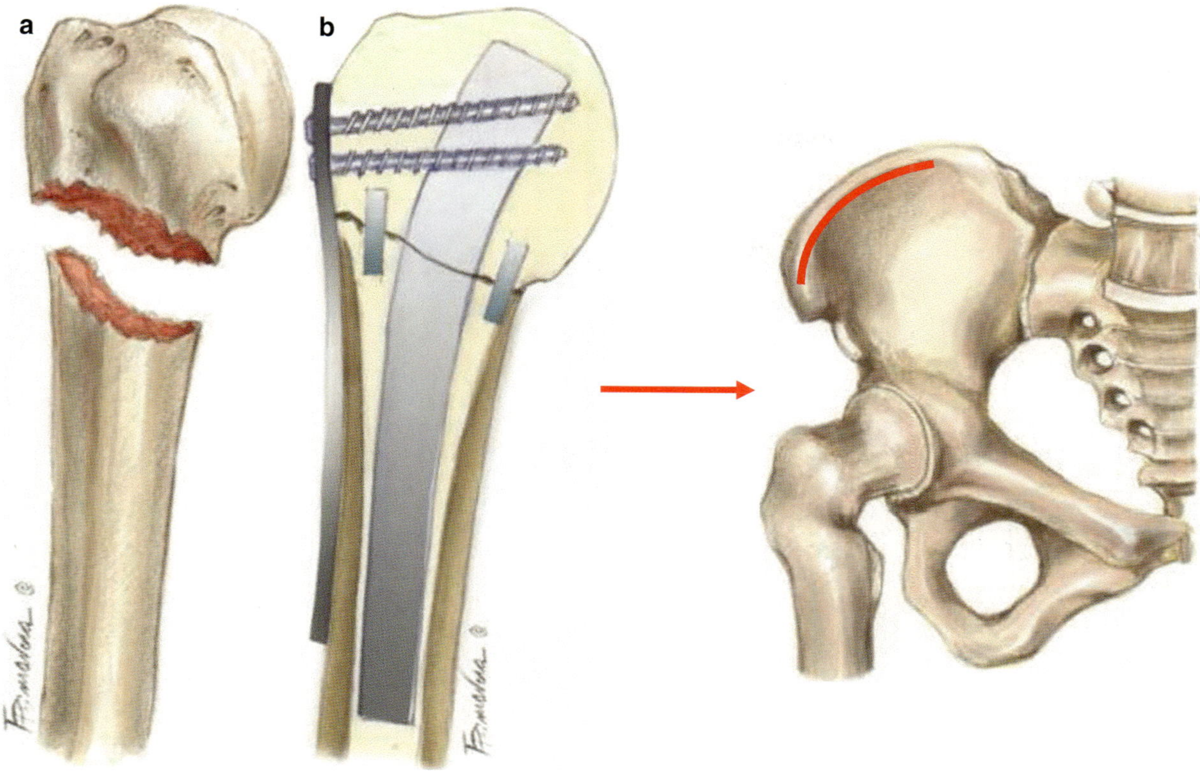

Fig. 1.60 (**a**) *Type 3*- Surgical neck fracture. (**b**) PEG bone graft

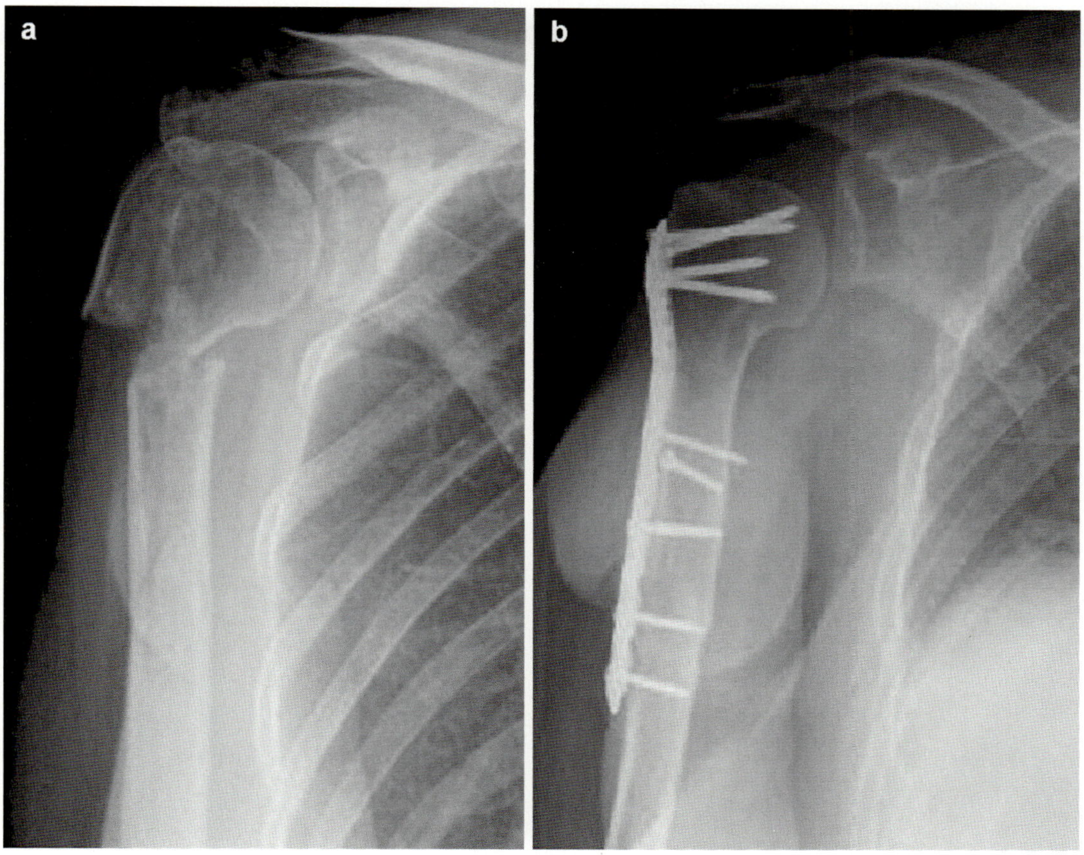

Fig. 1.61 (**a**) *Type 3*- sequelae of surgical neck fracture. (**b**) Surgical solution with ORIF

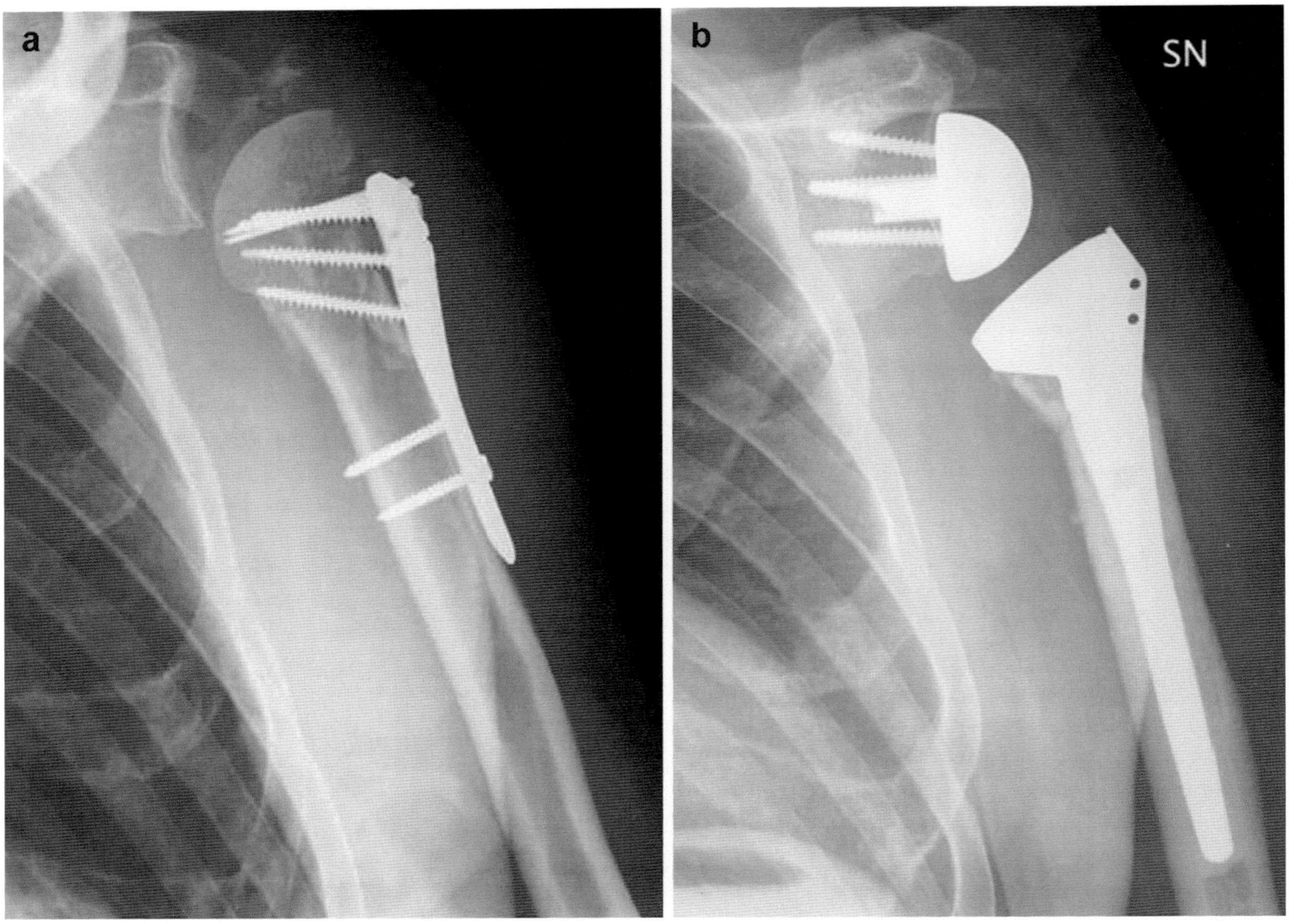

Fig. 1.62 (**a**) *Type 4*-fracture sequelae with severe tuberosity mal-union (loss of *Engine*). (**b**) Surgical solution Reverse. sn: left side

1.9 Rehabilitation Pearls

Rehabilitation and patient management after surgery for PHF are complex procedures, clearly illustrating the need for physiotherapy and orthopedic professionals to work in concert.

Post-op PHF patients are best managed by a team comprising the orthopedic surgeon, physiatrist, physiotherapist and radiologist specialist in these conditions.

Patient management is particularly delicate also from the emotional standpoint since patients may have often previously had unsuccessful surgery and/or undergone several months rehabilitation.

While the team must make it their business to encourage patients, a first essential step to ensuring good post-operative recovery and rehabilitation, care should also be taken to provide each patient with a realistic picture of potential complications and the possibility of achieving only partial functional results.

1.9.1 Information Strategy

Explain to the patient the complexity of the fracture he/she has suffered and that the complications of conservative and/or surgical treatment are due to biological reasons that are not always easy to predict or interpret.

Putting him/herself in the hand of a dedicated surgical and rehabilitation team allows the patient to best manage the recovery timeframes involved. Straightforward information given by professional in a simple manner is generally well understood and reinforces the relationship of trust between the patient and the healthcare team.

Feedback and exchange between the surgical and rehab team is key. The surgeon must inform the rehabilitator of the patient's clinical history, on the reasons for opting for surgery, patient bone and soft tissue quality, and the state of any fixation plates or prostheses. By the same token, the rehabilitator is required to keep the surgeon informed of any initial clinical signs that could signal infection, fibrous adhesions or neuromuscular disorders.

1.9.2 Rehabilitation Strategy

The surgical management options for sequelae are: open reduction internal fixation (ORIF), HEMI or Reverse.

Post-surgery rehab protocols align with the indications given in the specific chapters. It should, however, be borne in mind that poor quality bone and soft tissue are characteristic sequelae of fracture. It follows that the pace of the rehabilitation program must be patient specific, taking into account the need to balance the requirements of the biological deficit while preventing fibrous reactions and the formation of adhesions.

1.10 Correct Information Feedback

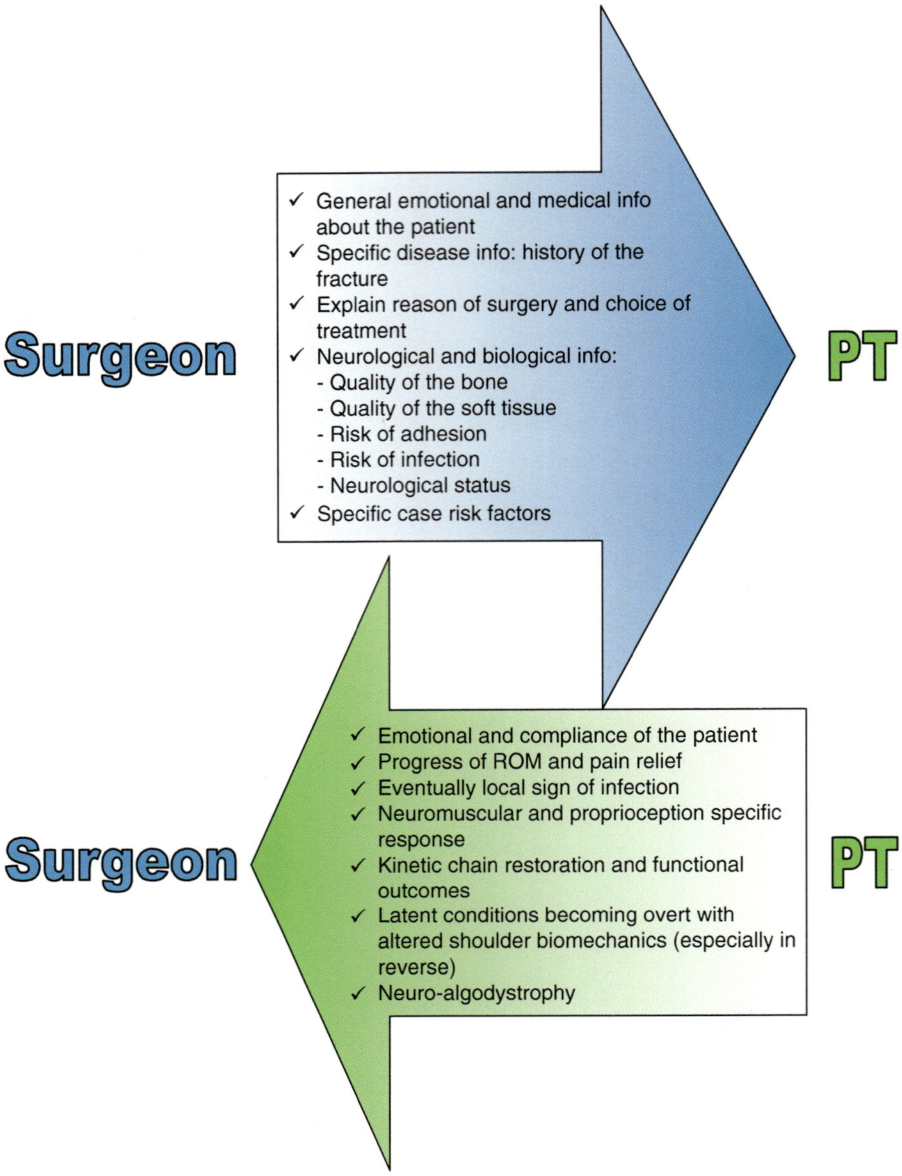

References

1. Horak J, NilssonBE (1975) Epidemiology of fracture of the upper end of the humerus. Clin Orthop Relat Res Vol 112, 250–253
2. Stimson B (1947) A manual of fractures and dislocations, 2nd edn. Lea & Febiger, Philadelphia
3. Court- Brown CM, Grag A, McQueen MM (2001) The epidemiology of proximal humeral fractures. Acta Orthop Scand 72:365–371
4. Roux A, Decroocq L, El Batti S, Bonnevialle N, Moineau G, Trojani C, Boileau P, de Peretti F (2012) Epidemiology of proximal humerus fractures managed in a trauma center. J Orthop Trauma Surg Res 98:715–719
5. Palaven M, Kannus P, Niemi S, Parkkari J (2006) Update in the epidemiology of proximal humerus fractures. Clin Orthop Relat Res 442:87–92
6. Gardner MJ, Weil Y, Barker JU, Kelly BT, Helfet DL, Lorich DG (2007) The importance of medial support in locked plating of proximal humerus fractures. J Orthop Trauma 21:185–191
7. Hertel R, Hempfing A, Stiehler M, Leunig M (2004) Predictors of humeral head ischemia after intracapsular fracture of proximal humerus. J Shoulder Elbow Surg 13:427–433
8. Resh H, Beck E, Bayley I (1995) Recostruction of the valgus-impacted humeral head fracture. J Shoulder Elbow Surg 4:73–80
9. Neer CS (1970) Dispiace proximal humerus fractures. Classification and evaluation. J Bone Joint Surg Am 52:1077–1089
10. Codman E (1934) The shoulder: rupture of the supraspinatus tendon and other lesion in or about the subacromial bursa. Privately Printed, Boston
11. Boileau P, Bicknell RT, Mazzoleni N, Walch G, Urien JP (2008) CT scan method accurately assesses humeral head retroversion. Clin Orthop Relat Res 466(3):661–669
12. Hernigou P, Duparc F, Hernigou A (2002) Determining humeral controversion with computed tomography. J Bone Joint Surg Am 84(10):1753–1762
13. Muller ME, Nazarian S, Koch P, Schatzker J (1990) The comprehensive classification of fractures of long bones. Springer, Berlin, pp 120–121
14. Hertel R (2005) Fractures of the proximal humerus in osteoporotic bone. Osteopors Int 16(Suppl2):S65–S72
15. Codman EA (1934) Fractures in relation to the subacromial bursa. In: Codman EA (ed) The shoulder, rupture of the supraspinatus tendon and others lesion in or about the subacromial bursa. Krieger Publishing, Malabar, pp 313–331
16. Majed A, Macleod I, Bull AMJ, Zyto K, Resh H, Hertel R, Reilly P, Emery RJH (2011) Proximal humeral fracture classification system revisited. J Shoulder Elbow 20:1125–1132
17. Solberg BD, Moon CN, Franco DP, Paiement GD (2009) Surgical treatment of three four part proximal humeral fractures. J Bone Joint Surg Am 91:1689–1697
18. Solberg BD, Moon CN, Franco DP, Paiement GD (2009) Locked plating of 3 and 4-part proximal humerus fractures in older patients: the effect of initial fracture pattern on outcome. J Orthop Trauma 23:113–119
19. Herbert Resh MD (2001) Proximal humeral fractures: current controversies. J Shoulder Elbow Surg 20:827–832
20. Gerber C, Schneeberger AG, Vinh TS (1990) The arterial vascularization of humeral head: An anatomical study. J Bone Joint Surg Am 72(10):1486–1494
21. Brooks CH, Revel WJ, Heatley FW (1993) Vascularity of the humeral head after proximal humeral fractures: an anatomic cadaver study. J Bone Joint Surg Br 75(1):132–136
22. Duparc F, Muller JM, Fregér P (2001) Arterial blood supply of the proximal humeral epiphysis. Surg Radiol Anat 23(839):185–190
23. Hettrich CM, Boraiah S, Dyke JP, Neviaser A, Helfet DL, Lorich DG (2010) Quantitative assessment of the vascularity of the proximal part of the humerus. J Bone Joint Surg Am 92(4):943–948
24. Edwin R, Cadet MD, Christopher S, Ahmad MD (2012) Hemiarthroplasty for three- and four- part proximal humerus fractures. J Am Acad Orthop Surg 20:17–27
25. Turpka A, Wiedemann E, Ruchholtz S et al (1997) Dislocated multiple fragment fractures of the head of the humerus. Does dislocation of the humeral head fragment signify a worse prognosis? Unfallchirurg 100:105–110
26. Coudane H, Fays J, De la Selle H, Nicoud C, Pilot L (2000) Arteriography after complex fractures of the upper extremity of the humerus bone. A prospective study- preliminary results. J Shoulder Elbow Surg 9:548
27. Esser RD (1994) Treatment of three and four-part fractures of the proximal humerus with a modified cloverleaf plate. J Orthop Trauma 8:15–22
28. Jakob RP, Miniaci A, Anson PS et al (1991) Four –part valgus impacted fractures of the proximal humerus. J Bone Joint Surg Br 73:295–298
29. Resh H, Povacz P, Frohlich R, Wambacher M (1997) Percutaneaos fixation of three- and four- part fractures of the proximal humerus. J Bone Surg Br 79:295–300
30. Vandenbussche E, Peraldi P, Naouri JF, Rougereau G, Augereau B (1996) Four part valgus impacted fractures of the upper extremity of the humerus: ilium graft reconstruction. Apropos of 8 cases. Rev Chir Orthop Reparatrice Appar Mot 82:658–662
31. Gerber C, Hersche O, Berberat C (1998) The clinical relevance of post-traumatic avascular necrosis of the humeral head. J Shoulder Elbow Surg 7:586–590
32. Burkhart Stephen S, Lo Ian D (2006) Arthroscopic rotator cuff repair. J Am Acad Orthop Surg 14:333–346
33. Hoffmeyer P (2002) The operative management of displaced fractures of the proximal humerus. J Bone Joint Surg Br 84(B):469–480
34. Poppen NK, Walker PS (1983) Force at the glenohumeral joint in abduction. Clin Othop 135:165–170
35. Poppen NK, Walker PS (1976) Normal and abnormal motion of the shoulder. J Bone Joint Surg Am 58-A:195–201
36. Widnall JC, Dheerendra SK, Jacob George Malal J, Waseem M (2013) Proximal humeral fractures: a review of current concepts. Open Orthop J 7(Suppl 3: M12):361–365
37. Kristiansen B, Christensen SW (1986) Plate fixation of Proximal humeral fractures. Acta Orthop Scand 57(4):320–323
38. Lefevre- Colau MM, Babinet A, Fayad F et al (2007) Immediate mobilization compared with conventional immobilization for the impacted nonoperatively treated proximal humeral fractures: a randomized controlled trial. J Bone Joint Surg Am 89(12):2582–2590
39. Deldycke J, Rommens PM, Heyvaert G, Broos PL (1993) Conservative study between the classical Desault- bandage and the new Gilchrist- bandage. Unfallchirurgie 232:145–146
40. Hutten TT, Launonen AP, Pihlajamaki H, Kannus P, Mattila VM (2012) Trends in the surgical treatment of proximal humeral fractures- a nationwide 23-year study in Finland. MBC Muscoloskeletal Disord 13:261
41. Ellenbecker TS (2004) Clinical examination of the shoulder. Elsevier Saunders, St. Louis. 2014
42. Nho SJ, Brophy RH, Barker JU, Cornell CN, MacGillivray JD (2007) Management of proximal humeral fractures based on current literature. J Bone Joint Surg 89(Suppl 3):44–58
43. Khmelnitskaya E, Lamont LE, Taylor SA, Lorich DG, Dines DM, Dines JS (2012) Evaluation and management of proximal humerus fractures. Hindawi Publ Corp Adv Othop; Art ID 861598
44. Cadet ER, Ahmad CS (2012) Hemiathroplasty for three- and four-part proximal humerus fractures. J Am Acad Orthop Surg 20(1):17–22

45. Olerud P, Ahrengart L, Ponzer S, Saving J, Tidermark J (2011) Hemiarthroplasty versus non operative treatment of displaced 4-part proximal humeral fractures in elderly patient: a randomized controlled trial. J Shoulder Elbow 20(7):1025–1033
46. Sudkamp NP, Audige L, Lambert S, Hertel R, Konrad G (2011) Path analysis of factors for functional outcome in one year in 463 proximal humerus fractures. J Shoulder Elbow Surg 18(8):1207–1216
47. Boileau P, Krishnan SG, Tinsi L, Walch G, Coste JS, Molè D (2002) Tuberosity malposition and migration : reason for poor outcomes after hemiarthroplasty for displaced fractures of the proximal humerus. J Shoulder Elbow Surg 11(5):401–412
48. Frankle MA, Ondrovic LE, Markee BA, Harris ML, Lee WE 3rd (2002) Stability of tuberosity reattachment in proximal humeral hemiarthroplasty. J Should Elbow Surg 11:413–420
49. Mighell MA, Kolm GP, Collinge CA, Frankle MA (2003) Outcomes of hemiarthroplasty for fractures of the proximal humerus. J Shoulder Elbow Surg 12:569–577
50. Kontakis GM, Damilakis J, Christoforakis J, Papadakis A, Katonis P, Prassopopulus P (2001) The bicipital groove as a landmark for orientation of the humeral prosthesis in cases of fractures. J Shoulder Elbow Surg 10:136–139
51. Christoforakis JJ, Kontakis GM, Katonis PG, Stergiopopulus K, Hadjipavlou AG (2004) Shoulder hemiarthroplasty in the management of the humeral head fractures. Acta Orthop Belg 70:214–218
52. Becker R, Pap G, Machner A, Neumann WH (2002) Strength and motion after hemiarthroplasty in displaced four-fragment fracture of the proximal humerus: 27 patient followed 1–6 years. Acta Orthop Scand 73:44–49
53. Parkash U, McGurty DW, Dent JA (2002) Hemiarthroplasty for severe fractures of the proximal humerus. J Shoulder Elbow Surg 11:428–430
54. Garrigues E, Johnston PS, Pepe MD, Tucker BS, Ramsey ML, Austin LS (2012) Hemiarthroplasty versus reverse total shoulder arthroplasty for acute proximal humerus fractures in elderly patients. Orthopaedics 35(5):703–708
55. Boyle MJ, Youn SM, Frampton CM, Ball CM (2013) (in press) Functional outcomes of reverse shoulder arthroplasty compared with hemiartroplasty for acute proximal humeral fractures. j shoulder and elbow surg 1:32–7
56. Kralinger F, Schwaiger R, Wambacher M, Farrel E, Menth-Chiari W, Lajtai G, Hubner C, Resch H (2004) Outcome after primary hemiartroplasty for fracture of the head of the humerus. A retrospective multicenter study of 167 patient. J Bone Joint Surg Br 86:217–219
57. Doetsch AM, Faber J, Lynnerup N et al (2004) The effect of calcium and vitamin D3 supplementation on the healing of the proximal humerus fracture: a randomized placebo- controlled study. Calcif Tissue Int 75:183–188
58. Healy WL, Jupiter JB, Kristiansen TK, White RR (1990) Non union of the proximal humerus: a review of 25 cases. J Orthop Trauma 4:424–431
59. Rooney PJ, Cockshott WP (1986) Pseudoarthrosis following proximal humeral fractures: a possible mechanism. Skeletal Radiol 15:21–24
60. Bigliani LU, Flatow EL, Cluskey M, Fisher RA (1991) Failed prosthetic replacement of displaced proximal humerus fractures. Orthop Trans 15:747–748
61. Kontakis G, Koutras C, Tosounidis T, Giannoudis P (2008) Early management of proximal humeral fractures with hemiartroplasty: a systematic review. J Bone Joint Surg 90(11):1407–1413
62. Mirzayan R, Itamura JM, Vangsness CT Jr, Holtom PD, Sherman R, Patzakis MJ (2000) Management of deep infection following rotator cuff repair. J Bone Joint Surg Am 82(8):1115–1121
63. Sperling JW, Kozak TK, Hanssen AD, Cofield RH (2001) Infection after shoulder arthroplasty. Clin Orthop Relat Res 382:206–216
64. Athwal GS, Sperling JW, Rispoli DM, Cofield RH (2007) Deep infection after rotator cuff repair. J Shoulder Elbow Surg 16(3):306–311
65. Herrera MF, Bauer G, Reynolds F, Wilk RM, Bigliani LU, Levine WN (2002) Infection after mini-open rotator cuff repair. J Shoulder Elbow Surg 11(6):605–608
66. Kalainov DM, Bisson LJ, Brause BD, Figgie MP, Weiland AJ (1996) Management of infected shoulder arthroplasties. Orthop Trans 20:411–412
67. Themistocleous G, Zalavars C, Stine I, Zachos V, Itamura J (2007) Prolonged implantation of an antibiotic cement spacer for the management of shoulder sepsis in compromised patients. J Shoulder Elbow Surg 16(6):701–705
68. Brems JJ (2002) Complication of shoulder arthroplasty: infection instability and loosening. Instr Course Lect 51:29–39
69. Coste JS, Regis S, Trojani C, Berg M, Walch G, Boileau P (2004) The management of infection in arthroplasty of the shoulder. J Bone Joint Surg Br 86(1):65–69
70. Kiber WB, Press J, Sciascia AD (2006) The role of the core stability in Athletic Function. Sports Med 36(3):189–198
71. McCann PD, Wootten MF, Kadaba MP, Bigliani LU (1993) A kinematic and electromyographic study of shoulder rehabilitation exercises. Clin Orthop Related Res 288:179–188
72. Codman EA (1934) The shoulder. Thomas Todd Company, Boston
73. Kisner C, Colby LA (1996) Therapeutic exercises: foundations and techniques, 3rd edn. FA Davis Co, Philadelphia, pp 283–284
74. Kibler WB (1991) Role of the scapula in the overhead throwing motion. Contemp Orthop 22(5):525–532
75. Kibler WB (1998) Shoulder rehabilitation. Principle and practice. Med Sci Sports Exerc 30(4):S40–S50
76. Levine WN, Marra G (2003) Fractures of the shoulder girdle. Marcel Dekker, New York, p 126
77. Inman VT, Saunders JB, Abbott LC (1944) Observation of the function of the shoulder joint. J Bone Joint Surg 26(1):1–30
78. Ellsworth AA, Mullaney M, Tyler TF, McHugh M, Nicholas SJ (2006) Electromyography of selected shoulder musculature during un-weighted and weighted pendulum exercises. North Am J Sports Phys Ther 1(2):73–74
79. Faulkner JA (2003) Terminology for contractions of muscles during shortening, while isometric, and during lengthening. J Appl Physiol 95(2):455–459
80. Faulkner JA, Larkin LM, Claffin DR, Brooks SV (2007) Age-related changes in the structure and function of skeletal muscles. Clin Exp Pharmacol Physiol 34:1091–1096
81. Hemmings B, Smith M, Graydon J, Dyson R (2000) Effects of massage on physiological restoration, perceived recovery, and repeated sports performance. Br J Sports Med 34:109–114
82. Crane JD, Ogborn DI, Cupido C, Melov S, Hubbard A, Bourgeois JM, Tarnopolsky MA (2012) Massage therapy attenuates inflammatory signaling after exercise-induced muscle damage. Sci Transl Med 4(119):119
83. Moreside JM, Vera-Garcia FJ, McGill SM (2007) Trunk muscle activation patterns, lumbar compressive forces, and spine stability when using the bodyblade. Phys Ther 87(2):153–163
84. Buteau JL, Eriksrud O, Hasson SM (2007) Rehabilitation of a glenohumeral instability utilizing the body blade. Physiother Theory Pract 23(6):333–349
85. Tidus PM (1997) Manual massage and recovery of muscle function following exercise: a literature review. J Orthop Sports Phys Ther 25(2):107–112
86. Boileau P, Trojani C, Walch G, Krishnan SG, Romeo A, Sinnerton R (2001) Shoulder arthroplasty for the treatment of the sequelae of fractures of the proximal humerus. J Shoulder Elbow Surg 10(4):299–308

87. Cofield RH (1987) Shoulder replacement:prognosis related to diagnosis. Shoulder Replace 157–161
88. Neer CS. Old trauma in genohumeral arthroplasty. Shoulder reconstruction. Philadelphia Saunders; 1990. pp 222–234
89. Tanner MW, Cofield RH (1983) Prosthetic arthroplasty for fractures and fractures dislocations of the proximal humerus. Clin Orthop 179:116–128
90. Mansat P (2006) Les sèquelles traumatiques ostéo-articulares de l'articulation gléno-humérale. Sauramps Mèdical, Montpellier
91. Moineau G, Mc Celland WB, Trojano C, Rumian A, Walch G, Boileau P (2012) Prognostic factors and limitations of anatomic shoulder arthroplasty for the treatment of post-traumatic cephalic collapse or necrosis (Type 1 proximal humeral fracture sequelae). J Bone Joint Surg Am 94:2186–2194
92. Boileau P, Walch G, Trojani C, Sinnerton R, Romeo AA, Veneau B (1999) Sequelae of fractures of the proximal humerus: surgical classification and limits of shoulder arthroplasty. In: Walch G, Boileau P (eds) Shoulder arthroplasty. Springer, Berlin/Heidelberg
93. Boileau P., Neyton L (2008) Reverse shoulder arthroplasty in proximal humerus fracture sequelae. Constrained or noncostrained prosthesis? In: Walch BG, Molé D, Favard L, Lévigne C, Sirveaux F, Kempf JF. "Shoulder concepts 2008- proximal humeral factures and sequelae" under the direction of p. Sauramps Médical. pp 265–269
94. Perlmutter GS (1999) Axillary nerve injury. Clin Orthop Relat Res (368):28–36
95. Rockwood C, Masten FA III, Wirth M, Lippitt S (2008) The shoulder, 4th edn. Saunders Elsevier, Philadelphia
96. Gardner MJ, Griffith MH, Dines JS, Briggs SM, Weiland AJ, Lorich DG (2005) The extended anterolateral acromial approach allows minimally invasive access to the proximal humerus. Clinical Orthop Relat Res (434):123–129
97. Kim SH, Szabo RM, Marder RA (2012) Epidemiology of proximal humerus fractures in the United States: nationwide emergency department sample, 2008. Arthritis Care Res 64(3):407–414
98. Cools AM, Dewitte V, Lanszweert F, Notebaert D, Roets A, Soetens B, Cagnie B, Witvrouw EE (2007) Rehabilitation of scapular muscle balance. Which exercises to prescribe? Am J Sports Med 35(10):1744–1751
99. Ishigaki T, Yamanaka M, Hirokawa M, Tai K, Ezawa Y, Samukawa M, Tohyama H, Sugawara M (2014) Rehabilitation exercises to induce balanced scapular muscle activity in an anti-gravity posture. J Phys Ther Sci 26(12):1871–1874

Shoulder Replacement

2

John E. Kuhn, Rebecca N. Dickinson, and Woodley Desir

Contents

J.E. Kuhn, MD, MS (✉)
Kenneth D. Schermerhorn Professor of Orthopedics and Rehabilitation, Chief of Shoulder Surgery, Director of the Division of Sports Medicine, Vanderbilt University Medical Center, Nashville, TN, USA
e-mail: j.kuhn@vanderbilt.edu

R.N. Dickinson, DPT, COMT
Department of Orthopedic Surgery and Rehabilitation, Vanderbilt University Medical Center, Nashville, TN, USA
e-mail: rebecca.n.dickenson@vanderbilt.edu

W. Desir, MD
Fellow, Division of Sports Medicine, Vanderbilt University Medical Center, Nashville, TN, USA
e-mail: woodley.desir@vanderbilt.edu

G. Di Giacomo, S. Bellachioma (eds.), *Shoulder Surgery Rehabilitation: A Teamwork Approach*,
DOI 10.1007/978-3-319-24856-1_2

2.1 Introduction

Arthroplasty of the glenohumeral joint has revolutionized the treatment for painful advanced degenerative diseases of the shoulder. Although shoulder joint replacement is less common than knee or hip replacement, it is just as successful in relieving joint pain for a variety of arthritic disorders. Shoulder pain is one of the most common complaints in primary care and in rheumatologic, orthopedic, rehabilitation, and other practice settings [1]. Shoulder pain originates from a range of pathoanatomic entities including involvement of the rotator cuff tendons, bursae, and glenohumeral joint structures. Most shoulder disorders respond to conservative management with medication and rehabilitation. Patients with advanced, symptomatic, disabling glenohumeral joint arthritis are typically candidates for total shoulder arthroplasty (Fig. 2.1a, b).

2.2 History of Shoulder Arthroplasty

The earliest documented report of prosthetic shoulder replacement dates back to 1893, when the French surgeon Jules-Émile Péan inserted a prosthesis composed of platinum and rubber for glenohumeral joint damaged by tuberculosis infection [2]. Advancement of modern-day shoulder replacement has evolved from both European and American influences. In Europe during the 1950s, at Royal National Orthopedic Hospital in Stanmore, surgeons used a prosthetic replacement for tumors of the proximal humerus. This prosthesis had poor function but the long-term survival was good [3]. The Stanmore group later designed a prosthetic shoulder replacement for patients with osteoarthritis and rheumatoid arthritis. This constrained prosthesis shared similar design with the hip replacement components at that time.

In the United States, Dr. Charles S. Neer II developed an unconstrained Vitallium (chrome-cobalt alloy) prosthesis for the treatment of complex proximal humerus fractures [4]. These devices improved the patient's level of function and reduced pain more effectively than resection arthroplasty, which was the standard treatment at the time.

The improved success of total hip arthroplasty during this era influenced Dr. Neer to design a total shoulder prosthesis for joints with advanced osteoarthritis (The Neer II Prosthesis). This prosthesis was composed of an all-polyethylene glenoid component and newly designed metal humeral component with a variety of humeral stem lengths and humeral head sizes.

During this time, a number of innovators developed variety of implants for the shoulder. These included constrained implants (where the glenoid fits tightly over the humeral head), and metal-backed and hooded glenoid components, and even early models of a reverse shoulder arthroplasty [5]. High failure rates of these different designs led to their abandonment and the adoption of the Neer II unconstrained implant.

The next advance in shoulder arthroplasty involved attempts at replicating the patient's anatomy, by making the implants more modular [6, 7]. These "Anatomic" prostheses became popular in the 1990s. In the current decade, newer implants are designed to improve glenoid fixation (center pegs to allow bone ingrowth), to preserve proximal humeral bone, and to use computer-assisted navigation to more accurately position the glenoid.

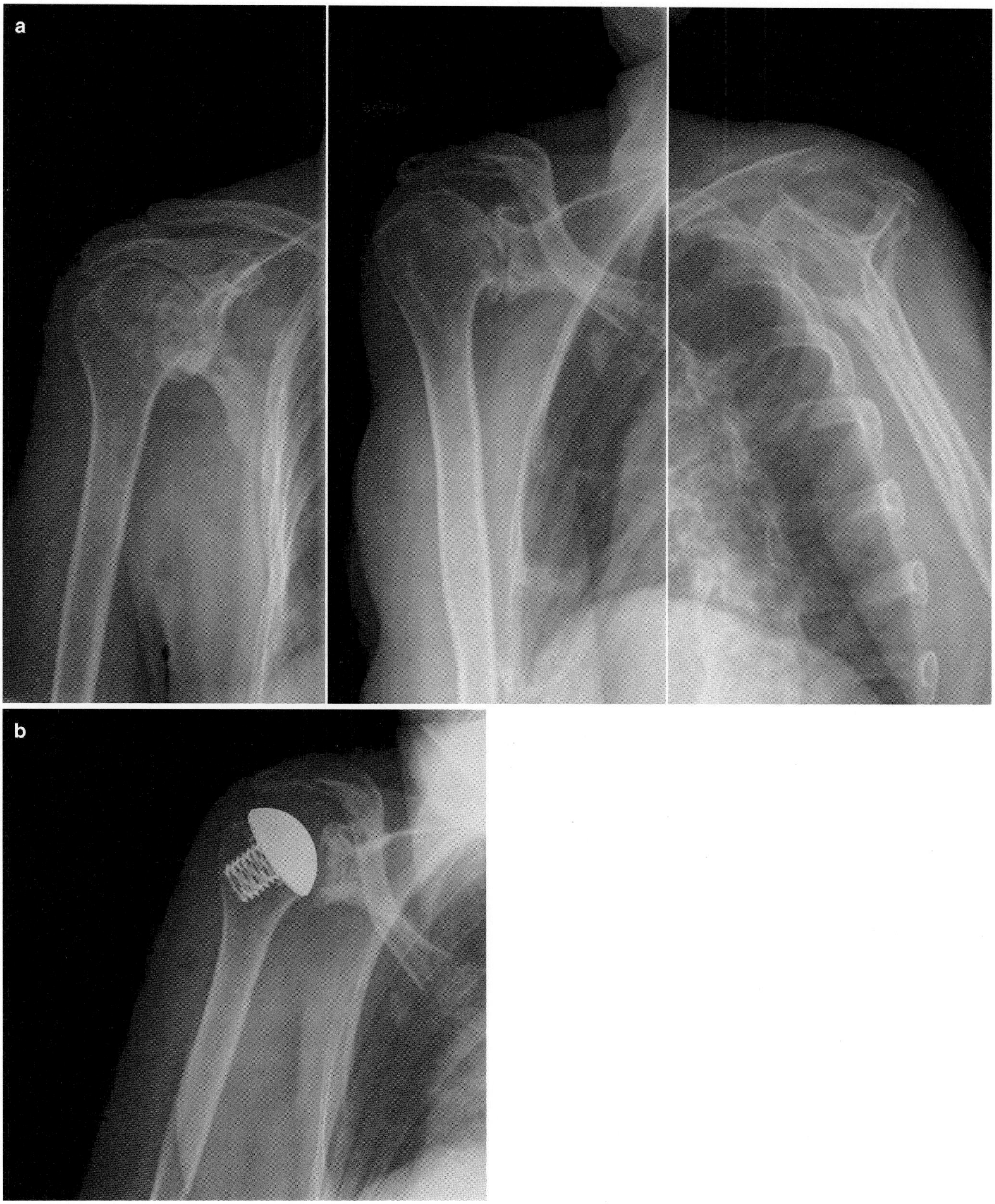

Fig. 2.1 (**a**) Osteoarthritis (**b**) Shoulder arthroplasty

2.3 Non-arthroplasty Management and Rehabilitation

Before surgery is considered, nonoperative management should be offered to patients with osteoarthritis. Medical management includes the use of nonsteroidal anti-inflammatory drugs (NSAIDs) that help relieve pain and inflammation. In general, trials comparing paracetamol or placebo to NSAIDs suggest that NSAIDs are more effective [8, 9]; however NSAIDs have more gastrointestinal and cardiac risk, which is especially concerning in the elderly patients with arthritis.

Intra-articular injections are commonly used. Corticosteroids have a limited effect [10] and should be limited to three or four per year. These may be best used for acute flares of symptoms, but not for long-term management. Intra-articular injections of hyaluronic acid have also been found to be helpful in patients with glenohumeral joint arthritis [10–12].

Rehabilitation for shoulder arthritis has not been studied well. Most authors recommend a program that includes improving glenohumeral joint motion, strengthening the rotator cuff, and strengthening the scapula-stabilizing muscles (lower trapezius and serratus anterior) [13–15]. Until more evidence is available, no standard protocol can be recommended.

Arthroscopic debridement and capsular releases for shoulder arthritis may have some benefit, but the data supporting arthroscopy is low level evidence and derived from case reports. While more cost-effective [16] and associated with fewer complications than arthroplasty [17], the clinical effectiveness of arthroscopic debridement is limited, and as such, arthroscopic treatment may not provide much benefit for patients with glenohumeral osteoarthritis [18, 19].

2.4 Indications for Shoulder Arthroplasty Osteoarthritis

Osteoarthritis of the shoulder is very common affecting over 30 % of people over age 60 [20, 21] (Fig. 2.2a, b). Osteoarthritis of the shoulder increases with age and women are more susceptible than men [22]. This is a very debilitating condition and patients perceive the impact of shoulder arthritis to be similar to other chronic medical ailments like diabetes, heart failure, and myocardial infarction [23].

The indications for surgery are essentially based on the severity of the patient's symptoms. Contraindications include younger age, higher activity levels, and patients with neuromuscular disease. Patients with irreparable rotator cuff tears are subject to higher rates of early glenoid loosening and should avoid standard total shoulder replacement, with reverse arthroplasty preferred.

Some patients may have dysplastic or biconcave glenoids. These circumstances make total shoulder arthroplasty less successful as stable fixation of the glenoid may be difficult to obtain, even in the face of eccentric reaming of the glenoid or bone grafting in severe cases [24].

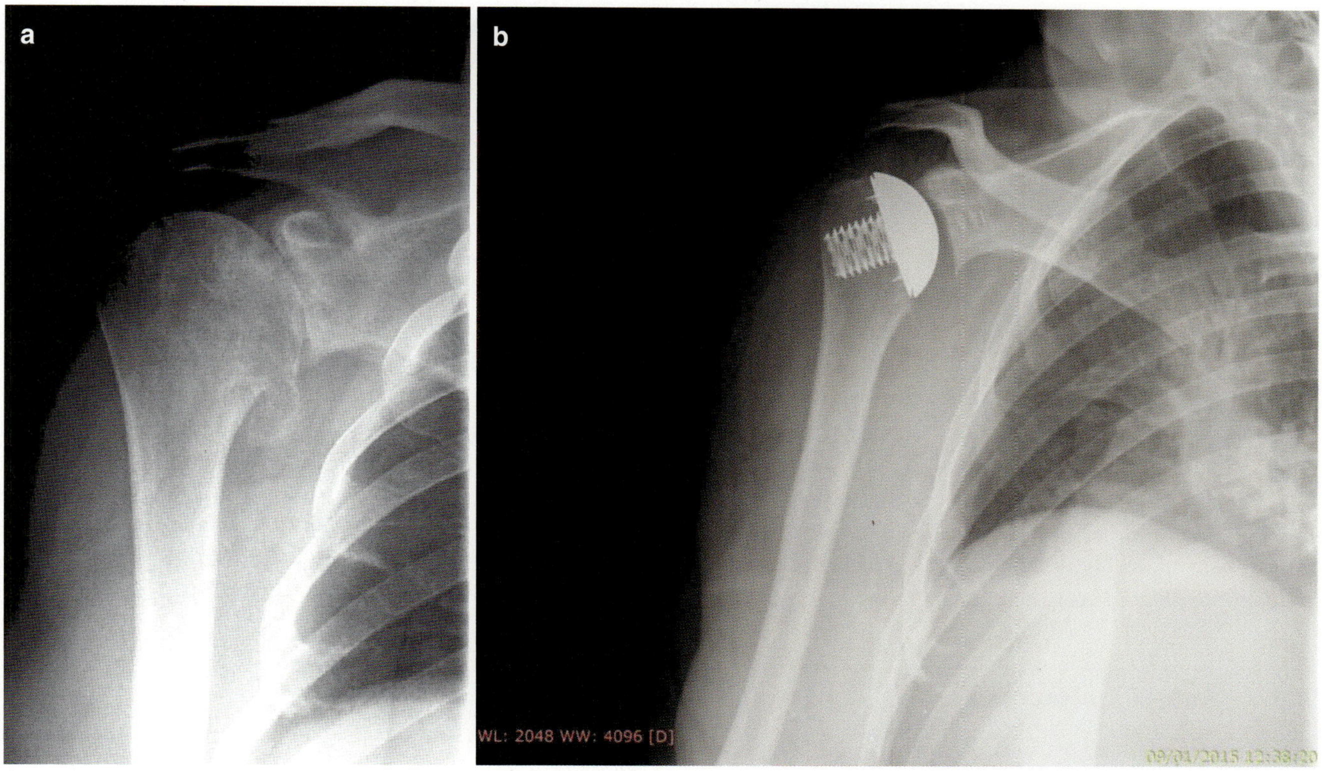

Fig. 2.2 (**a**) Severe osteoarthritis. (**b**) Total shoulder arthroplasty

2.5 Rheumatoid Arthritis

Rheumatologic diseases affect the shoulder commonly, and disease progression characterized by joint destruction and rotator cuff deterioration is expected [25]. Interestingly, the severity of the rotator cuff involvement seems to predict the patient status best [25].

Arthroscopic synovectomy with capsular release if needed can be helpful in relieving pain and restoring function [26]. Both hemiarthroplasty and total shoulder arthroplasty can be performed in patients with intact rotator cuffs, whose symptoms warrant arthroplasty. Results after arthroplasty demonstrate better pain relief and motion if total shoulder arthroplasty is performed [27]. When the rotator cuff is deficient, reverse arthroplasty can be very helpful in this population [28, 29]; however, patients with rheumatoid arthritis are more likely to be at risk for fracture and may have severe glenoid erosion requiring bone grafting.

2.6 Avascular Necrosis

Shoulder arthroplasty is an accepted treatment for patients with avascular necrosis of the humeral head. Avascular necrosis can develop after trauma or may be related to sickle cell disease, systemic lupus erythematosus, alcohol abuse, and oral corticosteroid use. Avascular necrosis is staged based on the severity of the disease, from stage I (no radiographic changes) to stage V (humeral head collapse and glenoid involvement) [30]. Humeral head replacement may be used as a treatment for avascular necrosis in patients with humeral head, but no glenoid involvement. When the disease has reached stage V, and the glenoid is involved, total shoulder arthroplasty is recommended. Generally, patients over age 65, those with posttraumatic avascular necrosis, postradiation avascular necrosis, and preoperative restrictions in motion have poorer outcomes after arthroplasty [31].

2.7 Posttraumatic Arthritis

While avascular necrosis is known to occur when fractures of the proximal humerus disrupt the blood supply, malunited intra-articular fractures or significant trauma to the cartilage of the glenoid or humeral head may produce posttraumatic arthritis (Fig. 2.3a, b). Glenohumeral joint arthritis is also known to occur as a result of frequent glenohumeral joint dislocations [32]. Additionally, patients who underwent instability surgery are at increased risk for developing glenohumeral joint osteoarthritis [33] (Fig. 2.4a, b).

All of these patients may be successfully treated with shoulder arthroplasty. It is important to recognize that patients who have had open anterior surgery for instability may have limited external rotation, and these patients may require lengthening of the anterior capsule and/or subscapularis tendon to improve their range of motion. As a result, additional protection of the subscapularis in the postoperative period may be required.

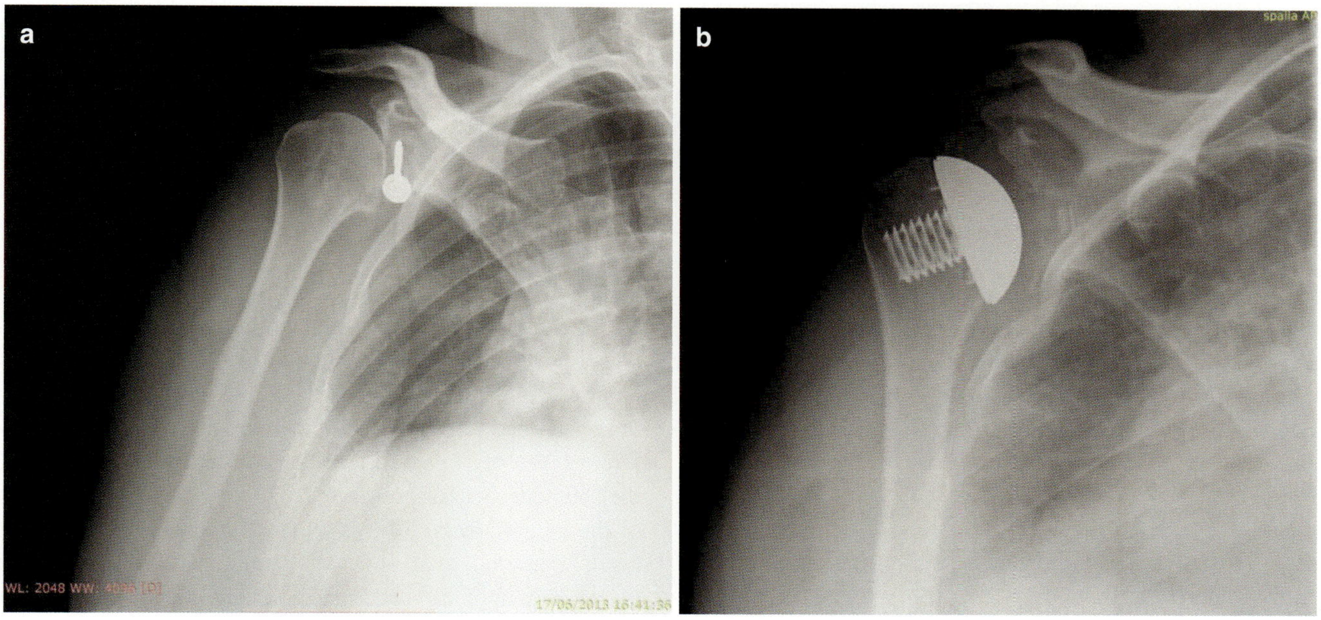

Fig. 2.3 (**a**) Iatrogenic arthritis. (**b**) Arthroplasty

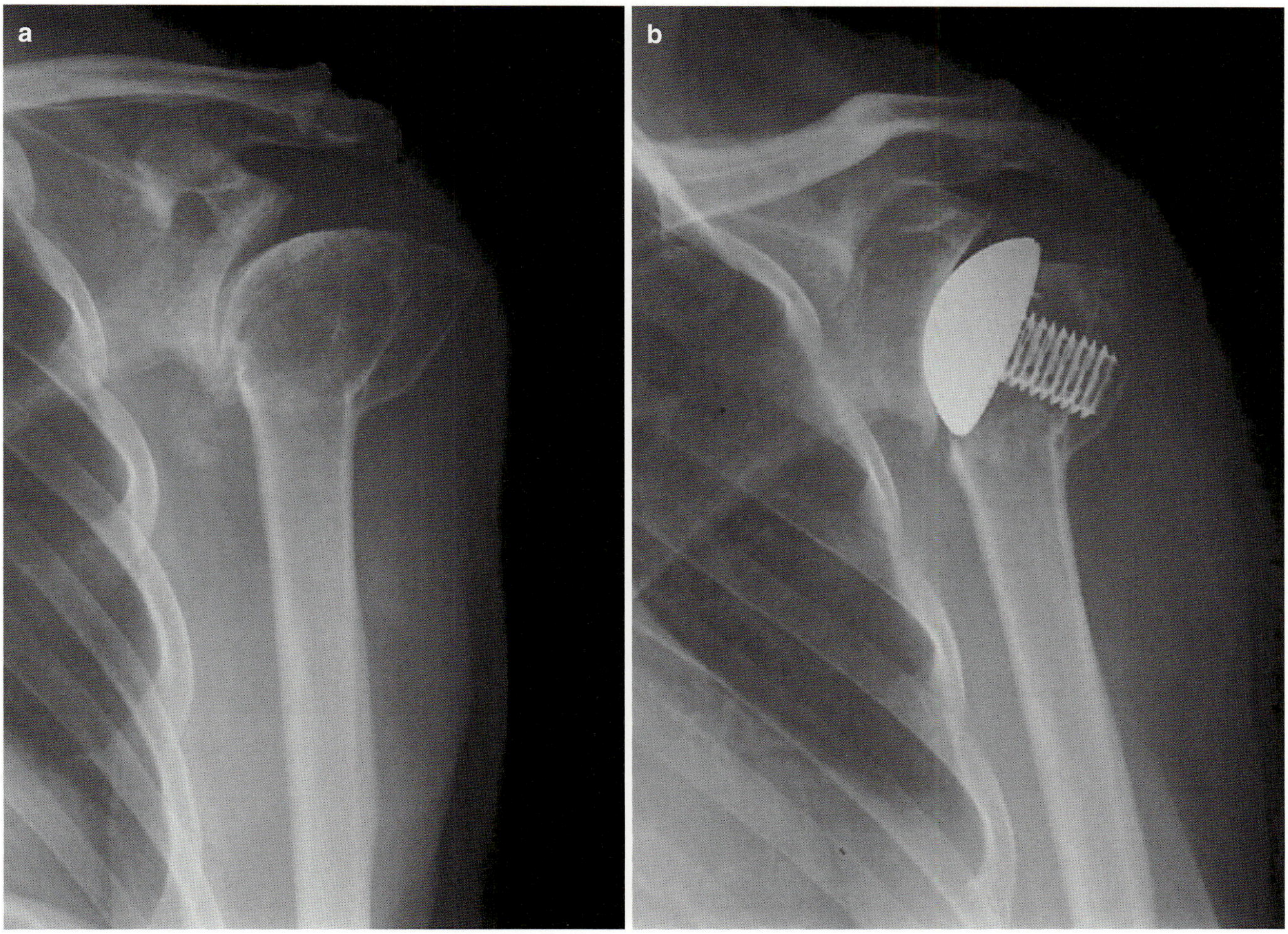

Fig. 2.4 (**a**) Posttraumatic arthritis. (**b**) Hemiarthroplasty

2.8 Rotator Cuff Tear Arthropathy

Rotator cuff tear arthropathy is a special type of arthritis that develops in conjunction with a massive rotator cuff tear. In this patient, the rotator cuff is unable to keep the humeral head centered in the glenoid, and the deltoid pulls the humeral head superiorly. Over time, the eccentric wear on the glenoid and humeral head leads to arthritis [34]. Because the rotator cuff tear in these patients is massive, a total shoulder arthroplasty would be contraindicated, as the eccentric loads on the superior prosthetic glenoid would lead to early failure. Instead, a hemiarthroplasty replacing the humeral head or a reverse shoulder arthroplasty would be recommended [35].

2.9 Contraindications for Shoulder Arthroplasty

Contraindications for shoulder arthroplasty include younger age, higher activity levels, active infection, and patients with neuromuscular disease and/or Charcot arthropathy [36]. Patients with irreparable rotator cuff tears are subject to higher rates of early glenoid loosening and should avoid standard total shoulder replacement, with reverse arthroplasty preferred.

2.10 Surgical Approaches for Shoulder Arthroplasty

The therapist charged with managing a patient after arthroplasty must have an understanding of the surgical approach and the implant design in order to protect the surgical procedure and obtain the best result. In general, there are three different types of approaches to the prosthetic replacement of the shoulder: hemiarthroplasty (Fig. 2.5a, b) where only part of the glenohumeral joint is replaced, typically the humeral head; anatomic total shoulder arthroplasty (Fig. 2.6a, b) where the humeral head and glenoid are replaced with implants that resemble the patient's normal anatomy; and reverse shoulder arthroplasty (Fig. 2.3) where the glenohumeral joint is flipped such that the ball is placed on the glenoid and the cup part of the joint is placed on the humerus.

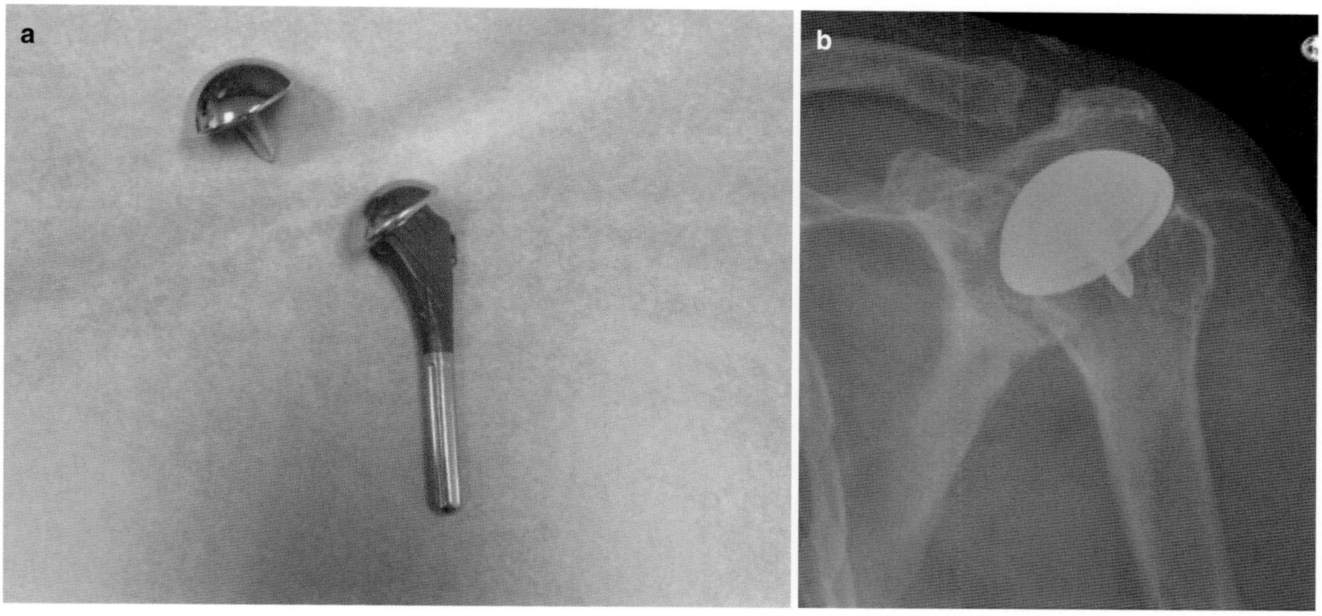

Fig. 2.5 (**a**) Two implants are shown. A stemmed implant (*Bottom*) and a resurfacing implant. (**b**) Radiograph of resurfacing hemiarthroplasty

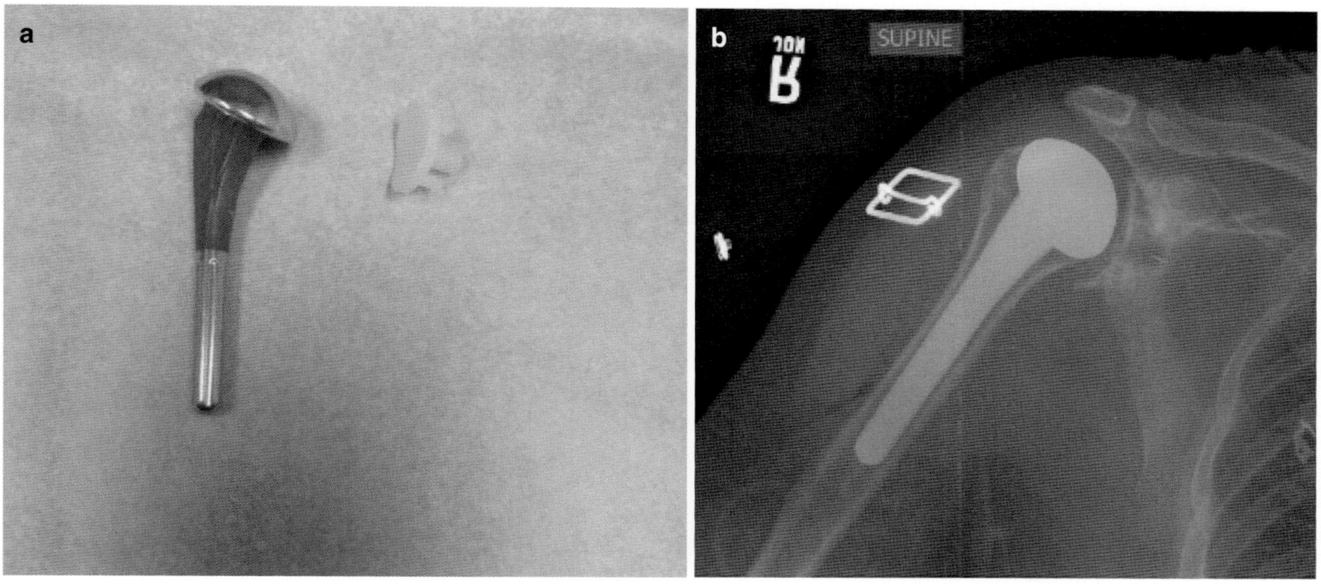

Fig. 2.6 (**a**) Implants. (**b**) Radiograph of implants

2.11 Hemiarthroplasty and Total Shoulder Arthroplasty

The deltopectoral approach is the most commonly used approach for exposing the glenohumeral joint. The anatomy and the different approaches to the subscapularis were recently reviewed by Gadea et al. [37]. The skin incision is made on the anterolateral aspect of the shoulder, directly above the coracoid process and toward the deltoid insertion, avoiding the axilla. The inter-nervous plane between the deltoid (axillary nerve) and pectoralis major (lateral and medial pectoral nerve) is then opened. The cephalic vein is a landmark that is typically found in this interval. The cephalic vein has many branches to the deltoid and is typically retracted laterally; however in large or muscular patients, the vein may be retracted with the pectoralis major to avoid injury from excessive retraction. At this point, the conjoined tendon is exposed. The fascia on its lateral border is released, exposing the subscapularis tendon and muscle.

2.11.1 Approach to the Subscapularis

In order to gain access to the glenohumeral joint, the subscapularis must be violated to some extent. There are a number of approaches to the subscapularis, but in general, it must be detached, then later repaired. This repair requires postoperative protection and directs much of the postoperative physical therapy restrictions (see below), as subscapularis failure is a devastating complication after total shoulder arthroplasty [38].

The subscapularis tendon can be peeled off of the lesser tuberosity, then later repaired with sutures through bone; it can be opened with a tenotomy, leaving a tendon stump on the lesser tuberosity requiring a tendon-to-tendon stump repair, or the tendon can be removed with a piece of the lesser tuberosity (lesser tuberosity osteotomy), which requires repair of the lesser tuberosity to the shaft of the humerus. Studies have failed to show a significant statistical difference between these techniques in terms of functional score, clinical outcome, or subscapularis fatty degeneration [39–41] (Fig. 2.7a, b).

Recently, some authors have experimented with a subscapularis-sparing approach by working above the subscapularis through the rotator interval, or below the subscapularis by opening the inferior capsule, but to date, the results have been disappointing as implants may be positioned poorly and/or osteophytes may be retained [42–45].

After the subscapularis has been taken down, the glenohumeral joint capsule is released. There are a number of ways to release the capsule, but exposure of the glenoid may require significant and nearly circumferential releases, particularly in the patient with severely restricted preoperative motion.

The implant is then inserted. Each implant maker has different tools for inserting the implant that are specific to their own implant design. The important considerations from a rehabilitation perspective relate to how the implant is secured to the bone. If the implant is cemented in place, the rehabilitation program does not require modification. If the implant is coated with materials such that bone ingrowth is expected, the surgeon may prefer waiting a few weeks—particularly with regard to loading the shoulder—to allow bony ingrowth to occur.

After the implant is inserted, the subscapularis is closed with nonabsorbable, strong suture to prevent its failure (Fig. 2.8a, b). The deltopectoral interval is re-approximated and the skin is closed.

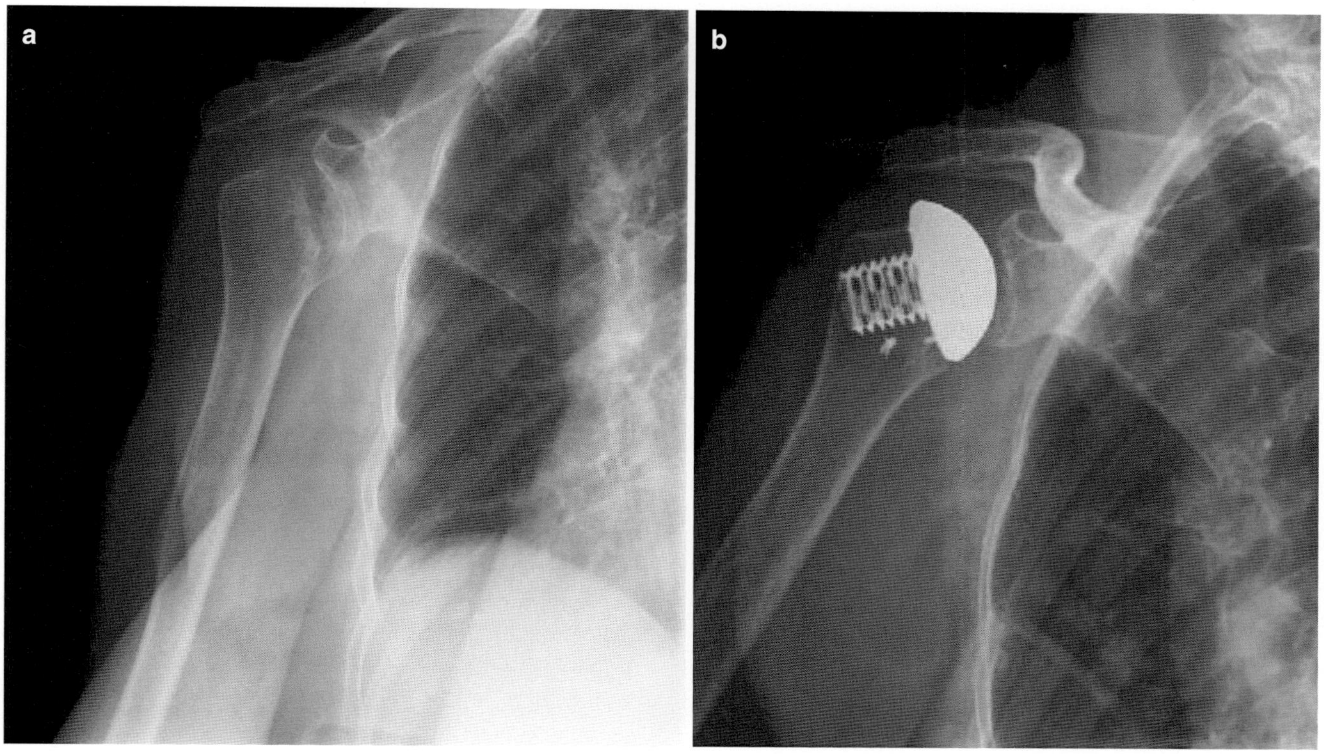

Fig. 2.7 (**a**) Posterior looked discretion. (**b**) Subscapularis reinsertion with suture anchor in hemiarthroplasty

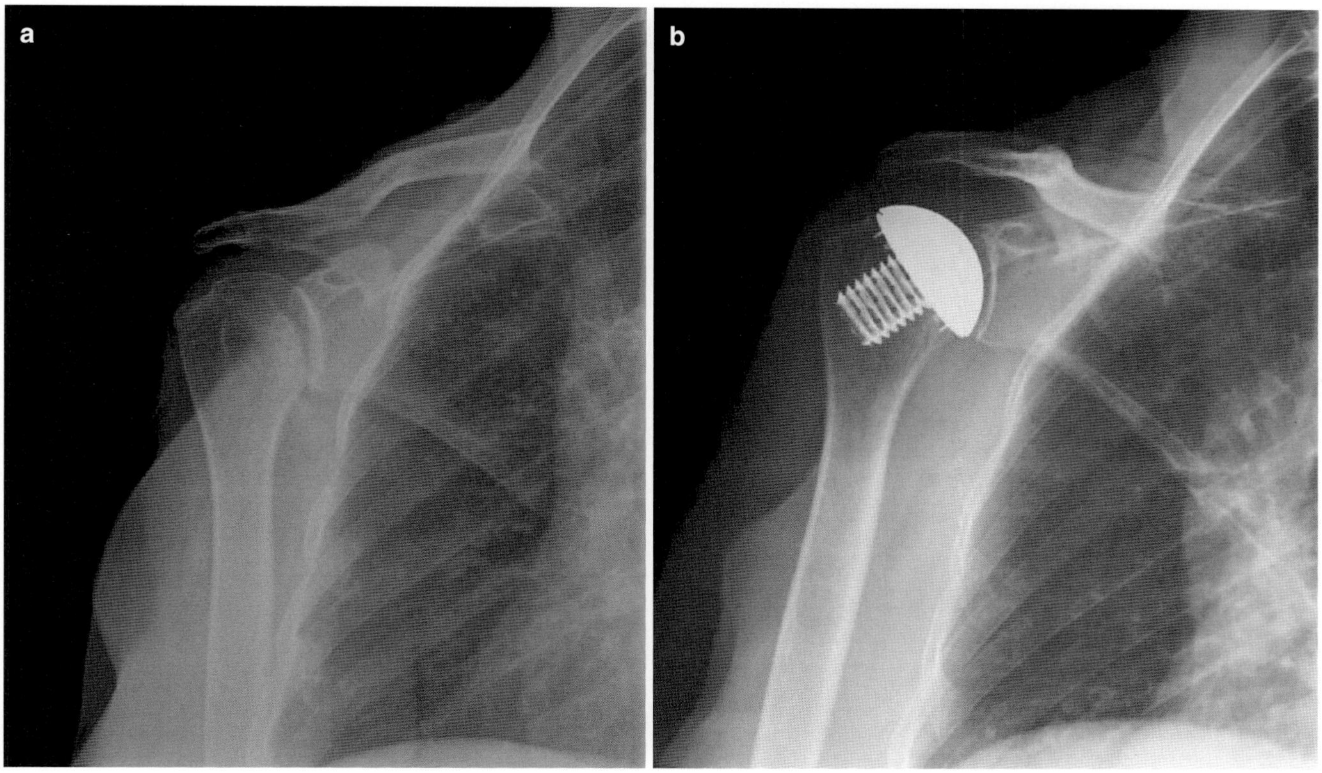

Fig. 2.8 (**a**) Chronic locked posterior dislocation. (**b**) hemiarthroplasty

2.12 Reverse Shoulder Arthroplasty

Two techniques are commonly used for inserting a reverse shoulder arthroplasty. These are the deltopectoral and the superior approach (Figs. 2.9a, b, 2.10a, b, 2.11a, b).

2.12.1 Deltopectoral Approach

The deltopectoral approach is described above. In patients with rotator cuff tear arthropathy, the subscapularis may be torn or may be unable to be repaired. In some implant designs, the failure to repair the subscapularis may lead to instability of the implant, and in other designs, a repair of the subscapularis is not as important [46].

2.12.2 Superior Approach

The anterosuperior approach utilizes for reverse total shoulder arthroplasty used by many surgeons [47]. In rotator cuff arthropathy, there may be significant superior escape of the humeral head; this procedure takes advantage of the defective supraspinatus and preserving the majority of subscapularis, therefore, allowing faster rehabilitation and improved postoperative stability [47].

A longitudinal or horizontal incision along the Langer lines is used, centered on a point just posterior to the anterolateral edge of the acromion. Skin flaps are developed, the deltoid raphe is identified, and the deltoid is split between the anterior and middle thirds distally up to 4 cm. Splitting deltoids beyond 4 cm increases the possibility of axillary nerve injury. The anterior deltoid can be damaged from excessive deltoid origin release or axillary nerve injury during the deltoid split. The axillary nerve can be within 2–2.5 cm from the anterior acromion, with some cadaveric studies showing 25 % shoulders can be less than 4 cm away for the axillary nerve [48, 49].

The coracoacromial ligament is taken with the deltoid off of the acromion as a single layer. The biceps tendon—if present—is tenotomized or tenodesed. The insertion of the subscapularis is preserved, but the anterior capsule along the glenoid may be released to facilitate exposure. This technique gives excellent exposure of the anterior and superior glenoid and the humeral head. It is generally recommended for patients with rotator cuff tear arthropathy as the rotator cuff is absent making visualization excellent. While many surgeons prefer the anterosuperior approach, the risk for component malpositioning (superior glenoid tilt and valgus stem insertion) is higher [50].

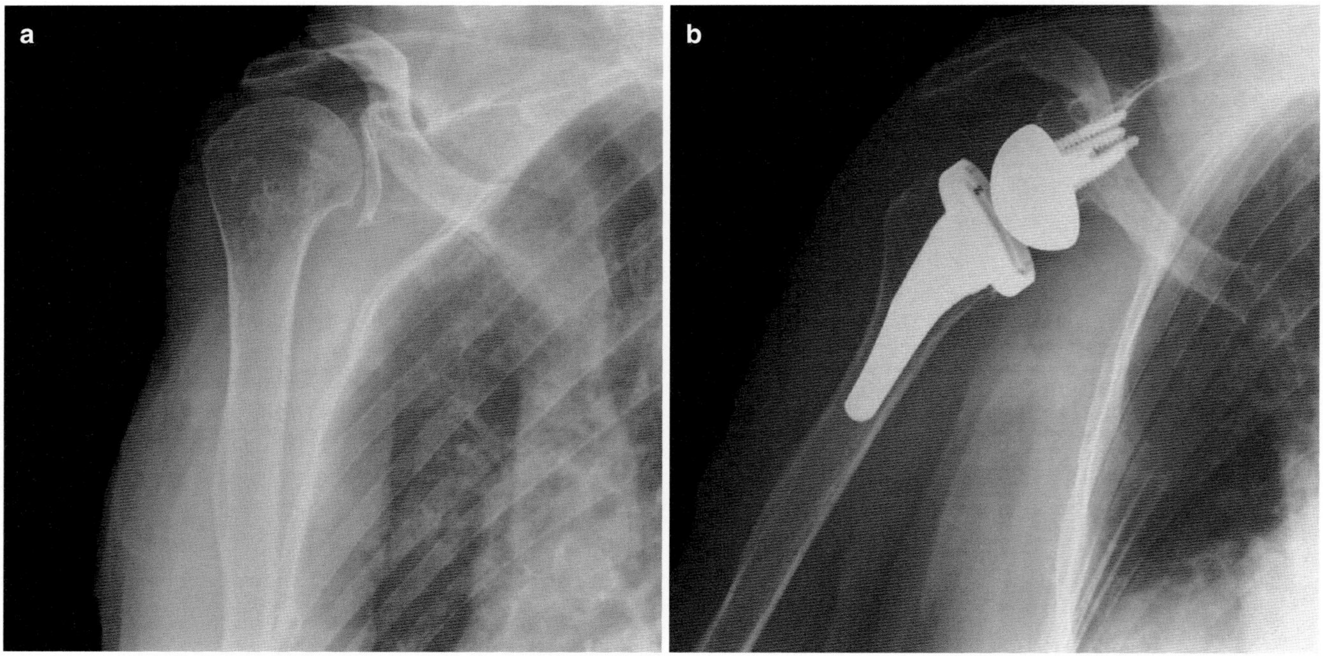

Fig. 2.9 (**a**) Cuff arthropathy. (**b**) Reverse arthroplasty

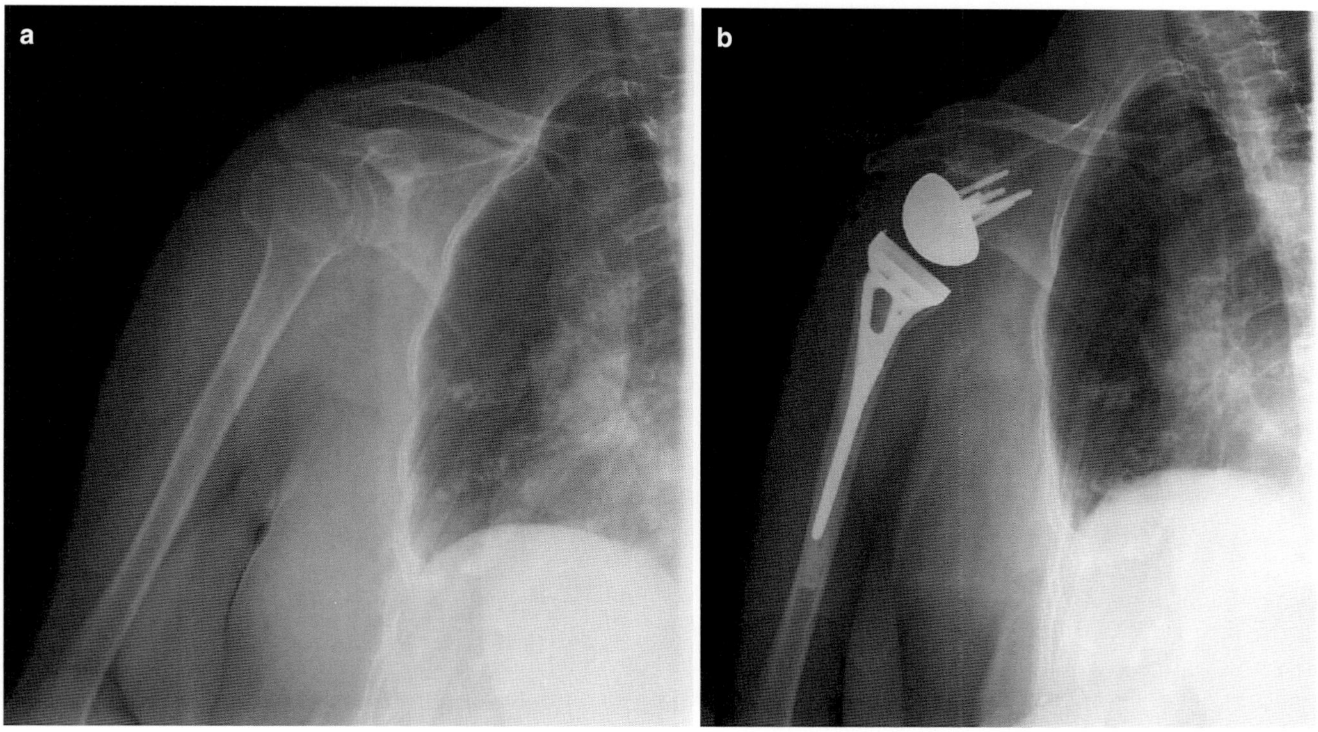

Fig. 2.10 (**a**) Acute fracture. (**b**) Trauma reverse arthroplasty

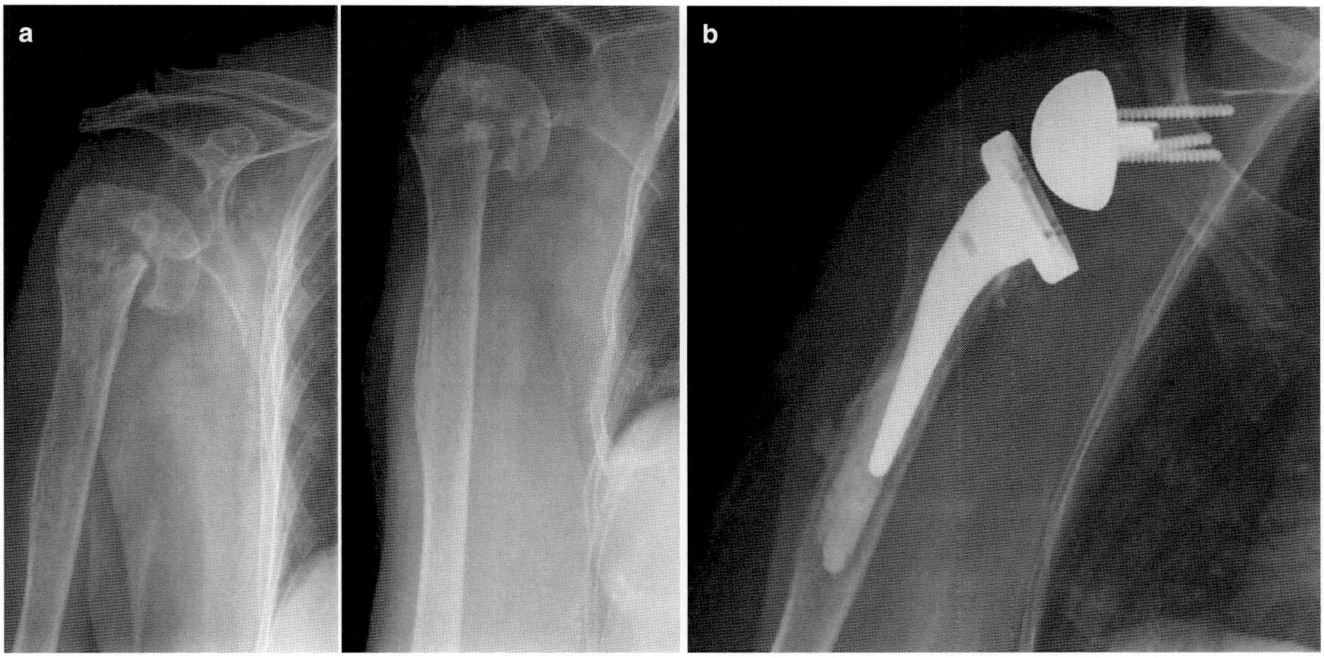

Fig. 2.11 (**a**) Fracture sequelae. (**b**) Reverse arthroplasty

2.12.3 Latissimus Transfer

Many patients with rotator cuff tear arthropathy have little or no rotator cuff function. This can severely limit the ability of the arm to externally rotate. To try to improve on this, some surgeons will transfer the tendon of the latissimus dorsi (an internal rotator) to the humeral shaft to make the muscle function as an external rotator [51]. Certainly, if this is done, the surgeon would require protection of this transferred muscle in the early phases of rehabilitation; resisted external rotation should be avoided as should extremes of internal rotation of the humerus.

2.13 Rehabilitation after Shoulder Arthroplasty: General Comments

Physical therapy is an essential element to allow patients to regain their range of motion. However, there is a lot of variation in the reported outcomes in the literature regarding patients' final shoulder movements [52, 53]. The rehabilitation program contributes significantly in reaching the optimal clinical outcome after shoulder arthroplasty.

There are few comparative trials to guide us with regard to finding the best postoperative protocol for treating patients who have undergone shoulder arthroplasty [54, 55]. Eriksson et al. compared two approaches to postoperative rehabilitation after shoulder arthroplasty in patients who lived far from their hospital [56]. One group had standard supervised physical therapy in the patient's hometown; the other did therapy at home while maintaining contact using videoconferencing with the surgeon's therapist. Interestingly, the telemedicine group had better Constant scores, shoulder function scores, and less pain than the other group [56]. In a population of patients who underwent total shoulder arthroplasty, Mulieri et al. [54] compared standard supervised physical therapy to a physician-directed home-based program with substantially fewer restrictions. They found no differences in ASES or SST score, or patient satisfaction, but interestingly the home therapy group had better motion [54]. These studies suggest that intensive, supervised physical therapy may not be required as long as the patient is able to follow a specific home program with appropriate instruction.

There are numerous published rehabilitation protocols for postoperative treatment of patients after shoulder arthroplasty [54, 57, 58]. It is widely accepted that a successful outcome depends on effective communication between the surgeon and the therapist. With regard to the postoperative physical therapy, most authors who offer their protocols in print provide similar postoperative restrictions.

2.13.1 Protect the Subscapularis

The standard surgical approach for shoulder hemiarthroplasty, total shoulder arthroplasty, and, for many surgeons, reverse arthroplasty is an anterior deltoid splitting approach (see above). To enter the joint, some method of violating the subscapularis is required. As such, rehabilitation efforts must protect the subscapularis to allow healing.

Most authors have their patients wear either a shoulder immobilizer or sling for 4–6 weeks postoperatively and recommend limitations in external rotation, which are eased over a 6–8-week period. Similarly, reaching behind the back—which places the subscapularis under tension—is restricted during this period as is any strengthening of the internal rotators of the rotator cuff.

2.13.2 Avoid Positions that Lead to Instability

In an anatomic shoulder arthroplasty, postoperative protocols limit abduction and external rotation for 6–8 weeks postoperatively.

The reverse arthroplasty is at risk for instability when the arm is adducted and extended. As such, many authors avoid this position in the first 6–8 weeks postoperatively. This may require the use of a sling or abduction sling. It is important to stress to reverse arthroplasty patients that they should not reach behind to push themselves out of a chair.

2.13.3 Sequence of Activity and Return to Sports or Work

Most authors recommend early mobilization (passive and active assisted), minimizing fulltime immobilization, and achieving maximal passive range of motion prior to advancing to the strengthening phase. The return to sporting activities or work is typically between 4 and 6 months after surgery. Healy et al. surveyed the American Shoulder and Elbow Surgeons to get their recommendations on return to sport after anatomic shoulder arthroplasty [59]. Football, gymnastics, hockey, and rock climbing were not recommended. Golf, ice skating, shooting sports, and downhill skiing were recommended in experienced players. Other sports, including cross-country skiing, swimming, doubles tennis, canoeing, and dancing, were allowed [59]. It is important to note that surgeon variation is extensive with regard to participation [60], and as such, recommendations should come from the surgeon on what is permissible and what is not.

2.14 Total Shoulder Arthroplasty Rehabilitation: Author's Protocol

Shoulder arthroplasty is performed to reduce pain in the arthritic shoulder to allow for improved functional mobility. Rehabilitation following shoulder arthroplasty should be focused on improving range of motion and increasing strength, motor control, and proprioception of the upper quadrant to restore the best possible return to functional mobility and activities of daily living.

Time for recovery following shoulder arthroplasty is generally 9–12 months. In this procedure, the subscapularis is detached for exposure of the glenohumeral joint and then reattached after the surgery is complete. This reattachment must be protected for 6 weeks. During this time, strengthening activities that stress the subscapularis such as resisted internal rotation or excessive stretching into external rotation must be avoided.

A sling should be worn for the first 48–72 h for protection while the effects of anesthesia, possible nerve blocks, and other medications wear off. After 3 days, the sling can be removed for light activity such as deskwork as long as the hand is kept in front of the body. Sling should be worn as needed during the day, whenever the patient is active or in an unprotected environment; it should always be worn at night for the first 6 weeks. The sling can be discontinued completely at 6 weeks postoperatively. Active range of motion of the glenohumeral joint is allowed starting around week 4.

2.14.1 Postoperative (Weeks 0–4)

Initial rehabilitation goals include pain control, restoration of range of motion of the glenohumeral joint through both passive and active-assistive exercises, and light muscle activation of the glenohumeral and scapulothoracic joints.

In the first postoperative visit, the dressing is removed and wound inspection is performed. The patient should be educated in sling donning/doffing and icing. A home exercise program is started including pendulum exercises (all motions), active range of motion exercises of the wrist and elbow, and active-assistive exercises of the glenohumeral joint into flexion, abduction, and external rotation up to 20° to protect the subscapularis repair. These active-assistive exercises can be performed with cane exercises (Figs. 2.12 and 2.13) or table walkouts (Fig. 2.14). The patient should also start scapular mobility in the sling including elevation and depression (Fig. 2.15) and scapular retraction (Fig. 2.16).

At 1 week, the patient may start submaximal isometric exercises into flexion, extension, abduction, and external rotation (Figs. 2.17, 2.18, and 2.19). No internal rotation is performed at this time for continued protection of the subscapularis. Patient may also begin prone scapular retraction (Fig. 2.20). Use of the upper body ergometer and overhead pulleys may be added as patient tolerance allows (Fig. 2.21).

Passive range of motion is performed in the clinic by the physical therapist, taking care not to place stress on the surgical implant or soft tissue structures that have been affected by the procedure.

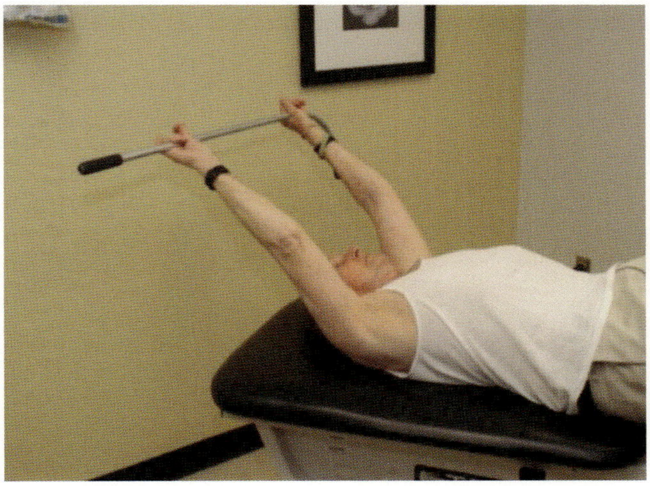

Fig. 2.12 Supine cane flexion

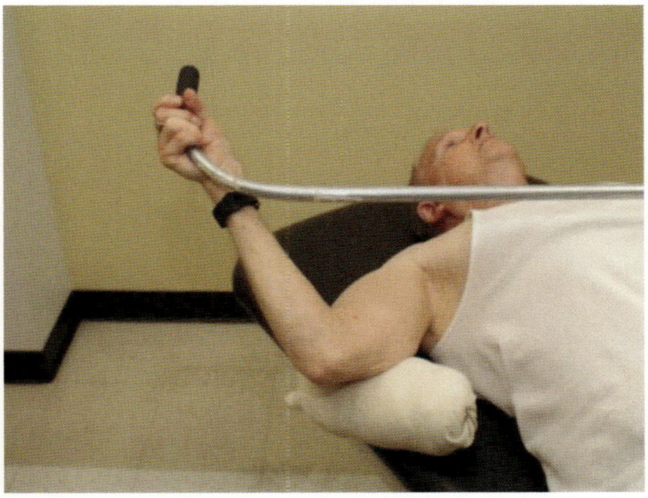

Fig. 2.13 Supine cane external rotation—towel roll to maintain motion in the scapular plane

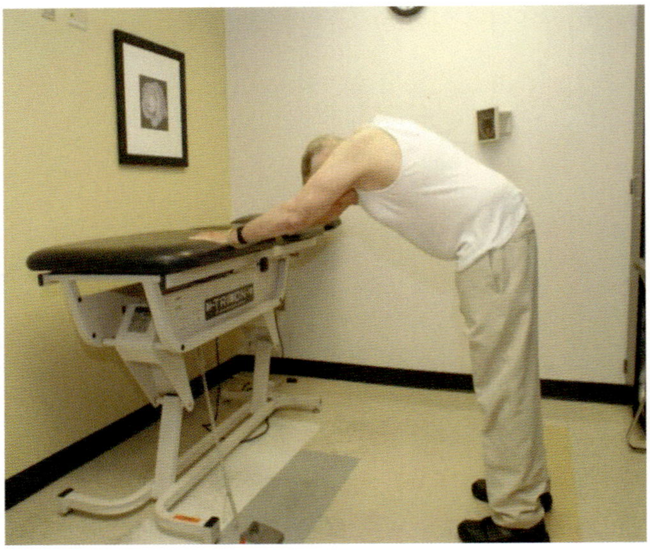

Fig. 2.14 Table walkouts—with hands on the table, slowly walk backward and lean forward for passive shoulder flexion to tolerance

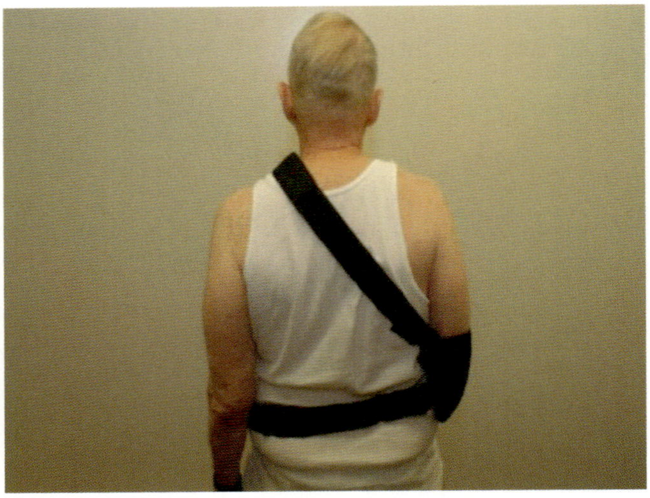

Fig. 2.16 Scapular retraction

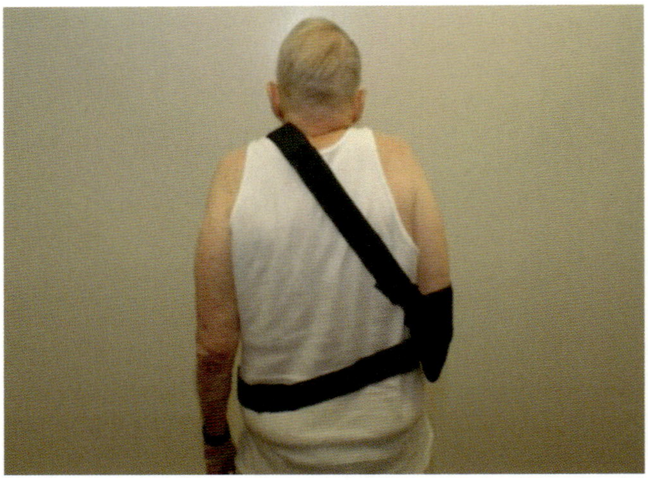

Fig. 2.15 Scapular elevation and depression can be performed in or out of the sling

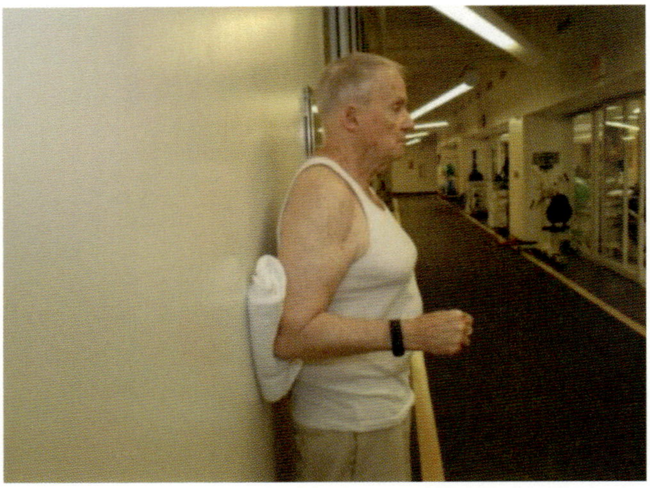

Fig. 2.17 Isometric shoulder flexion

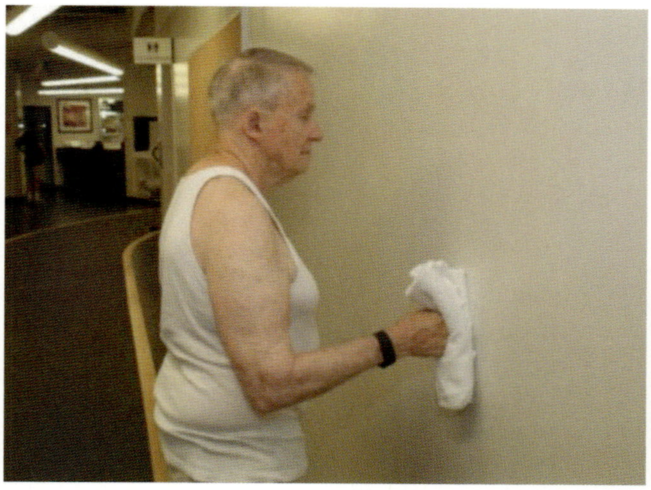

Fig. 2.18 Isometric shoulder extension

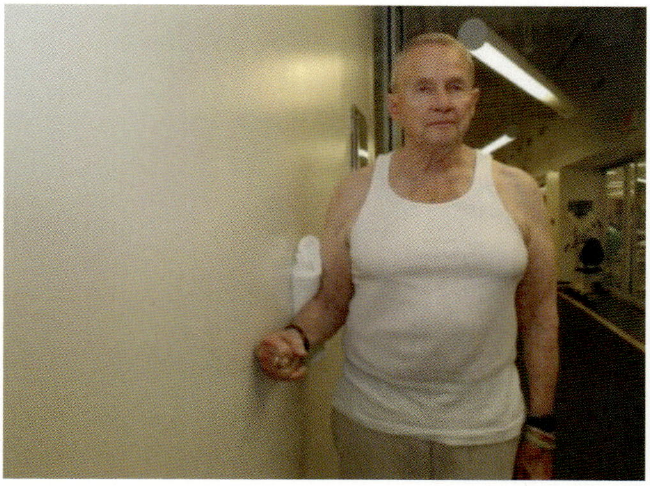

Fig. 2.19 Isometric shoulder abduction/external rotation

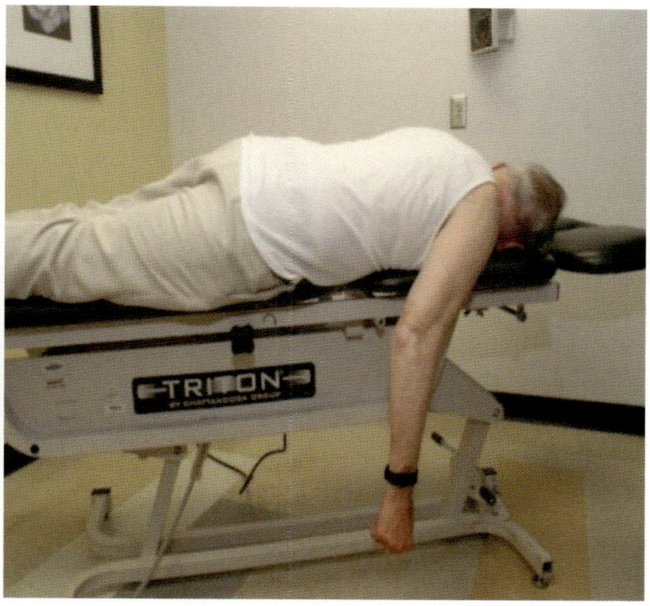

Fig. 2.20 Prone scapular retraction—with arm suspended off edge of table—scapula is retracted

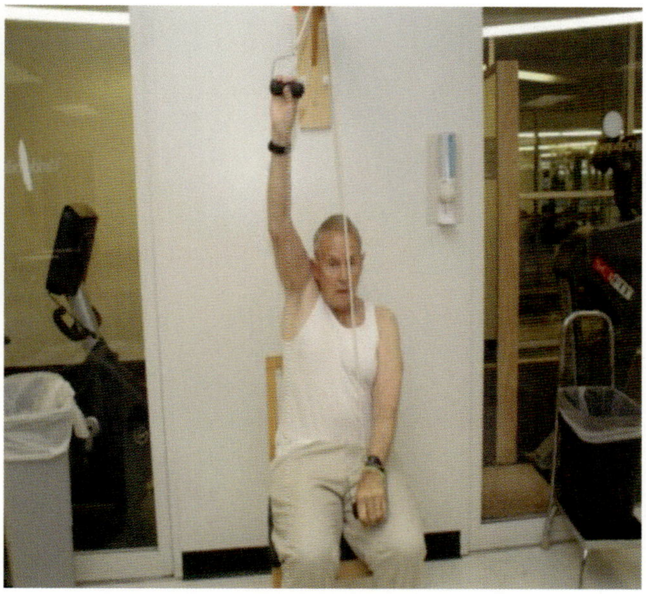

Fig. 2.21 Pulley flexion

2.14.2 Postoperative (Weeks 4–8)

At 4 weeks, the patient may start active range of motion on the glenohumeral joint. Suggested exercises include but are not limited to supine serratus punches (Fig. 2.22), prone rows, abduction and extension with focus on middle and lower trapezius recruitment with motion (Figs. 2.23, 2.24, and 2.25), lawn mower exercise for scapular stabilization (Figs. 2.26 and 2.27), and side-lying external rotation with towel roll under arm (Fig. 2.28). Patient will also need to initiate active flexion and scaption. This may be better accomplished starting in supine or side-lying position with focus on good motor control, with progression into upright position (Figs. 2.29, 2.30, and 2.31). Any active external rotation should be limited to 30° or as directed by physician based on operative technique. Passive range of motion should be continued until full range is achieved in all other motions.

At 6 weeks, the patient may continue all active range of motion with external rotation allowed to 45° or as directed based on repair. Internal and external rotation may be initiated at low resistance with a towel roll under the arm to eliminate the wringing out effect to the rotator cuff (Figs. 2.32 and 2.33). The patient may also begin wall push-ups plus for serratus strengthening (Fig. 2.34), as well as dynamic stabilization exercises either through body blade exercises in neutral (Fig. 2.35) and double arm at 90° flexion (Fig. 2.36) or through manual rhythmic stabilization exercises with therapist in supine flexion (Figs. 2.37 and 2.38) with progressions in speed, intensity, and angulation of flexion as tolerated.

At this point in their recovery, the patient may begin work on proprioceptive exercise. For example, a laser pointer can be attached to the arm and the patient is asked to perform tasks such as moving between two set positions marked on the wall, tracing previously drawn circles, etc. (Fig. 2.39).

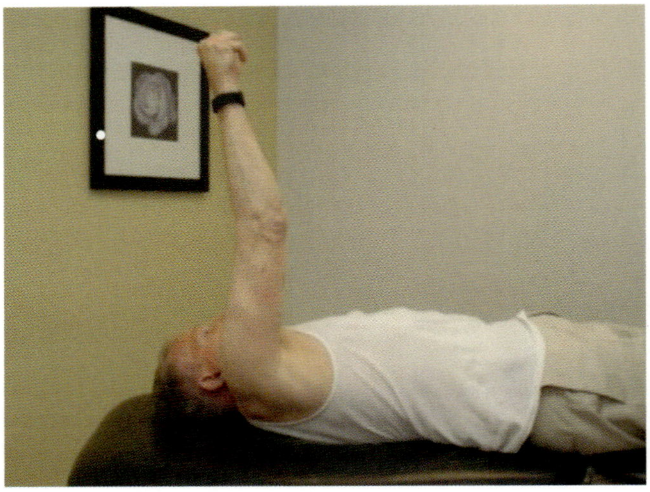

Fig. 2.22 Supine serratus punches

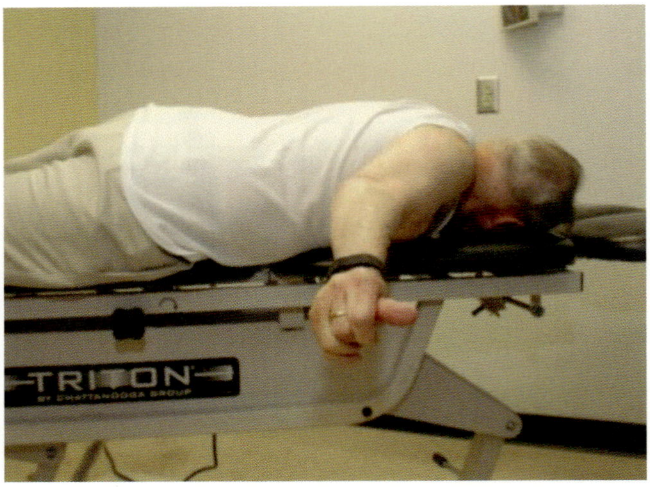

Fig. 2.24 Prone abduction with focus on middle and lower trapezius

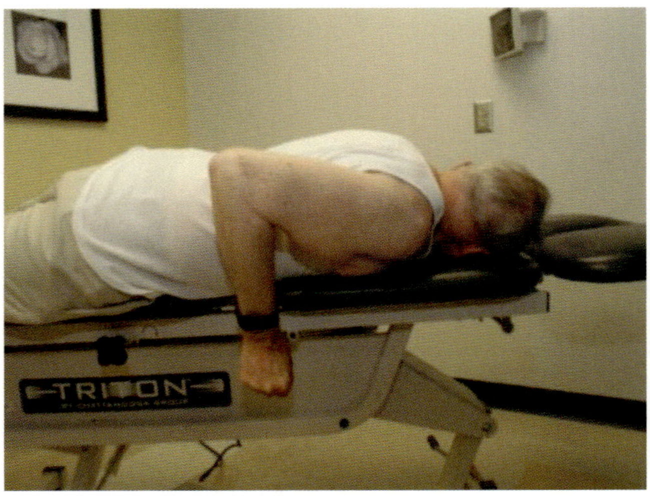

Fig. 2.23 Prone row with focus on good middle trapezius recruitment

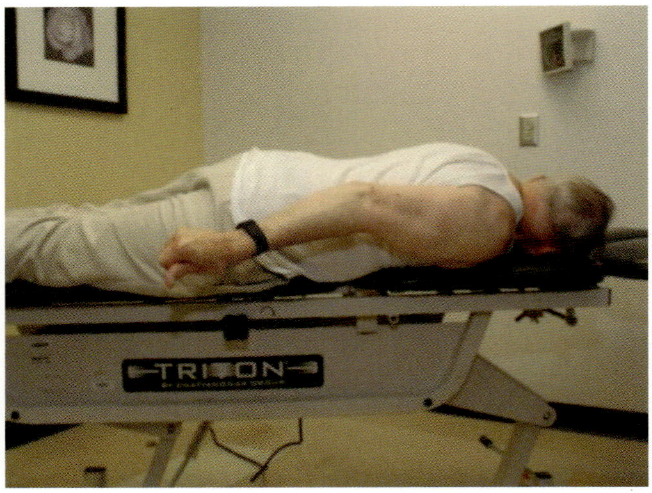

Fig. 2.25 Prone extension with focus on middle and lower trapezius

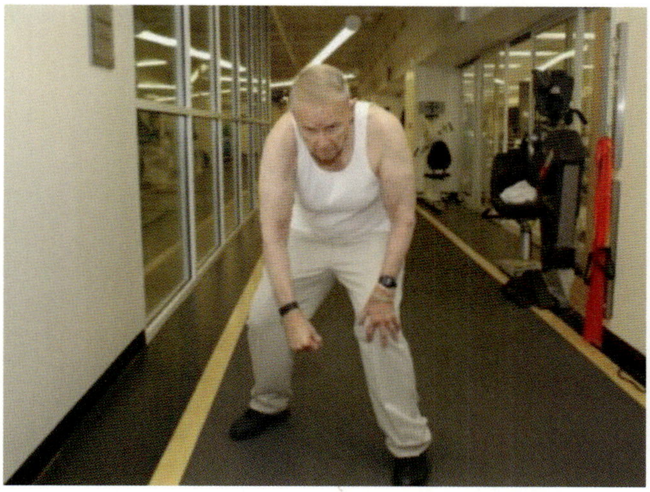

Fig. 2.26 Lawnmower starting position—cue to pull up like starting a lawn mower

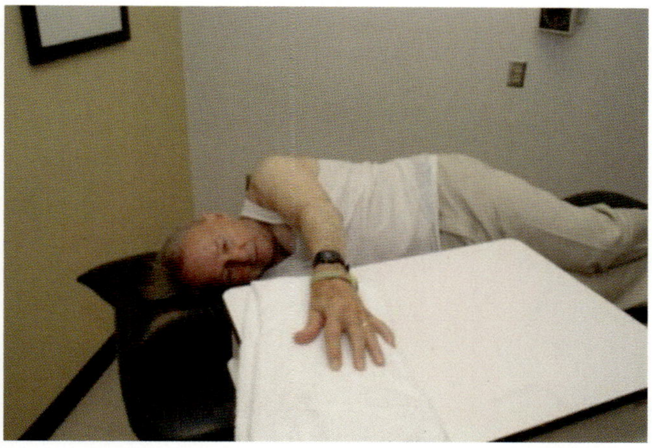

Fig. 2.29 Side-lying active-assistive flexion

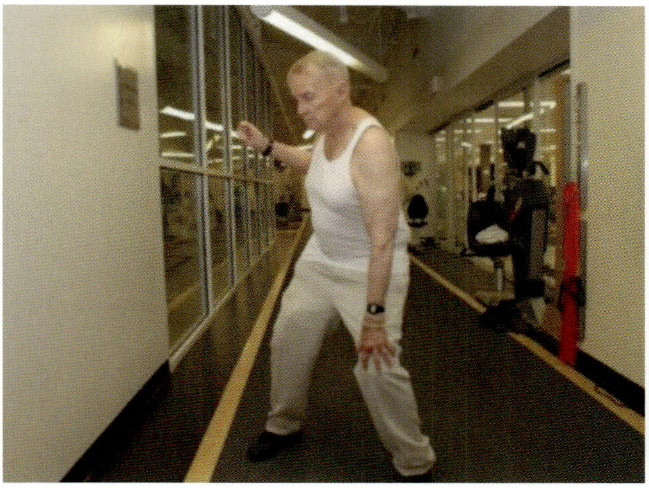

Fig. 2.27 Lawn mower ending position—with scapula retraction

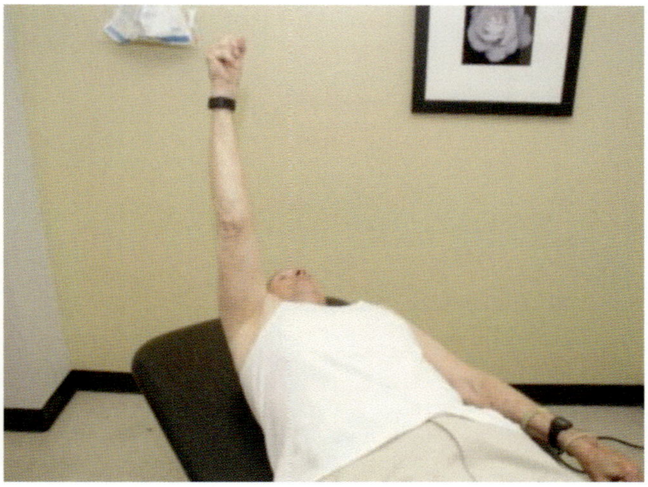

Fig. 2.30 Supine shoulder flexion

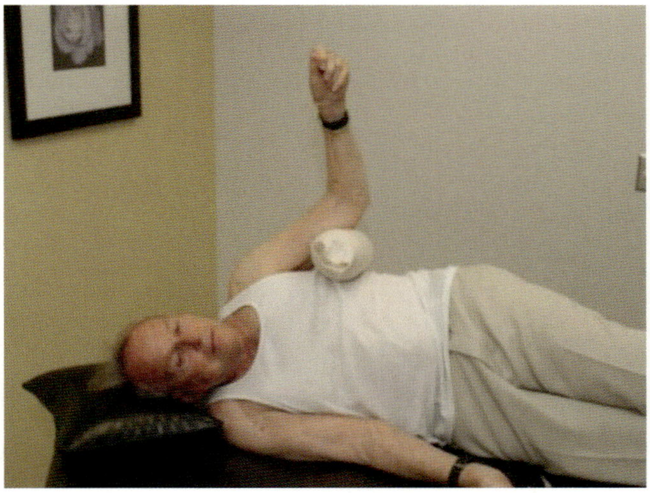

Fig. 2.28 Side-lying external rotation

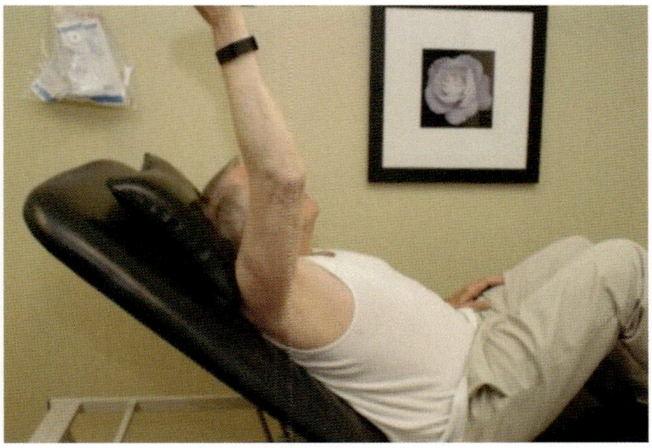

Fig. 2.31 Supine active flexion on incline—initial incline at 20–30° with progression to upright

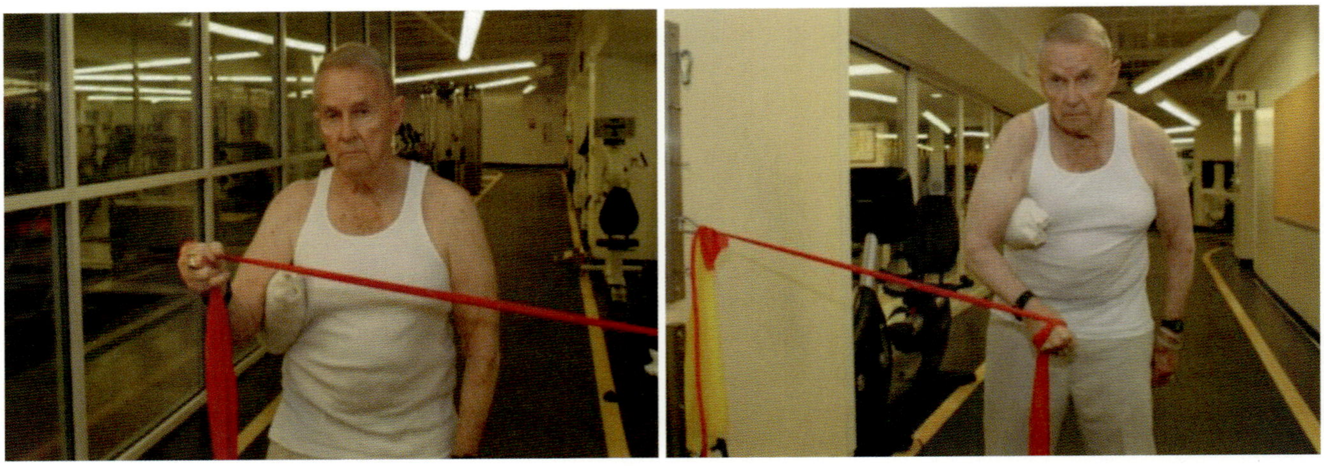

Figs. 2.32 and 2.33 Resisted external rotation with towel roll

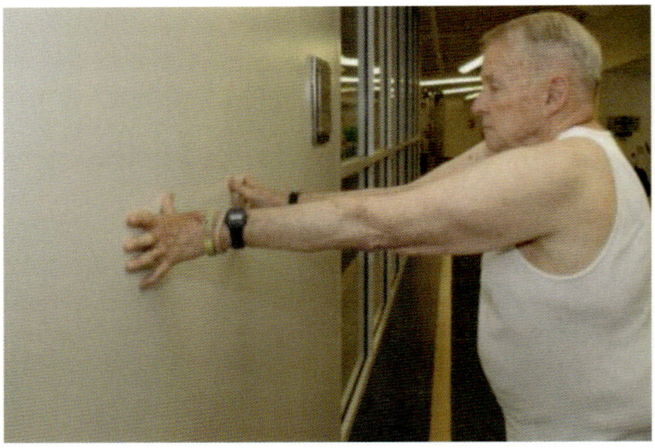

Fig. 2.34 Wall push-ups with serratus plus

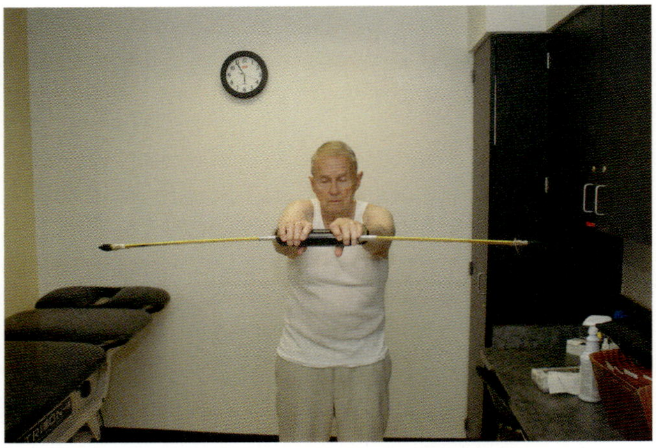

Fig. 2.36 Bodyblade in 90° flexion—double hand

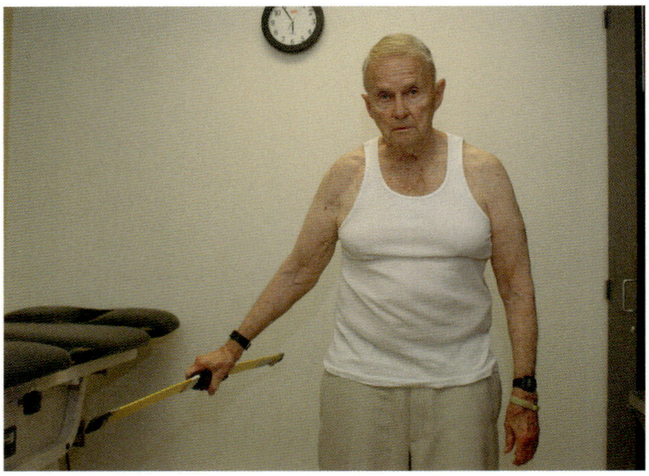

Fig. 2.35 Bodyblade in neutral at side

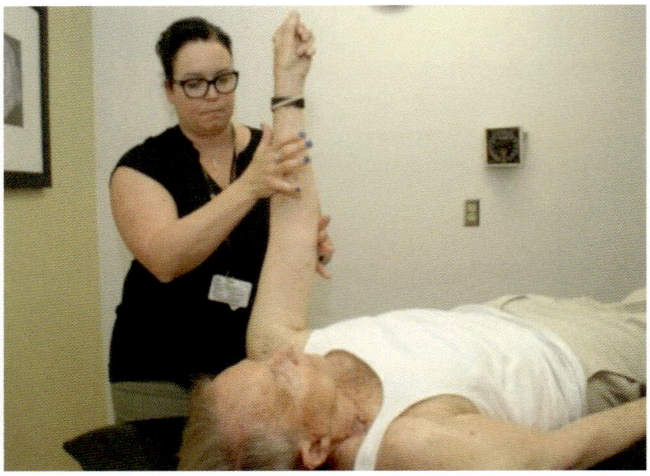

Fig. 2.37 Rhythmic stabilization—patient holds arm still in serratus plus—therapist changes direction of pressure

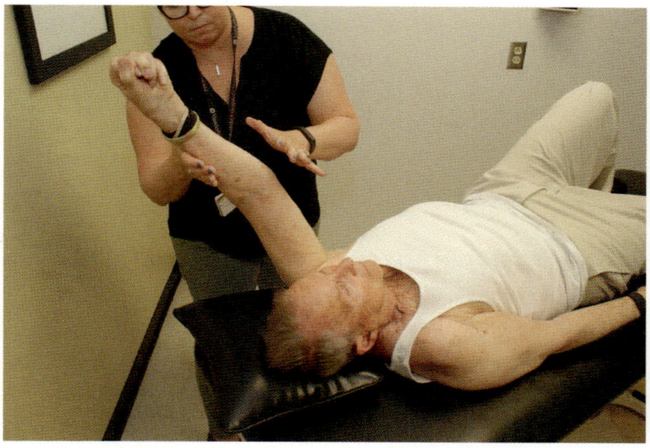

Fig. 2.38 Rhythmic stabilization progression into increased flexion

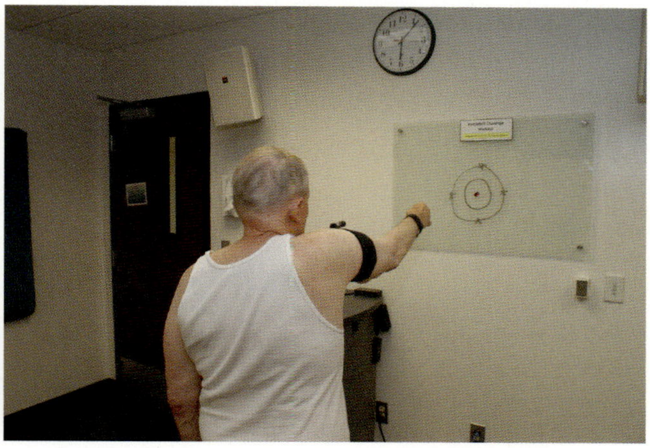

Fig. 2.39 Proprioception exercises with laser pointer

2.14.3 Postoperative (Weeks 8–12)

At this point, full passive and active range of motion with the restriction of 60° of exercise rotation should be obtained. If more aggressive stretching or mobilization is indicated, it may be done as long as attention is paid to the postoperative integrity of the anterior structures. Progressive resistive exercises and proprioceptive activities continue for the rotator cuff and periscapular musculature with body blade exercises progressing into higher angles of elevation. Scapular control exercises in closed-chain position should be initiated as well (Fig. 2.40). As the patient shows improved strength and motor control, closed chained activities can be moved into quadruped (Fig. 2.41). Weakness may still be present in the subscapularis if it was resected during surgery, so attention should be paid to restore strength with dynamic hug-type exercises (Fig. 2.42). Exercises should also reflect more functional movement strength such as diagonal patterns (Figs. 2.43 and 2.44). Bodyblade exercises can also be progressed into higher angles of elevation (Figs. 2.45 and 2.46).

2.14.4 Postoperative (Weeks 12+)

Focus at this point should be returning the patient to their individual goals, recreational activity, and job duties if applicable. Patient will most likely be on a home program by this point for gradual return to full strength and regular daily activities. Sport- or recreational activity-specific exercises should be part of the overall program.

Postoperative Exercises—Weeks 8–12

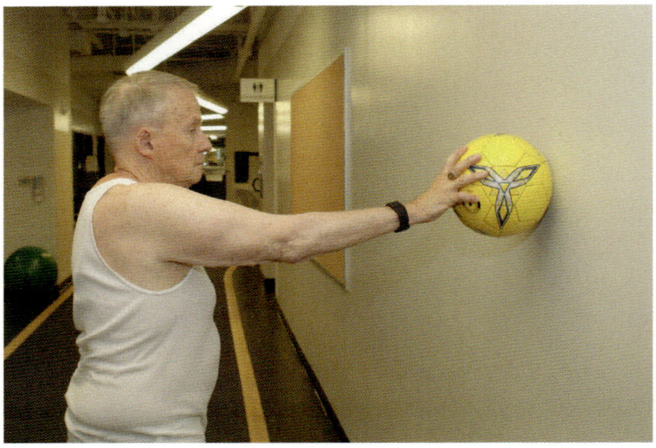

Fig. 2.40 Patient can perform circles, serratus press/scapular retraction, or rhythmic stabilization with therapist

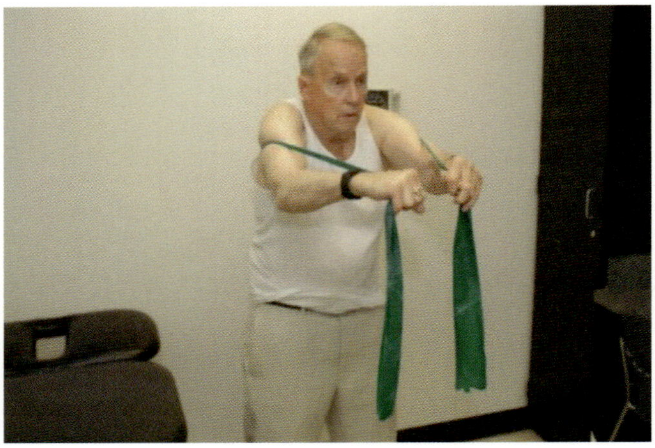

Fig. 2.42 Dynamic hug exercise—cue is to reach around like a hug

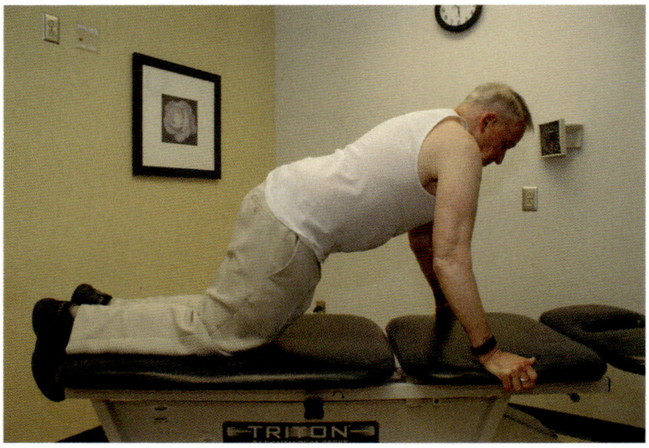

Fig. 2.41 Quadruped position for serratus plus or rhythmic stabilization with therapist

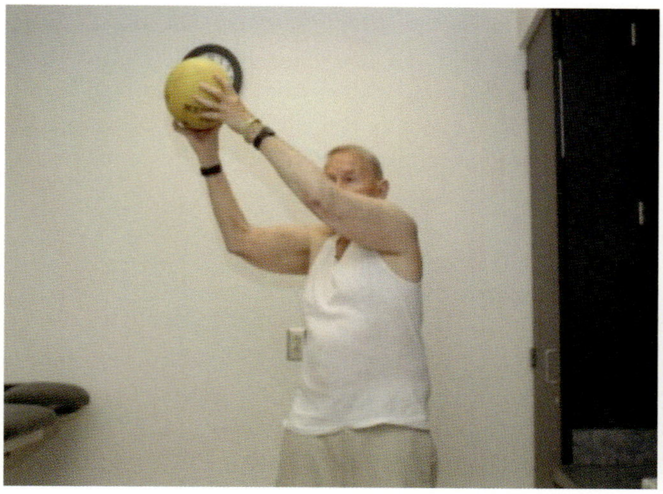

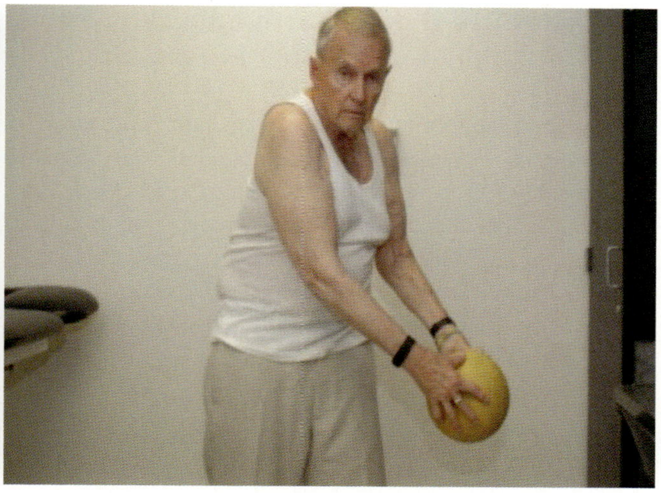

Figs. 2.43 and 2.44 Medicine ball diagonals

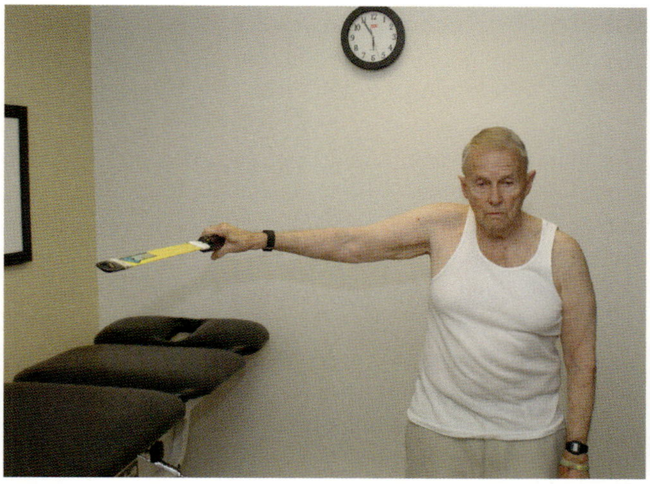

Fig. 2.45 Bodyblade at 90° abduction—single hand

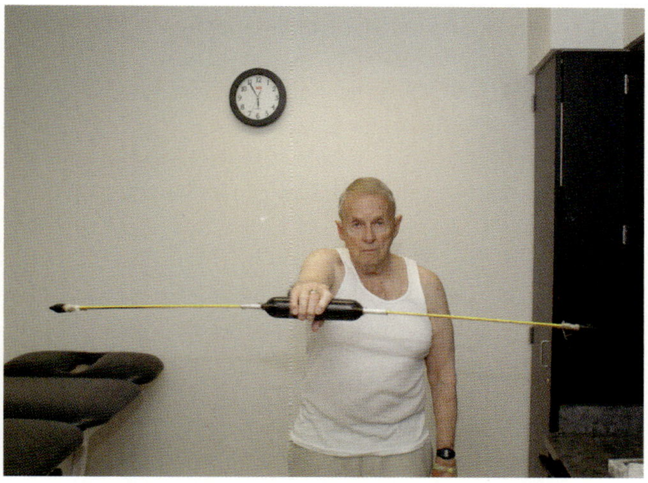

Fig. 2.46 Bodyblade at 90° flexion—single hand

2.15 Reverse Shoulder Arthroplasty Rehabilitation: Author's Protocol

Reverse shoulder arthroplasty is most commonly performed in the painful shoulder that has significant nonoperative rotator cuff damage. Postoperative guidelines for the reverse arthroplasty are similar to those for the shoulder arthroplasty in terms of when to introduce passive, active-assistive, and active range-of-motion activities and when is it safe to start progressive-resistive exercises. The previous arthroplasty guidelines and exercises may be followed for the reverse arthroplasty except for the following specific considerations.

Dislocation is a real concern due to the shape and mechanics of the implant. Avoidance of shoulder extension past neutral and the combination of shoulder adduction and internal rotation should be avoided for 12 weeks postoperatively. Activities such as tucking in a shirt or performing bathroom/personal hygiene with the operative arm should be avoided. Care during passive range of motion and exercises such as prone rows past neutral extension should be avoided as well.

The shoulder will now have to rely on the deltoid for elevation. More time will most likely be spent going through gradual incline shoulder elevation exercises with this procedure. Once active range of motion can be initiated, shoulder elevation can start in supine, and once this position is performed with ease, the incline of the table can be raised 20–30° and the patient performs active-assistive exercises at this level until active elevation can be performed. Again, once this becomes easy, the incline can be raised again and so on until the patient is upright or standing.

Due to rotator cuff damage, the patient will most likely have decreased or no external rotation strength so some exercises listed in the arthroplasty guidelines would therefore be inappropriate. A latissimus dorsi and/or teres major transfer may be performed in some cases to help restore external rotation strength. If this is the case, special precautions will need to be taken to protect the transferred musculature during healing phases.

2.16 Complications

Shoulder arthroplasty is one of the fastest growing areas in joint replacement surgery, and the prospects for future growth appear assured as the population of elderly expands rapidly over the next few decades.

As with other total joint replacement procedures, total shoulder arthroplasty can have a number of complications [61]. The literature reports great variations in complication rates (0–55 %), with a mean complication of 10–15 % [62]. For total shoulder arthroplasty, the number of reported complications has decreased tremendously in recent decades [63]. The most common complications include glenoid loosening (11.5 %), secondary rotator cuff pathology (4.6 %), glenohumeral instability (3.1 %), stiffness (1.6 %), neurological complications (1.6 %), humeral loosening (1.5 %), intraoperative fracture (1.4 %), infection (1.2 %), and postoperative humeral fracture (0.9 %) [64].

Complications for reverse arthroplasty can be similar to anatomic shoulder arthroplasty and include neurologic injury, periprosthetic fracture, hematoma, infection, loosening of the implant, and dislocation. Unique to reverse shoulder arthroplasty are the complications of scapular notching and acromion fracture [65].

References

1. Rekola KE, Keinanen-Kiukaanniemi S, Takala J (1993) Use of primary health services in sparsely populated country districts by patients with musculoskeletal symptoms: consultations with a physician. J Epidemiol Community Health 47:153–157
2. Lugli T (1978) Artificial shoulder joint by Pean (1893): the facts of an exceptional intervention and the prosthetic method. Clin Orthop Relat Res 133:215–218
3. Burrows HJ, Wilson JN, Scales JT (1975) Excision of tumours of humerus and femur, with restoration by internal prostheses. J Bone Joint Surg Br 57-B:148–159
4. Neer CS (1955) Articular replacement for the humeral head. J Bone Joint Surg Am 37-A:215–228
5. Lee DH (2009) History of shoulder arthroplasty. Chapter 1. In: Total shoulder arthroplasty. American Society for Surgery of the Hand, Rosemont, pp 1–15
6. Boileau P, Walch G (1997) Three-dimensional geometry of the proximal humerus: implications for surgical technique and prosthetic design. J Bone Joint Surg Br 79-B:857–865
7. Walch G, Boileau P (1999) Prosthetic adaptability: a new concept for shoulder arthroplasty. J Shoulder Elbow Surg 8(5):443–451
8. Zhang W, Jones A, Doherty M (2004) Does paracetamol (acetaminophen) reduce the pain of osteoarthritis?: a meta-analysis of randomised controlled trials. Ann Rheum Dis 63(8):901–907
9. Pincus T, Koch G, Lei H et al (2004) Patient Preference for Placebo, Acetaminophen (paracetamol) or Celecoxib Efficacy Studies (PACES): two randomised, double blind, placebo controlled, crossover clinical trials in patients with knee or hip osteoarthritis. Ann Rheum Dis 63(8):931–939
10. Merolla G, Sperling JW, Porcellini G (2011) Efficacy of Hylan G-F 20 versus 6-methylprednisolone acetate in painful shoulder osteoarthritis: a retrospective controlled trial. Musculoskelet Surg 95(3):215–224
11. Silverstein E, Leger R, Shea KP (2007) The use of intra-articular hylan G-F 20 in the treatment of symptomatic osteoarthritis of the shoulder: a preliminary study. Am J Sports Med 35(6):979–985
12. Kwon YW, Eisenberg G, Zuckerman JD (2013) Sodium hyaluronate for the treatment of chronic shoulder pain associated with glenohumeral osteoarthritis: a multicenter, randomized, double-blind, placebo-controlled trial. J Shoulder Elbow Surg 22(5):584–594
13. Boselli KJ, Ahmad CS, Levine WN (2010) Treatment of glenohumeral arthrosis. Am J Sports Med 38(12):2558–2572
14. McCarty LP III, Cole BJ (2005) Nonarthroplasty treatment of glenohumeral cartilage lesions. Arthroscopy 21(9):1131–1142
15. Maybach A, Schlegel TF (1995) Shoulder rehabilitation for the arthritic glenohumeral joint: preoperative and postoperative considerations. Semin Arthroplasty 6(4):297–304
16. Spiegl UJ, Faucett SC, Horan MP, Warth RJ, Millett PJ (2014) The role of arthroscopy in the management of glenohumeral osteoarthritis: a Markov decision model. Arthroscopy 30(11):1392–1399
17. Sayegh ET, Mascarenhas R, Chalmers PN, Cole BJ, Romeo AA, Verma NN (2015) Surgical treatment options for glenohumeral arthritis in young patients: a systematic review and meta-analysis. Arthroscopy 31(6):1156–1166.e8
18. Skelley NW, Namdari S, Chamberlain AM, Keener JD, Galatz LM, Yamaguchi K (2015) Arthroscopic debridement and capsular release for the treatment of shoulder osteoarthritis. Arthroscopy 31(3):494–500
19. Namdari S, Skelley N, Keener JD, Galatz LM, Yamaguchi K (2013) What is the role of arthroscopic debridement for glenohumeral arthritis? A critical examination of the literature. Arthroscopy 29(8):1392–1398
20. Kerr R, Resnick D, Pineda C, Haghighi P (1985) Osteoarthritis of the glenohumeral joint: a radiologic-pathologic study. Am J Roentgenol 144(5):967–972
21. Petersson CJ (1983) Degeneration of the gleno-humeral joint. An anatomical study. Acta Orthop Scand 54(2):277–283
22. Cushnaghan J, Dieppe PA (1991) Study of 500 patients with limb joint osteoarthritis. I. Analysis by age, sex, and distribution of symptomatic joint sites. Ann Rheum Dis 50(1):8–13
23. Gartsman GM, Brinker MR, Khan M, Karahan M (1998) Self-assessment of general health status in patients with five common shoulder conditions. J Shoulder Elbow Surg 7(3):228–237
24. Denard PJ, Walch G (2013) Current concepts in the surgical management of primary glenohumeral arthritis with a biconcave glenoid. J Shoulder Elbow Surg 22(11):1589–1598
25. van der Zwaal P, Pijls BG, Thomassen BJ, Lindenburg R, Nelissen RG, van de Sande MA (2014) The natural history of the rheumatoid shoulder: a prospective long-term follow-up study. Bone Joint J 96-B(11):1520–1524
26. Kanbe K, Chiba J, Inoue Y, Taguchi M, Iwamatsu A (2015) Analysis of clinical factors related to the efficacy of shoulder arthroscopic synovectomy plus capsular release in patients with rheumatoid arthritis. Eur J Orthop Surg Traumatol 25(3): 451–455
27. Barlow JD, Yuan BJ, Schleck CD, Harmsen WS, Cofield RH, Sperling JW (2014) Shoulder arthroplasty for rheumatoid arthritis: 303 consecutive cases with minimum 5-year follow-up. J Shoulder Elbow Surg 23(6):791–799
28. Holcomb JO, Herbert DJ, Mighell MA, Dunning PE, Pupello DR, Pliner MD, Frankle MA (2010) Reverse shoulder arthroplasty in patients with rheumatoid arthritis. J Shoulder Elbow Surg 19(70):1076–1084
29. Young AA, Smith MM, Bacle G, Moraga C, Walch G (2011) Early results of reverse shoulder arthroplasty in patients with rheumatoid arthritis. J Bone Joint Surg Am 93(20):1915–1923
30. Cruess RL (1985) Corticosteroid-induced osteonecrosis of the humeral head. Orthop Clin North Am 16:789–796
31. Harreld KL, Marker DR, Wiesler ER, Shafiq B, Mont MA (2009) Osteonecrosis of the humeral head. J Am Acad Orthop Surg 17(6):345–355
32. Brophy RH, Marx RG (2005) Osteoarthritis following shoulder instability. Clin Sports Med 24(1):47–56
33. Papalia R, Osti L, Del Buono A, Denaro V, Maffulli N (2010) Glenohumeral arthropathy following stabilization for recurrent instability. Br Med Bull 96:75–92
34. Macaulay AA, Greiwe RM, Bigliani LU (2010) Rotator cuff deficient arthritis of the glenohumeral joint. Clin Orthop Surg 2(4):196–202
35. Ramirez MA, Ramirez J, Murthi AM (2012) Reverse total shoulder arthroplasty for irreparable rotator cuff tears and cuff tear arthropathy. Clin Sports Med 31(4):749–759
36. Caniggia M, Fornara P, Franci M, Maniscalco P, Picinotti A (1999) Shoulder arthroplasty. Indications, contraindications and complications. Panminerva Med 41(4):341–349
37. Gadea F, Bouju Y, Berhouet J, Bacle G, Favard L (2015) Deltopectoral approach for shoulder arthroplasty: anatomic basis. Int Orthop 39:215–225
38. Miller BS, Joseph TA, Noonan TJ, Horan MP, Hawkins RJ (2005) Rupture of the subscapularis tendon after shoulder arthroplasty: diagnosis, treatment, and outcome. J Shoulder Elbow Surg 14(5):492–496
39. Krishnan SG, Stewart DG, Reineck JR, Lin KC, Buzzell JE, Burkhead WZ (2009) Subscapularis repair after shoulder arthroplasty: biomechanical and clinical validation of a novel technique. J Shoulder Elbow Surg 18(2):184–192
40. Scalise JJ, Ciccone J, Iannotti JP (2010) Clinical, radiographic, and ultrasonographic comparison of subscapularis tenotomy and lesser tuberosity osteotomy for total shoulder arthroplasty. J Bone Joint Surg Am 92(7):1627–1634

41. Lapner PLC, Sabri E, Rakhra K, Bell K, Athwal GS (2010) Comparison of lesser tuberosity osteotomy to subscapularis peel in shoulder arthroplasty: a randomized controlled trial. J Bone Joint Surg Am 94(24):2239–2246
42. Lafosse L, Schnaser E, Haag M, Gobezie R (2009) Primary total shoulder arthroplasty performed entirely thru the rotator interval: technique and minimum two-year outcomes. J Shoulder Elbow Surg 18(6):864–873
43. Savoie FH 3rd, Charles R, Casselton J, O'Brien MJ, Hurt JA 3rd (2015) The subscapularis-sparing approach in humeral head replacement. J Shoulder Elbow Surg 24(4):606–612
44. Ding DY, Mahure SA, Akuoko JA, Zuckerman JD, Kwon YW (2015) Total shoulder arthroplasty using a subscapularis-sparing approach: a radiographic analysis. J Shoulder Elbow Surg 24(6):831–837
45. Simovitch R, Fullick R, Zuckerman JD (2013) Use of the subscapularis preserving technique in anatomic total shoulder arthroplasty. Bull Hosp Jt Dis (2013) 71 Suppl 2:94–100
46. Routman HD (2013) The role of the subscapularis repair in reverse total shoulder arthroplasty. Bull Hosp Jt Dis (2013) 71 Suppl 2:108012
47. Molé D, Wein F, Dézaly C, Valenti P, Sirveaux F (2011) Surgical technique: the anterosuperior approach for reverse shoulder arthroplasty. Clin Orthop Relat Res 469(9):2461–2468
48. Loukas M, Grabska J, Tubbs RS, Apaydin N, Jordan R (2009) Mapping the axillary nerve within the deltoid muscle. Surg Radiol Anat 31(1):43–47
49. Gurushantappa PK, Kuppasad S (2015) Anatomy of axillary nerve and its clinical importance: a cadaveric study. J Clin Diagn Res 9(3):AC13–AC17
50. Gillespie RJ, Garrigues GE, Chang ES, Namdari S, Williams GR Jr (2015) Surgical exposure for reverse total shoulder arthroplasty: differences in approaches and outcomes. Orthop Clin North Am 46(1):49–56
51. Puskas GJ, Catanzaro S, Gerber C (2014) Clinical outcome of reverse total shoulder arthroplasty combined with latissimus dorsi transfer for the treatment of chronic combined pseudoparesis of elevation and external rotation of the shoulder. J Shoulder Elbow Surg 23(1):49–57
52. Sperling JW, Cofield RH, Rowland CM (1998) Neer hemi- arthroplasty and Neer total shoulder arthroplasty in patients fifty years old or less: long-term results. J Bone Joint Surg Am 80:464
53. Torchia ME, Cofield RH, Settergren CR (1997) Total shoulder arthroplasty with the Neer prosthesis: long-term results. J Shoulder Elbow Surg 6:495
54. Mulieri PJ, Holcomb JO, Dunning P, Pliner M, Bogle RK, Pupello D, Frankle MA (2010) Is a formal physical therapy program necessary after total shoulder arthroplasty for osteoarthritis? J Shoulder Elbow Surg 19(4):570–579
55. Fusaro I, Orsini S, Stignani S, Creta D, Cava FC, Benedetti MG, Società Italiana di Chirurgia della Spalla e del Gomito (2013) Proposal for SICSeG guidelines for rehabilitation after anatomical shoulder prosthesis in concentric shoulder osteoarthritis. Musculoskelet Surg 97 Suppl 1:31–37
56. Eriksson L, Lindström B, Gard G, Lysholm J (2009) Physiotherapy at a distance: a controlled study of rehabilitation at home after a shoulder joint operation. J Telemed Telecare 15(5):215–220
57. Friedman RJ (1994) Biomechanics of total shoulder arthroplasty. In: Friedman RJ (ed) Arthroplasty of the shoulder. Thieme, New York, pp 27–40
58. Brems JJ (1994) Rehabilitation following shoulder arthroplasty. In: Friedman RJ (ed) Arthroplasty of the shoulder. Thieme, New York, pp 99–112
59. Healy WL, Iorio R, Lemos MJ (2001) Athletic activity after joint replacement. Am J Sports Med 29(3):377–388
60. Golant A, Christoforou D, Zuckerman JD, Kwon YW (2012) Return to sports after shoulder arthroplasty: a survey of surgeons' preferences. J Shoulder Elbow Surg 21(4):554–560
61. Cox CL, Kuhn JE (2009) Complications in shoulder arthroplasty surgery. Chapter 10. In: Total shoulder arthroplasty. American Socity for Surgery of the Hand, Rosemont, pp 1–15
62. Bohsali KI, Wirth MA, Rockwood CA Jr (2006) Complications of total shoulder arthroplasty. J Bone Joint Surg Am 88:2279–2292
63. Chin PY, Sperling JW, Cofield RH, Schleck C (2006) Complications of total shoulder arthroplasty: are they fewer or different? J Shoulder Elbow Surg 15:19–22
64. Boileau P, Sinnerton RJ, Chuinard C, Walch G (2006) Arthroplasty of the shoulder. J Bone Joint Surg 88B:562–575
65. Cheung E, Willis M, Walker M, Clark R, Frankle MA (2011) Complications in reverse total shoulder arthroplasty. J Am Acad Orthop Surg 19:439–449

Traumatic Anteroinferior Instability

3

Giovanni Di Giacomo, Todd S. Ellenbeker, Elena Silvestri, and Silvia Bellachioma

Contents

G. Di Giacomo (✉) • S. Bellachioma
Concordia Hospital for Special Surgery, Rome, Italy
e-mail: concordia@iol.it; sissybll@hotmail.it

T.S. Ellenbeker, DPT, MS, SCS, OCS, CSCS
Clinic Director, Physiotherapy Associates Scottsdale Sports Clinic,
National Director of Clinical Research, Physiotherapy Associates
Vice President, Medical Services ATP World Tour,
Scottsdale, Arizona, USA
e-mail: ellenbeckerpt@cox.net

E. Silvestri
Fisiosmart, Rome, Italy
e-mail: elena.silvestri@email.it

G. Di Giacomo, S. Bellachioma (eds.), *Shoulder Surgery Rehabilitation: A Teamwork Approach*,
DOI 10.1007/978-3-319-24856-1_3

3.1 Introduction

Treatment of patients with glenohumeral joint instability is a complex process and involves a complete understanding of the functions and role of both the static and dynamic stabilizers of the glenohumeral joint. Additionally, a thorough knowledge of the surgical concepts and procedures outlined throughout this fine text to address the compromised anatomical structures in the patient with glenohumeral instability is of critical importance as well. The purpose of this chapter is to review the rehabilitative concepts and protocol for the treatment of the patient following arthroscopic Bankart reconstruction and latarjet technique.

3.1.1 Key Concepts in Shoulder Rehabilitation for Instability

One of the key concepts in upper extremity rehabilitation is the scapular plane concept. The scapular plane has ramifications in treatment, in evaluation, and even in functional activity in sports. According to Saha, the scapular plane is defined as being 30° anterior to the coronal or frontal plane of the body [1]. This plane is formed by the retroversion of the humeral head, which averages 30° relative to the shaft of the humerus, coupled with the native anteversion of the glenoid, which is also 30° in relation to the scapular plane [2, 3].

It is important for clinicians to recognize this relationship during humeral head translation testing and exercise positioning because of the inherent advantages of this position (Fig. 3.1). With the glenohumeral joint placed in the scapular plane, bony impingement of the greater tuberosity against the acromion does not occur because of the alignment of the tuberosity and the acromion in this orientation [1]. In addition to the optimal bony congruency afforded in the scapular plane, this position decreases stress on the anterior capsular components of the glenohumeral joint and enhances activation of the posterior rotator cuff through length-tension enhancement compared with function in the coronal plane [1, 2]. Placement of the glenohumeral joint in the scapular plane optimizes the osseous congruity between the humeral head and the glenoid and is widely recommended as an optimal position for the performance of various evaluation techniques and for the use during many rehabilitation exercises [1, 4].

Another important general concept of relevance for this chapter is that of muscular force couples. One of the most important biomechanical principles in shoulder function is the deltoid rotator cuff force couple [5]. This phenomenon, known as a *force couple*, can be defined as two opposing muscular forces working together to enable a particular motion to occur, with these muscular forces being synergists or agonist/antagonist pairs [5]. The deltoid muscle provides force primarily in a superior direction when it contracts unopposed during arm elevation [6]. The muscle-tendon units of the rotator cuff must provide a compressive force, as well as an inferiorly or caudally directed force, to minimize superior migration and to minimize contact or impingement of the rotator cuff tendons against the overlying acromion [5].

Failure of the rotator cuff to maintain humeral congruency leads to glenohumeral joint instability, rotator cuff tendon pathology, and labral injury [7]. Imbalances in the deltoid rotator cuff force couple, which primarily occur during inappropriate and unbalanced strength training, as well as during repetitive overhead sports activities, can lead to development of the deltoid without concomitant increases in rotator cuff strength and can increase the superior migration of the humeral head provided by the deltoid, leading to rotator cuff impingement.

Additionally, the serratus anterior and trapezius force couple is the primary muscular stabilization and prime mover of upward rotation of the scapular during arm elevation.

Bagg and Forrest have shown how the upper trapezius and the serratus anterior function during the initial 0–80° of arm elevation, providing upward scapular rotation and stabilization [8]. Because of a change in the lever arm of the lower trapezius that occurs during the lateral shift of the scapulothoracic instantaneous center of rotation with arm elevation, the lower trapezius and the serratus anterior function as the primary scapular stabilizer in phases II and III (80–140°) of elevation [8].

Knowledge of the important muscular force couples in the human shoulder and scapulothoracic region is imperative and can lead to proper evaluation and ultimately treatment provided via strengthening and monitoring of proper strength balance in these important muscular pairings. Finally, the concept of glenohumeral resting position deserves discussion in this section of the chapter because of its relevance both in evaluation of the shoulder and in the application of treatment, specifically mobilization and interventions performed to improve glenohumeral motion. The resting position of the human glenohumeral joint generally is considered to be the position where there is maximum range of motion (ROM) and laxity, caused by minimal tension or stress in the supportive structures surrounding the joint [9]. This position has been referred to as the *loose-pack* position of the joint as well. Kaltenborn and Magee both have reported that the resting position of the glenohumeral joint ranges between 55° and 70° of abduction (trunk-humeral angle) in the scapular plane [10, 11].

This loose-pack position is considered to be a "midrange" position, but only recently has it been subjected to experimental testing. Hsu et al. measured maximal anterior posterior displacements and total rotation ROM in cadaveric specimens, with altering positions of glenohumeral joint elevation in the plane of the scapula [9]. Their research identified the loose-pack position, where maximal anterior posterior humeral head excursion and maximal total rotation ROM occurred within the proposed range of 55–70° of humeral elevation in the scapular plane (trunk-humeral angle) at a mean trunk-humeral angle of 39.33°. This corresponded to 45 % of the available ROM of the cadaveric specimens.

Anterior posterior humeral head translations and maximal total rotation ranges of motion were significantly less at 0° of abduction and near 90° of abduction, respectively, in the plane of the scapula, and were greatest near the experimentally measured resting position of the glenohumeral joint (39.3°).

This study provides key objective evidence for the clinician to obtain the maximal loose-pack position of the glenohumeral joint by using the plane of the scapula and approximately 40° of abduction. This information is important to clinicians who wish to evaluate the glenohumeral joint in a position of maximal excursion or translation and to determine the underlying accessory mobility of the joint.

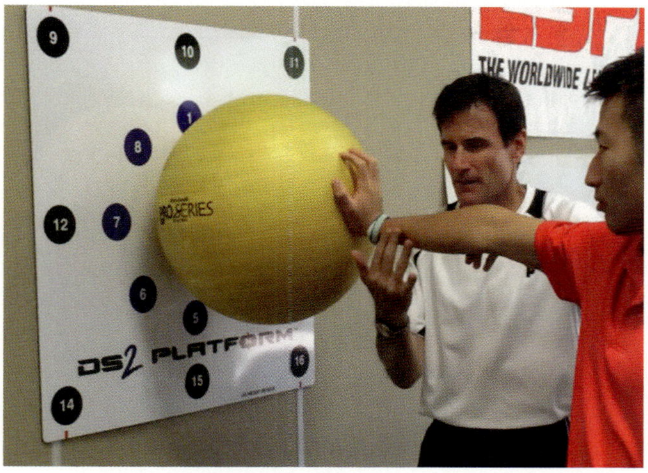

Fig. 3.1 Scapular plane position: Rehabilitation application using a physioball with rhythmic stabilization and perturbation applies in a position 30° anterior to the coronal plane of the body

3.2 Traumatic Anteroinferior Instability

3.2.1 Understanding Stability Mechanisms

The design of the shoulder makes it the most mobile and least constrained joint of the musculoskeletal system.

The forces acting on it may be divided into *static* and *dynamic* constraints [12].

It is important to consider the instability which may arise in the *midrange* or *end range* of shoulder motion [13].

- In the midrange, the lax capsule-ligamentous structures do not contribute to stabilization of the joint, which is instead achieved either by negative intra-articular pressure (hanging-arm position without muscle contraction) or by the concavity-compression effect caused by muscle contraction force against the glenoid concavity (Fig. 3.2) [14].
  Any pathological process which compromises these stabilizing mechanisms will lead to midrange instability, for example, a large bony defect of the glenoid, resulting in an insufficient concavity-compression effect; muscle imbalance, which makes it difficult to keep the humeral head centered in the glenoid socket; and enlarged joint volume with a thin joint capsule, which makes maintaining negative intra-articular pressure difficult are all causes of midrange instability.
- In the end range of shoulder motion, in abduction and maximum external rotation and maximum horizontal extension, the anteroinferior capsule becomes tight and plays a role as a stabilizer (Fig. 3.3).
  Hence, disruption of this capsule, for example, in a Bankart lesion, will result in a reduction in end-range stability. Another important pathology in the context of end-range stability is the large Hill-Sachs lesion which engages with the anterior rim of the glenoid; this concept is very important for a proper understanding of the pathophysiology associated with bony defects of the glenoid and the humeral head.

It is well established that patients with soft tissue incompetence [15, 16], humeral head deficiencies [17–19], and/or glenoid bone loss [15, 20–22] have higher failure in conservative and surgical rates than those in which these lesions are not present.

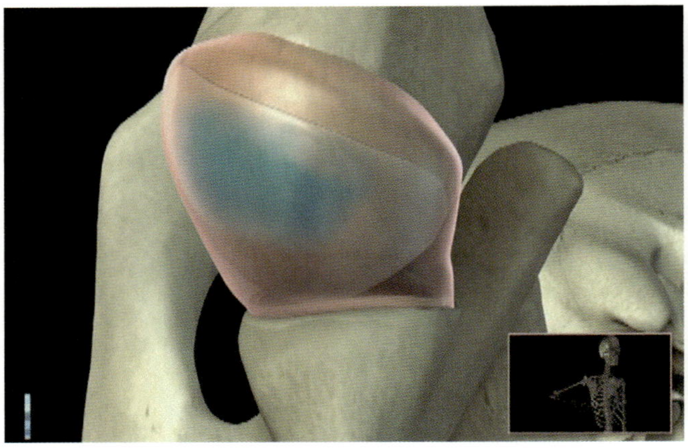

Fig. 3.2 In the *midrange* the capsule-legamentous structures do not contribute to the stabilization of the joint

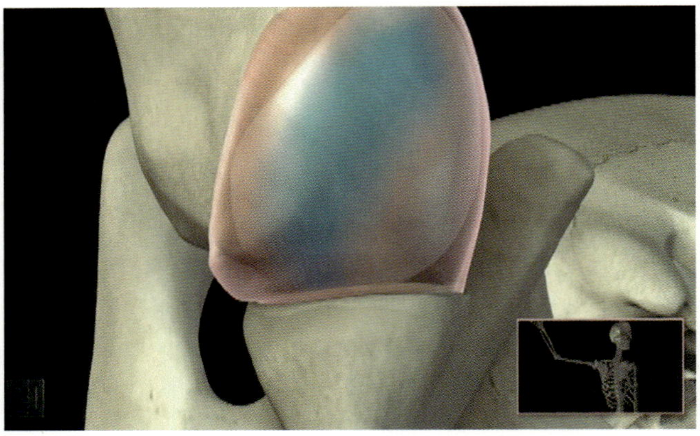

Fig. 3.3 At the *end of range* of motion, the anteroinferior capsule becomes tight and stabilizes the joint

3.3 Bone Loss

3.3.1 Glenoid Bone Loss

The prevalence of glenoid rim fracture or erosion in anterior shoulder instability has been reported to range from 8 to 95 % [21, 23–30].

In surgical observations of 158 cases of anteroinferior shoulder dislocation, 116 (73 %) were found to have a bony defect of the glenoid rim, 65 (41 %) had an *erosion*-type defect, and 51 (32 %) had a *fragment*-type defect [21, 23].

In patients with recurrent anterior shoulder dislocation studied with 3D (best-fit circle), 40 % -> had an *erosion*-type bone loss, 50 % had a *fragment*-type bone loss, and 10 % had intact bone [24, 30].

Burkhart and De Beer have suggested that acute glenoid rim fractures seen in rugby players may be the result of excessive axial load on the glenoid when the injury takes place (Fig. 3.4) [31].

Smaller rim avulsions, on the other hand, may occur following episodes of low-energy trauma associated with less axial load and more translation and shearing of the humeral head over the glenoid rim, a mechanism which may also be responsible for the compression fractures without bony fragments associated with attritional or erosive bone loss due to repeated or recurrent episodes of instability [32, 33].

Although there are no natural history studies of glenoid bone loss, the basic science literature suggests that a bony Bankart lesion and subsequent resorption may precede attritional bone loss [34].

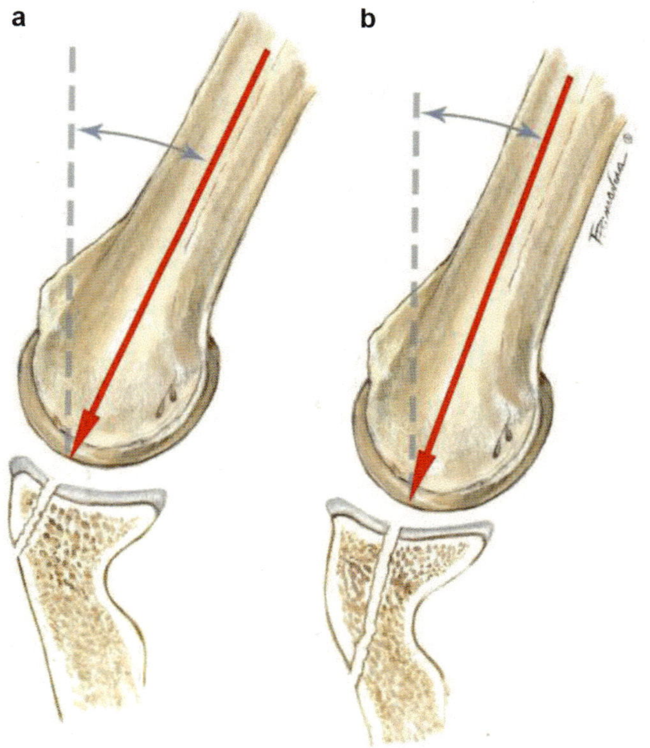

Fig. 3.4 (**a**) Excessive axial load on the glenoid can lead to glenoid fracture. (**b**) different angles of stress at the glohumeral joint on the axial plan (orizontale extension) a>b

According to Boileau et al. [15], an episode of instability will lead to rim avulsion (Fig. 3.5) without significant stretching of the joint capsule provided that the latter is "strong" and of "good" quality, whereas a "weak" capsule will be subject to elongation and thus recurrent subluxations or dislocations will lead to compression and erosion of the glenoid rim (Fig. 3.6). This means that in the clinical context, traumatic anterior instability is likely to lead to only *two types* of glenoid lesion: *rim fractures or avulsions* and *compression fractures* or *erosive* bone loss. A wide range of noninvasive imaging methods have been used to evaluate glenoid bone loss quantitatively but determining the extent of a rim avulsion or compression fracture remains difficult irrespective of the method adopted and may in any case be meaningless. Measurement of surface area is one of the methods which have gained the widest acceptance and is currently used to quantify glenoid bone loss of all types [35, 36].

In a study carried out by Sugaya et al. [36], 3D CT was used to evaluate bony Bankart lesions in 50 cases of recurrent anterior instability: one large fragment (>20 % of the glenoid fossa), 27 medium fragments (5–20 %), and 22 small fragments (<5 %) were found. A more recent study (d'Elia et al. [37]) found a glenoid rim lesion in the preoperative 2D CT results of 64 (80 %) of 80 patients with recurrent anterior instability.

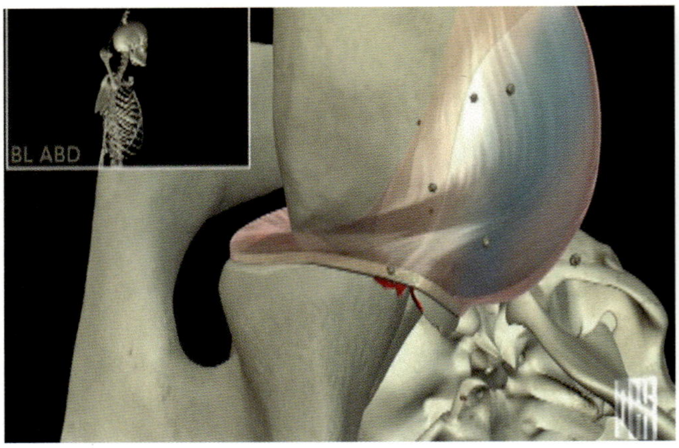

Fig. 3.5 An episode of instability with "strong" and of "good" quality ligaments can lead to rim *avulsion*

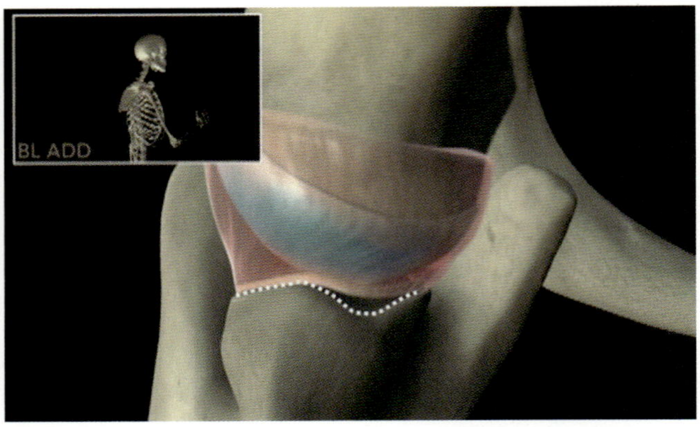

Fig. 3.6 Recurrent subluxations or dislocations will lead to *compression* and *erosion* of the glenoid rim

3.3.2 Hill-Sachs Lesion

In 1861, the "anatomical lesion" found on the articular humeral head posterior to the greater tuberosity in cases of anterior dislocation was described by Flower as a "groove" [38].

In 1880 Eve reported a case of subcoracoid dislocation with formation of a "groove" on the posterior surface of the humeral head; this became known as the "typical defect" [39].

The first well-documented cases of a "typical defect" occurring after initial anterior dislocation were described in 1934 by Hermodsson [40], who noted that (a) the defect occurs frequently; (b) the longer the humeral head is dislocated, the larger the defect will be; (c) the defect is generally larger with anteroinferior dislocation than with anterior dislocation; and (d) the defect is generally larger in recurrent dislocations [19, 40, 41].

Calandra et al. [17] established a classification of these defects based on arthroscopic evaluation: *grade I* is a defect in the articular surface down to, but not including, the subchondral bone; a *grade II* lesion includes the subchondral bone; and a *grade III* lesion signifies a large defect in the subchondral bone. This study also found that the true incidence of the Hill-Sachs lesion in young patients with an initial anterior shoulder dislocation was 47 %.

The incidence of this lesion is also known to increase with the number of dislocations: it ranges from 65 to 67 % after the first dislocation and rises to 84–93 % in cases of recurrent dislocations [17, 42–45].

When the humeral head is driven anteriorly, the capsulelabral structures of the shoulder become stretched and often tear, the humeral head translates further anteriorly, and a compression fracture occurs along the postero-supero-lateral aspect of the humeral head as it impinges on the dense cortical bone of the anterior glenoid rim. Hill and Sachs also described [8] the "line of condensation," which is a sharp line detectable on x-ray with the arm in internal rotation; this line represents "the compression or compaction into a narrow medial border of the spongy bone previously occupying the space of the defect" (Fig. 3.7) [19].

It is important to be able to distinguish between the normal anatomical structures of the posterior humeral head and the characteristic features of Hill-Sachs lesions. As Richards et al. [23] have described, the "bare spot" of the humeral head has no direct attachment of the rotator cuff tendons; it is the anatomical groove of the humeral head and flattening of the head as it progresses caudally to become the shaft.

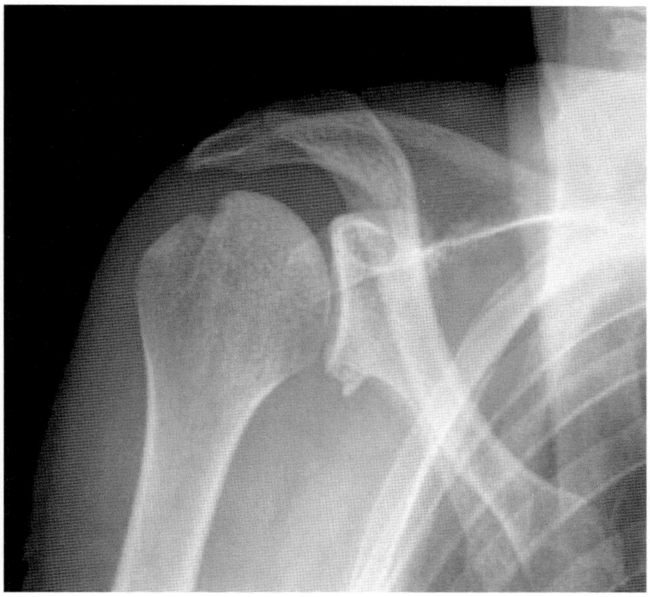

Fig. 3.7 Note "line of condensation" on the humeral head with the internal rotation

Recurrent instability renders the damaged anterior soft tissue structures particularly problematic as the static glenohumeral constraints (i.e., capsule, labrum) are progressively weakened with each episode. This attenuation makes it more likely that the relatively softer cancellous bone of the humeral head will sustain continued damage as it impacts repeatedly with the harder cortical bone of the glenoid [24], with specific orientation, location, and size (Fig. 3.8).

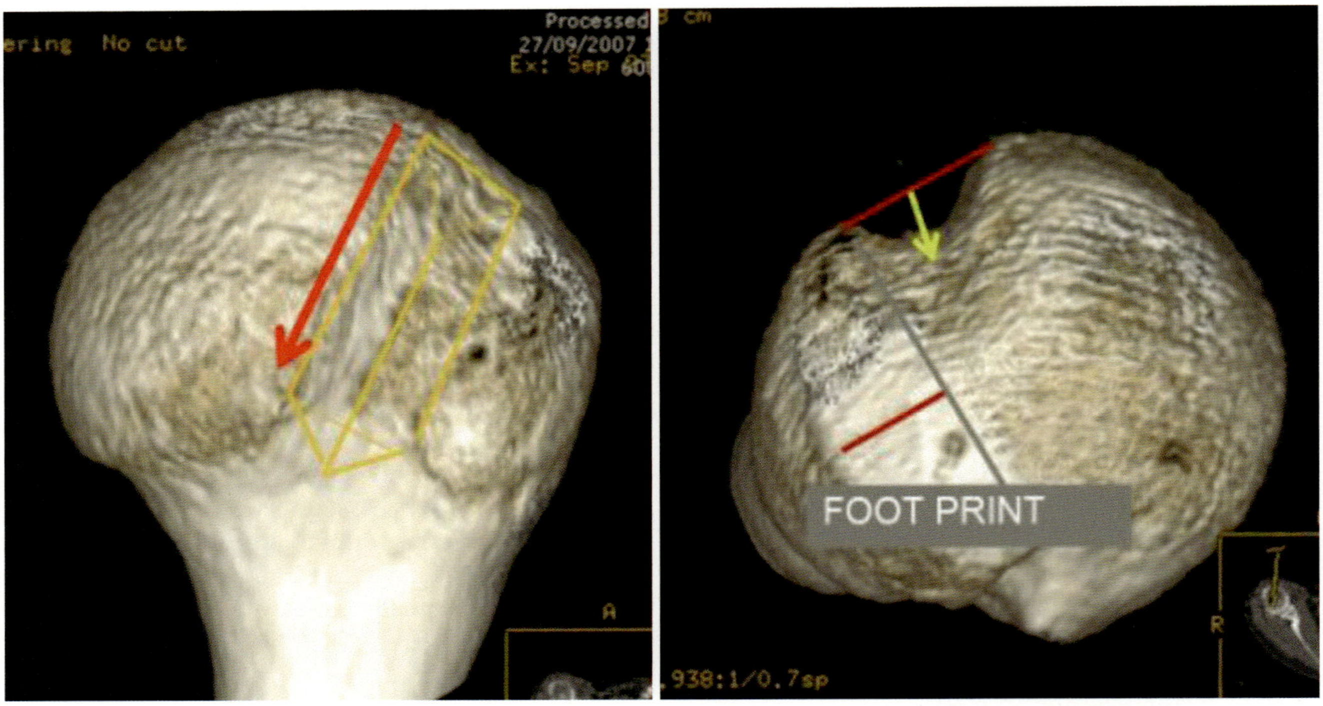

Fig. 3.8 Orientation, location (*red arrow*), and size of Hill-Sachs lesion (*yellow arrow*) (*Courtesy of Paolo Baudi*)

3.3.3 Hill-Sachs Orientation

A *non-engaging* Hill-Sachs lesion (Fig. 3.9) was defined by Burkhart and De Beer [31] as having its long axis at a diagonal, nonparallel angle to the anterior glenoid with the shoulder in a functional position of abd/ext. In this situation the articular surfaces are in continual contact, and the Hill-Sachs lesion does not engage with the anterior glenoid. Unless there is significant glenoid bone loss or poor soft tissue quality, there will be no functional articular-arc deficit, and therefore the lesion will be amenable to arthroscopic Bankart repair.

Conversely, it's *engaging* if the long axis of the Hill-Sachs lesion (Fig. 3.10) is parallel to the anterior glenoid with the shoulder in a functional position of abd/ext, so that the lesion engages with the corner of the glenoid. This kind of fracture makes the shoulder susceptible to recurrent dislocation and subluxation even after arthroscopic repair and tends to be especially if a glenoid defect is also present or if there is medial extension of the lesion beyond the medial margin of the *glenoid track*.

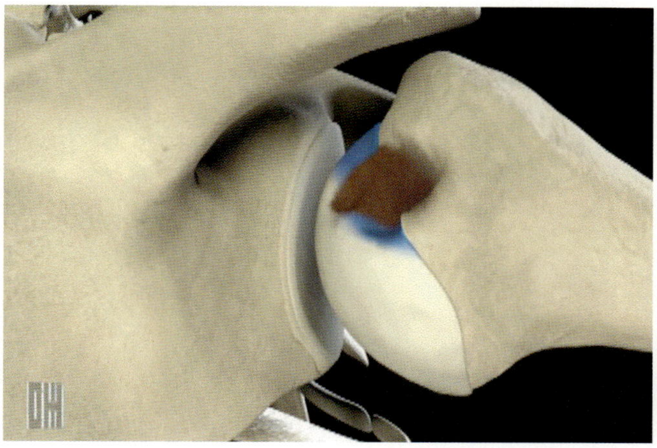

Fig. 3.9 The long axis of the Hill-Sachs lesion in the "non-engaging" pattern is *not parallel* to the glenoid with the shoulder in a functional position of abduction and external rotation

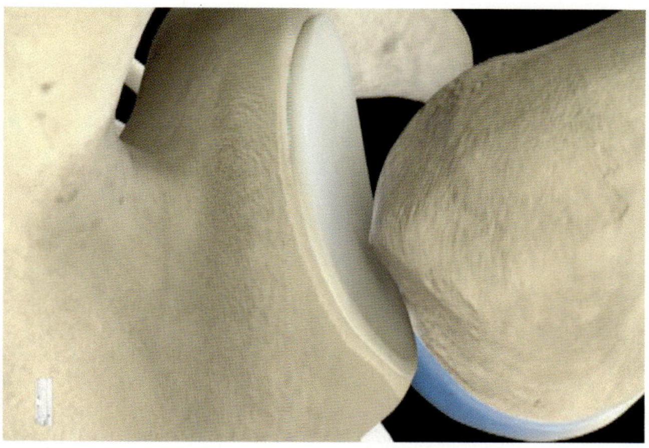

Fig. 3.10 The long axis of the Hill-Sachs lesion in the "engaging" pattern is *parallel* to the glenoid with the shoulder in a functional position of abduction and external rotation

3.3.4 Hill-Sachs Location

The *glenoid track* concept was first proposed by Yamamoto et al. [46] following their three-dimensional (3D) computed tomography (CT) study of the area of contact between the humeral head and the glenoid with regard to shoulder dislocation. They found that the area of contact moved from the infero-medial to the superolateral aspect of the posterior articular surface of the humeral head when the arm was raised and defined the zone of contact thus created as the *glenoid track*. Bone stability is guaranteed when there is no significant bone loss and the glenoid tract is intact (Fig. 3.11a).

The distance from the medial margin of the contact area to the medial margin of the rotator cuff attachment onto the humerus was 18.4 ± 2.5 mm or 84 ± 14 % of the glenoid width with the arm at 60° of abduction to the scapula or 90° of abduction to the trunk (Fig. 3.11b, c).

Both the integrity of the *glenoid track* and the location of the Hill-Sachs lesion with respect to its medial margin are of vital importance in the identification of those bipolar bone lesions which are at risk when Bankart repair or other standard stabilization procedures are being considered ("on-track" and "off-track" lesions are discussed in greater detail in Sect. 3.3.6) [47, 48].

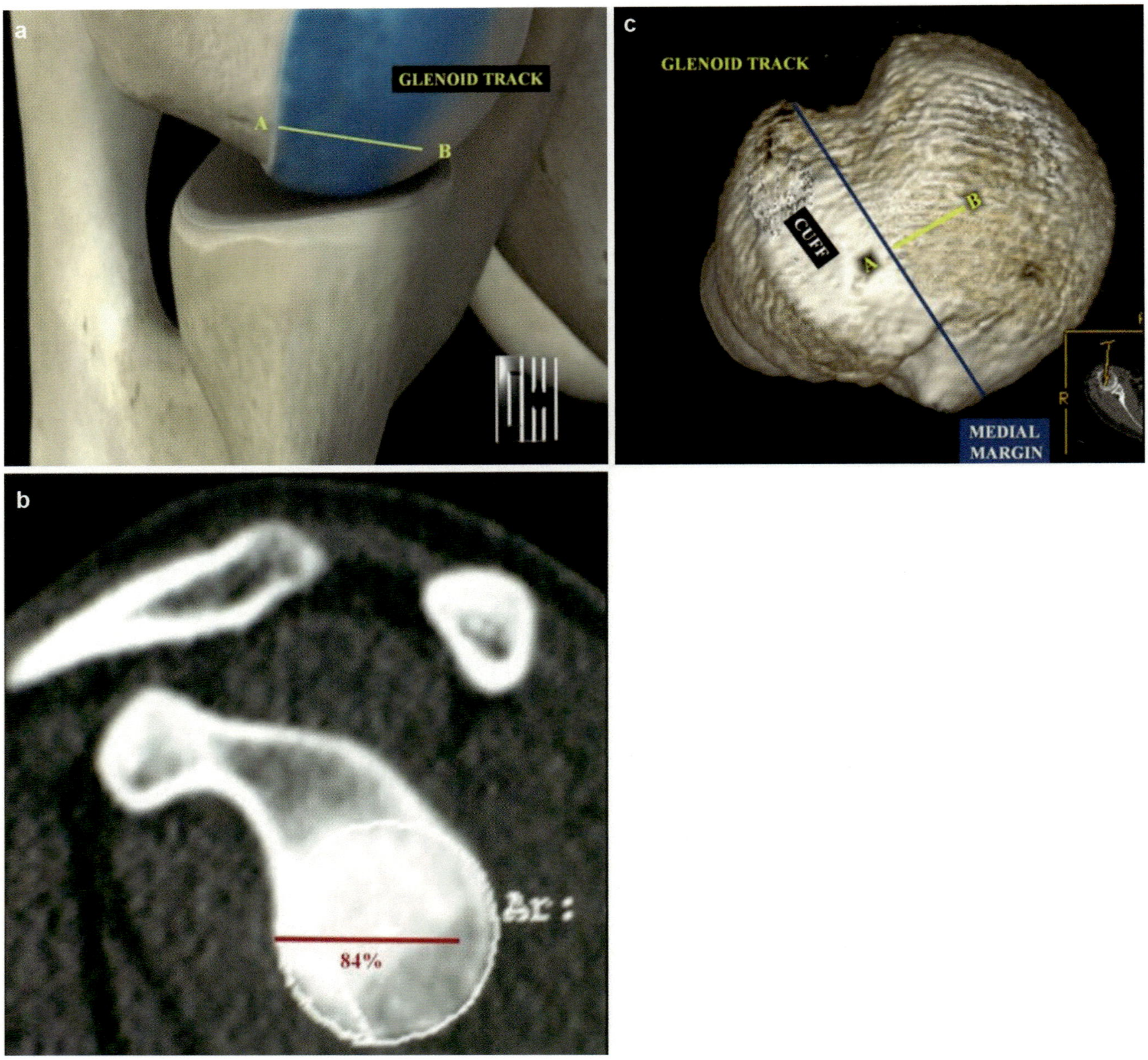

Fig. 3.11 (**a**) *AB* is the *glenoid track*; it guarantees the bone stability when the arm is raised. (**b**) The *glenoid track* is 84 ± 14 % of the glenoid width (*Courtesy of Paolo Baudi*). (**c**) The *glenoid track* on the humeral head (*AB*) is medial to the medial margin of the rotator cuff attachments (*Courtesy of Paolo Baudi*)

3.3.5 Size of Hill-Sachs Lesions

Both Boileau et al. [15] and Rowe et al. [18, 21] identified large Hill-Sachs lesions as a risk factor for recurrent shoulder instability, but did not elaborate further on possible quantitative definitions of "large." In biomechanical studies, Kaar et al. [49] showed that glenohumeral stability is substantially decreased by defects of five-eighths of the humeral head radius, while Sekiya et al. [50] demonstrated that a defect of 25 % of the radius of the humeral head decreased the stability.

Cho et al. [51] observed that *engaging* Hill-Sachs lesions were significantly wider and deeper than *non-engaging* lesions, demonstrating a close correlation between the size of the Hill-Sachs lesion and its engagement.

3.3.6 Bipolar Bone Loss Lesion

Both the integrity of the *glenoid track* and the location of the Hill-Sachs lesion with respect to its medial margin are of vital importance in the identification of those bipolar bone lesions, which are at risk when Bankart repair or other standard stabilization procedures are being considered (Fig. 3.12a, b).

Although we believe that the definition of engaging versus non-engaging Hill-Sachs lesions remains very important in discerning significant bone loss, it is also our opinion that it requires clarification in terms of how these lesions relate to the *glenoid track* and their behavior after capsular labral repair.

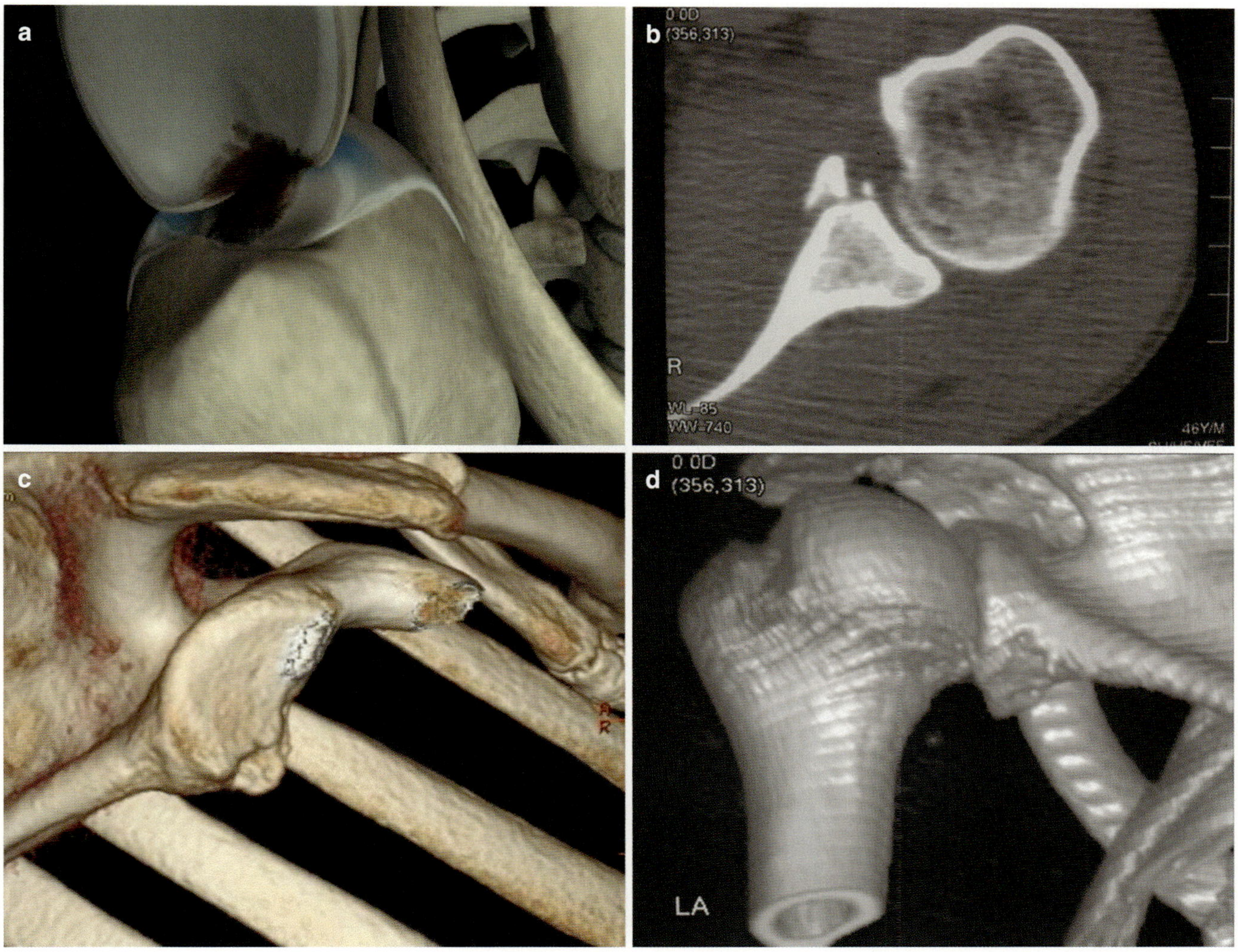

Fig. 3.12 (**a**) The "bipolar" bone loss lesion. (**b**) The "bipolar" bone loss lesion in TC axial view. (**c**) Glenoid bone loss with sottraction of the humeral head. (**d**) Bone loss on humeral head 3D recostruction posterior view (Hill-Sachs lesion)

Burkhart and De Beer's concept [31] of engaging versus non-engaging lesions is consistent with and complimentary to that of the *glenoid track* proposed by Itoi et al. [46], as each evaluates the interaction of bipolar bone loss during dynamic shoulder function.

Both Warner et al. [52] and Provencher et al. [53] maintain that as engagement is required for the formation of the Hill-Sachs lesion, all Hill-Sachs lesions would engage provided that the exact mechanism and sufficient energy were reproduced.

Kurokawa et al. [54] supported this idea, recommending that evaluation of engaging Hill-Sachs lesions should be performed using the *glenoid track* concept rather than dynamic intraoperative assessment. Although the latter is almost always carried out prior to Bankart lesion repair, its use may lead to overdiagnosis of engaging Hill-Sachs lesions because of excessive anterior translation of the humeral head permitted by ligament insufficiency, which would facilitate engagement of the humeral defect with the glenoid rim. Such anterior translation of the humeral head during motion in the horizontal plane has been shown experimentally [55]. According to Kurokawa et al. [54], a "true engaging Hill-Sachs lesion" is one which either engages after Bankart repair or extends over the *glenoid track*.

Arthroscopic evaluation of the dynamic interaction of bipolar bone loss carried out before repairing a Bankart lesion may reproduce a less than entirely reliable situation, which does not correspond either anatomically or biochemically to the context of a shoulder with an intact capsule-ligamentous complex. On the other hand, post-repair arthroscopic assessment of engagement, despite being more correct from anatomical and functional points of view, risks compromising the repair itself by overstressing the newly repaired capsule-labral complex in abduction and external rotation.

The arthroscopic assessment currently carried out prior to Bankart repair in order to distinguish engaging from non-engaging Hill-Sachs lesions should therefore be replaced by a *new approach* which does not consider the anterior translation related to the Bankart lesion and involves assessment of the *glenoid track*, including the effect of associated glenoid bone loss and the role of the location of the Hill-Sachs lesion with respect to the *glenoid track* itself.

Glenoid bone loss will result in a reduction of the width of the *glenoid track*. Under these circumstances, *glenoid track* width can be determined by subtracting the width of the defect from 83 % of the glenoid width, which is the width of the *glenoid track* in the absence of a glenoid defect [35]. In this way, the bone defects of the glenoid and humeral head can be assessed with regard to each other. When the medial margin of a Hill-Sachs lesion lies within the *glenoid track*, the lesion has adjacent bone support and is *on track*; conversely, a Hill-Sachs lesion with a medial margin which is medial to the *glenoid track* will lack bone support and is *off track* (Figs. 3.13, 3.14, and 3.15).

Having established that the orientation of the Hill-Sachs lesion (*engaging* or *non-engaging*) and its position on the humeral head (*on track* or *off track*) are crucial in guaranteeing bone stability, it is essential to understand how this lesion is created (if it occurs after the first dislocation), its relationship to the mechanism of lesion formation, and, in particular, how it evolves morphologically and topographically with subsequent episodes of dislocation.

We will therefore focus our attention on the orientation and location of the Hill-Sachs lesion and its relationship to the first mechanism of lesion formation, characteristics with an important predictive value in the identification of cases following a first traumatic anteroinferior dislocation which have a risk of recurrence or are amenable to tailored surgical techniques.

Most published decision analysis studies in the field of orthopedics are intended to serve as a guide for both physicians' recommendations and patients' treatment decisions.

A key aspect of modern patient-centered care is shared decision-making, with active involvement of patients in the decision-making process.

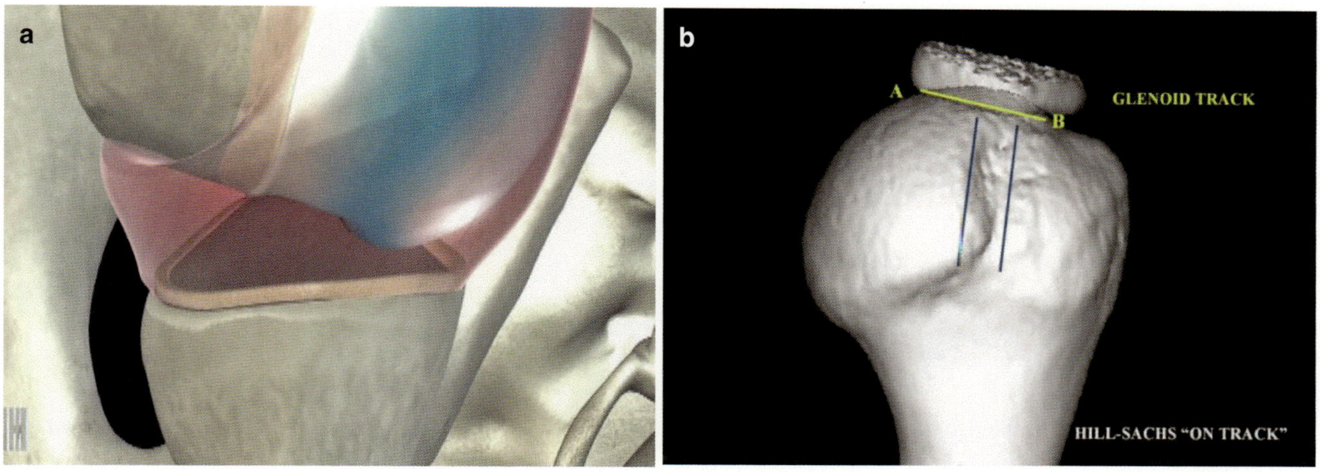

Fig. 3.13 (**a**) When the medial margin of the Hill-Sachs lies within the "glenoid track," the lesion has adjacent bone support and is *on-track*. (**b**) 3D reconstruction of Hill-Sachs *on-track* . The *blue line* is medial of lateral borders of Hill-Sachs (*Courtesy of Paolo Baudi*)

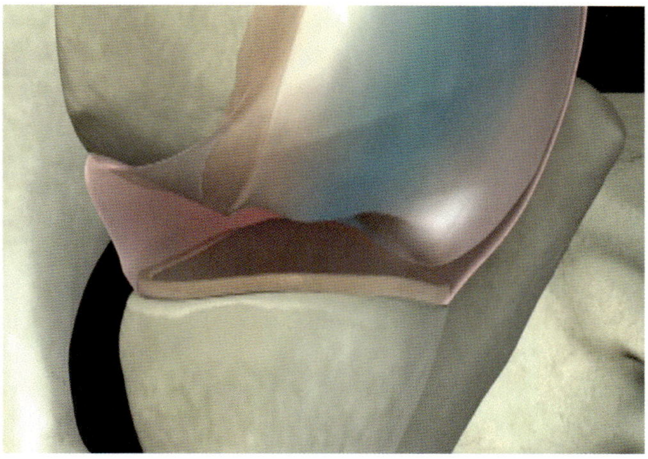

Fig. 3.14 When the medial margin of the Hill-Sachs lies medial to the "glenoid track," the lesion has not adjacent bone support and is *off track*

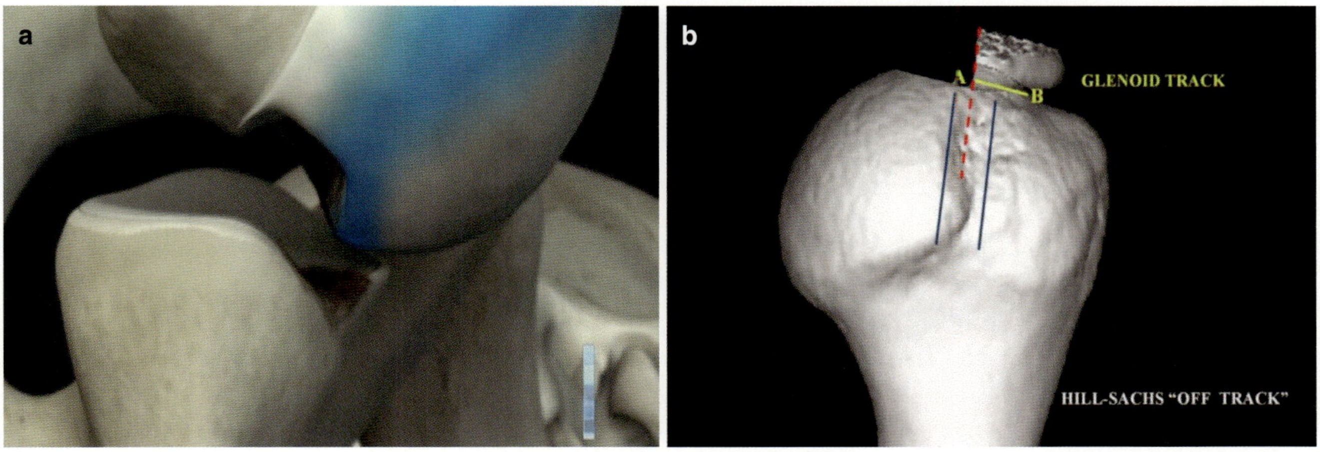

Fig. 3.15 (**a**) The bone loss on the glenoid reduces the width of the "glenoid track," and a "on-track" lesion can be transformed in a "off-track" lesion. (**b**) 3D reconstruction of Hill-Sachs off track. The *blue line* is medial of lateral borders of Hill-Sachs *red dotted line* is medial margin of the glenoid track (*Courtesy of Paolo Baudi*)

3.4 First-Time Anterior Shoulder Dislocation

Traumatic first-time anterior shoulder dislocation (*FTASD*) does not lead to recurrent instability in all patients; indeed, there is increasing evidence that early surgical stabilization in young, active individuals, collision sports, the military context, and extreme activities may achieve excellent results [56].

However, initial non-operative treatment should be seriously considered in many patients with anterior shoulder instability, including selected cases in seasonal athletes, older low-demand patients, and those who prefer to adopt appropriate activity modification, as well as cases in which there is no obvious history of trauma.

It is important to establish *elements* which may assist in the identification of patients susceptible to recurrence after FTASD, as repeated episodes may compromise *soft tissue stabilizers*, *lead to further attritional glenoid bone loss*, and *enlarge Hill-Sachs lesions*; essentially the *severity of the lesions* which accompany the first episode may be increased by further dislocations and subluxations of the joint.

Following FTASD, it is therefore necessary to furnish the epidemiological, clinical, anatomical, and pathological elements which, according to their various combinations, can be used to tailor treatment to the specific circumstances of the case and the requests of the patient.

A correct interpretation of the *risk factors* for recurrence will make it possible to identify patients who may benefit from conservative treatment rather than surgery following FTASD.

It is generally accepted that the rate of recurrence of instability after first-time dislocation is higher in *younger patients*, *males*, those who participate in *contact sports*, and in cases where there are *other associated pathological conditions*.

Recurrence rates as high as 90–95 % have been reported in patients younger than 25 years of age [57–60].

In a 2003 study of 32 pure traumatic anterior dislocations in adolescents aged 11–18 years, Deitch et al. [61] found the recurrence rate to be 75 %, while the recurrence rates reported by Rowe [62] were 100 % for patients under the age of 10, 94 % for those aged between 10 and 20, and 79 % for those aged between 20 and 30.

It is increasingly the case that athletes dedicate themselves to only one sports and sub-specialize in that sports progressively earlier in their careers. Exceptional demands may therefore be placed on the musculoskeletal systems of these young athletes, especially on the shoulders of those who participate in high-energy sports which involve physical contact or an overhead position of the arm [63].

In a study designed to investigate lesions accompanying primary anterior dislocation, Doo-Sup Kim et al. [64] observed that 24.2 % of patients in the study group had Bankart lesions, 27.2 % had free ALPSA lesions, 12.1 % had bony Bankart lesions, 57.5 % had Hill-Sachs lesions, and 12.1 % had fractures of the greater tuberosity of the humerus.

It has been reported that lesions of the humeral head, which are usually larger are more likely to lead to subsequent redislocations [54], account for up to 80 % of all first-time dislocations [6, 7, 55].

These lesions are important both from the standpoint of their influence on treatment options for recurrent dislocations and also as a risk factor after first-time dislocations.

In fact, the size of humeral head bony defects, their orientation, their location, and dynamic interaction with glenoid bone loss, if present (on/off track), all have an effect on glenohumeral stability [43, 47], which has been shown to worsen with further instability events.

In order to identify high-risk patients, we must improve our knowledge concerning prognostic factors following FTASD, besides age, sex, traumatic sport, professional, and hyperlaxity [65]. One way to learn more about acute dislocations and to optimize treatment, when bipolar bone loss is suspected, may be to evaluate bone lesions of the intra-articular head of the humerus according to the mechanism of the lesion.

An in-depth study of the mechanism of the lesion, accurately described in the capsule-ligamentous pathologies of the knee, elbow, and ankle, allows the best possible interpretation and determination of the location of soft tissue problems and any associated lesions. The literature concerning FTASD reports lesion mechanisms as the history of traumatic events in contexts such as military training, tackling and falls when playing football, falling from motorcycles, etc., but these descriptions are too generic and inaccurate.

According to Broca and Hartmann [66], periosteal stripping occurs in shoulder dislocations brought about by direct trauma mechanisms (with external force applied to the shoulder like a tackle or a fall), and shoulder dislocation with capsular tearing can only occur due to indirect trauma (without any external force applied to the shoulder like ABER position during throwing) with the arm abducted or elevated, with failure of the posteroinferior capsular structures when this is associated with internal rotation, but failure of the anteroinferior capsular structures when external rotation occurs as well. Delorme [67] maintained that the state of humeral rotation when trauma occurs determines the type of lesion that is caused by an indirect trauma mechanism in hyperabduction. When the arm is rotated internally, the greater tubercle impinges on the coracoid process, which acts as a fulcrum for levering the humeral head downward out of the joint through a lesion of the inferior glenohumeral ligament. In the case of external rotation, movement is limited by inferior glenohumeral ligament tension, and the greater tubercle is thus prevented from touching the coracoid process. The inferior glenohumeral ligament itself acts as a fulcrum and tears, usually from its glenoid insertion; tearing of the middle glenohumeral ligament only occurs when sudden extension is added to abduction and external rotation.

As the likelihood of further dislocations following an initial anteroinferior episode also depends on the topographic and morphological characteristics of the Hill-Sachs lesion, it is essential to determine in each case whether the mechanism of lesion (ABD vs ADD) is related to a specific humeral bone loss. If this were to be demonstrated, an accurate patient history of the trauma which provoked the initial or recurrent episode, combined with CT imaging, could provide the physician with another useful prognostic tool [68].

We performed a multicentric consecutive patient retrospective review of all first-time traumatic anterior shoulder dislocations, during a period from 2010 to 2014.

The initial injury lesion mechanism was classified according to Burkhart and De Beer [31] in *ABD* (a position defined as 90° abduction combined with external rotation in the range between 0° and 135°) and *ADD* (with the arm in adduction and some extension).

Inclusion criteria consisted of first-time anterior shoulder instability, a complete set of radiographic images, studies (3D CT scan of the shoulder with the humeral head digitally disconnected), documented physical examination confirming anterior shoulder instability, and patient able to fully describe the lesion mechanisms that caused the dislocation, *ABD* position versus *ADD*.

With this method, 102 patients met the inclusion criteria: 89 male (87.2 %) and 13 female (12.8 %), the mean age being 32 years (range 17–38, SEM 0.50). [In regard to mechanism, a total of 45 (44.1 %) attributed it to a movement in a functional position (*ABD*) and 57 (55.9 %) to a fall with the arm at the side.]

Hill-Sachs lesion occurs during the dislocation at a specific angle (α angle) between the anterior glenoid (A–B) and the humeral diaphysis (C–D); the same angle is between the long axis of the Hill-Sachs (A–B) and humeral diaphysis (C–D), so if we measure this angle (α), we know at what glenohumeral angle the Hill-Sachs lesion is created (Fig. 3.16a, b).

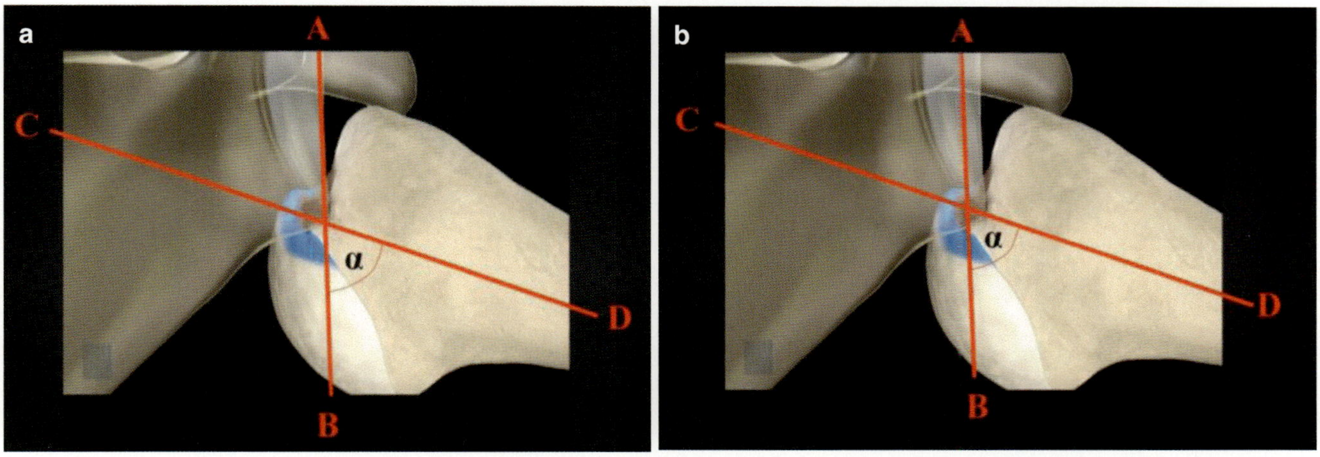

Fig. 3.16 (**a**, **b**) The angle between axis of the humerus (*CD*) and anterior glenoid margin (*AB*) at which the Hill-Sachs is created is the same angle between the long axis of the Hill-Sachs (*AB*) and the axis of the humerus (*CD*)

We have found that when the first episode occurs with the ADD mechanism, the Hill-Sachs lesion is formed with a glenohumeral angle of approximately ±16° (Fig. 3.17a) and therefore tends to be relatively parallel to the axis of the humeral diaphysis; thus in the ABD position, the lesion becomes diagonal to the glenoid and *non-engaging*. On the other hand, when the mechanism of the first episode is ABD, the Hill-Sachs lesion is formed at a glenohumeral angle of approximately 31° (Fig. 3.17b), and it is more oblique with respect to the diaphyseal axis; it is therefore more parallel to the anterior margin of the glenoid in the ABD position and *engaging*.

The high percentage of "on-glenoid-track" Hill-Sachs lesions observed in our cases is related to the fact that we only assessed first episodes. Comparing our results with the value of 7 % for "off-track" lesions in recurrent cases reported in the literature, we may infer that the recurrent episodes are responsible for reducing the *glenoid track*, as a result of concurrent glenoid bone loss, which increases with each recurrence, and greater medial extension of the Hill-Sachs lesions [54].

These phenomena may be related to the fact that patients with a first lesion mechanism in ADD acquire anteroinferior instability, supported by the subequatorial capsule-ligamentous lesion and may therefore also redislocate more easily in ABD, thus creating a greater confluent Hill-Sachs. At the same time, further dislocations and the total dislocation time both tend to medialize the Hill-Sachs lesion and produce increased glenoid bone loss, thus increasing the possibility that the Hill-Sachs lesion may become off track [54].

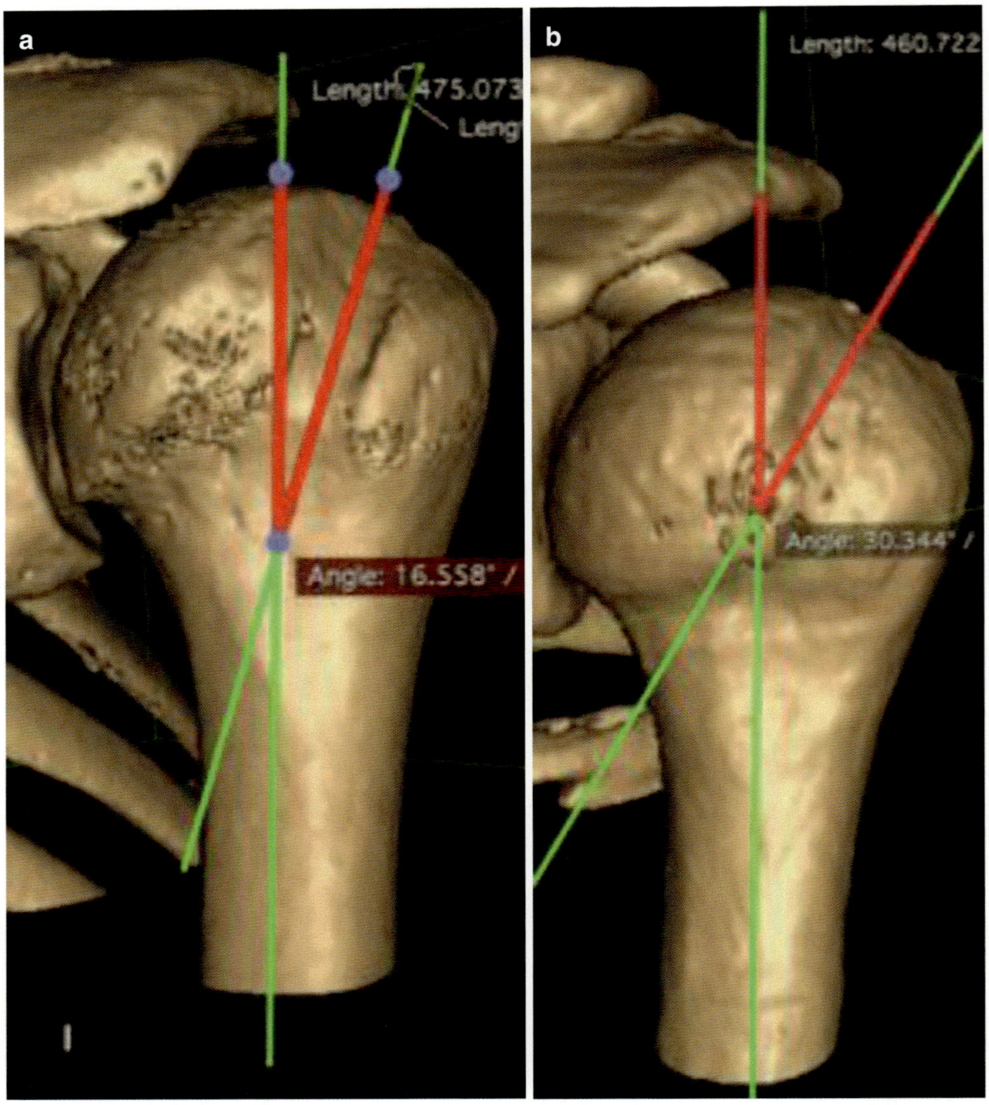

Fig. 3.17 (**a**) With ADD mechanism of lesion, the Hill-Sachs lesion is oriented 16.1° ± 2.9° with respect to the axis of the humerus and is in a less engaging position. (**b**) With ABD mechanism of lesion, the Hill-Sachs lesion is oriented 32.4° ± 4.7° with respect to the axis of the humerus and is in a more engaging position

Having confirmed that, after an initial episode, the Hill-Sachs lesion is formed in ADD at around 16.1° ± 2.9°, and in ABD at around 32.4° ± 4.7°, *we were able to break the dislocation times down into four phases:*

- *Phase 1*: is dynamic. It depends strictly on the mechanism of the lesion. It is the time period in which dislocation of the humeral head from the center of rotation of the glenoid to its anterior margin takes place (when Bankart and/or bony Bankart lesions are created); the posterosuperior head could potentially engage with the anteroinferior glenoid.
  If a Hill-Sachs lesion is present, this is its *starting point* (Fig. 3.18).
- *Phase 2*: is the reposition phase. Aided by gravity, patients with dislocation of the humeral head gradually take the arm from the point of dislocation to a less painful position closer to the side (Fig. 3.19a, b). The specific characteristics will, however, depend on the mechanism of dislocation.
  If dislocation occurs in *abduction*, in the repositioning phase a Hill-Sachs engages with the anteroinferior glenoid and induces protraction and internal rotation of the scapula, in an appearance of adduction. The humeral head rotates like a fan on the anteroinferior glenoid rim (the "hand fan effect") resulting in latero-medial and supero-inferior enlargement of the Hill-Sachs lesion, with abduction to adduction on the frontal plane and external to internal rotation on the axial plane, usually patients present at the emergency room holding the involved arm in varying degrees of abduction by supporting it at the elbow with the contralateral hand. If the trauma occurs in *adduction*, the repositioning phase is obviously limited, and the patient's arm is in true adduction.

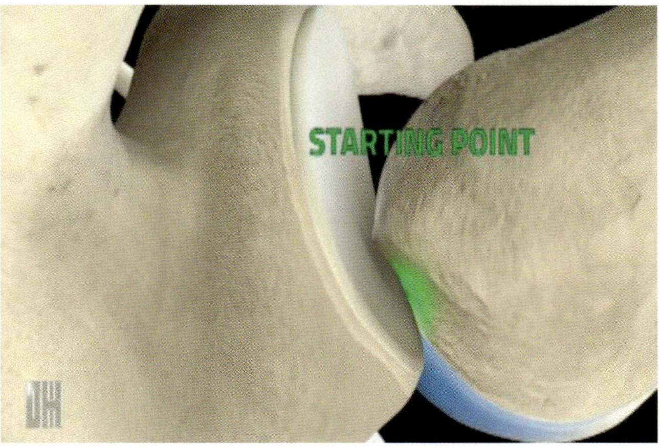

Fig. 3.18 *Phase 1* → starting position of the Hill-Sachs

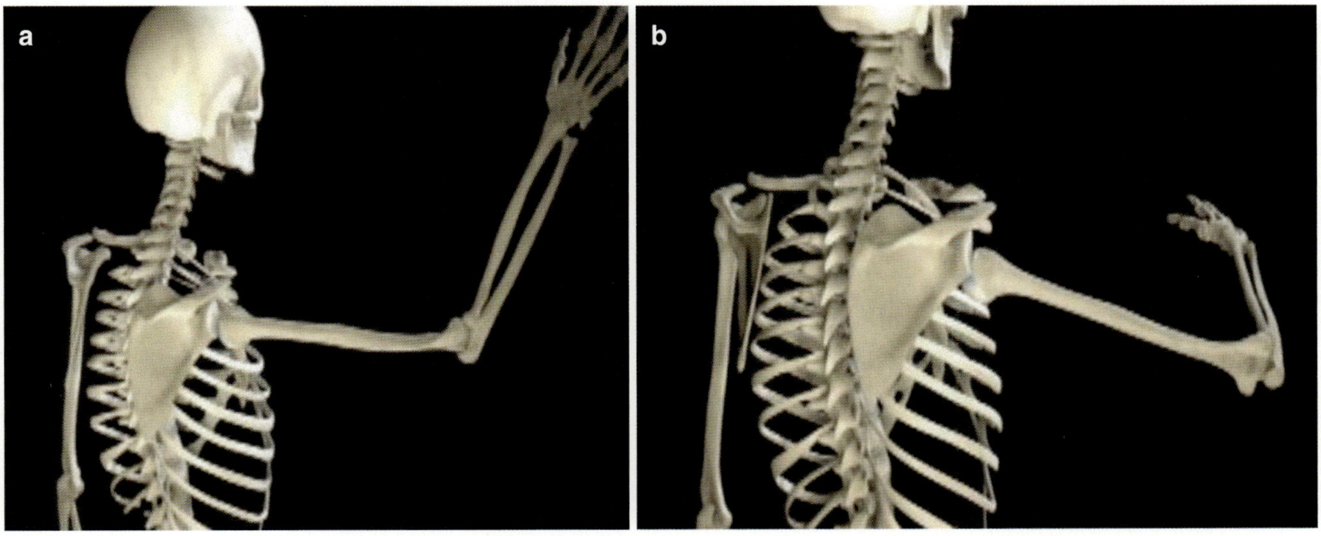

Fig. 3.19 (**a**, **b**) *Phase 2* → reposition phase

- *Phase 3*: is relatively static. At the conclusion of phase 2, with the patient in the "dislocated position," there are two important considerations. The first of these is *the orientation* of the humerus to the anterior glenoid (H-S angle), which will remain unchanged at 16.1° ± 2.9° in the ADD and 32.4° ± 4.7° in the ABD until the dislocation is reduced (the true clinical relationship of the humerus to the glenoid is obscured by changes in position of the scapula). The second consideration is the length of time for which the compressive force of the humerus acts against the anterior glenoid, which would appear to be the most important determinant of the depth of the Hill-Sachs lesion (Fig. 3.20).
- *Phase 4:* is dynamic. The reduction time (Fig. 3.21).

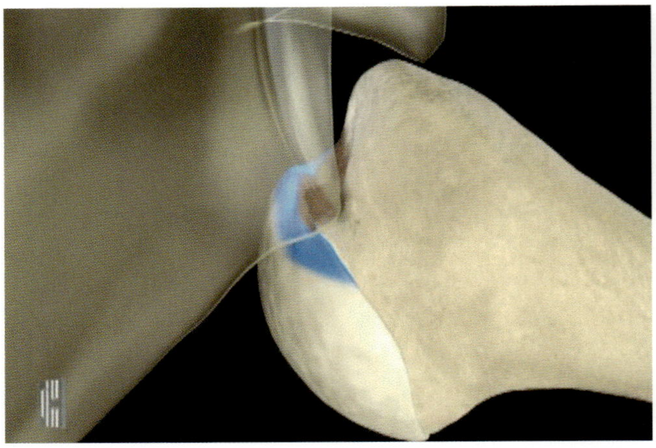

Fig. 3.20 *Phase* 3 → static phase during which the Hill-Sachs is really formed

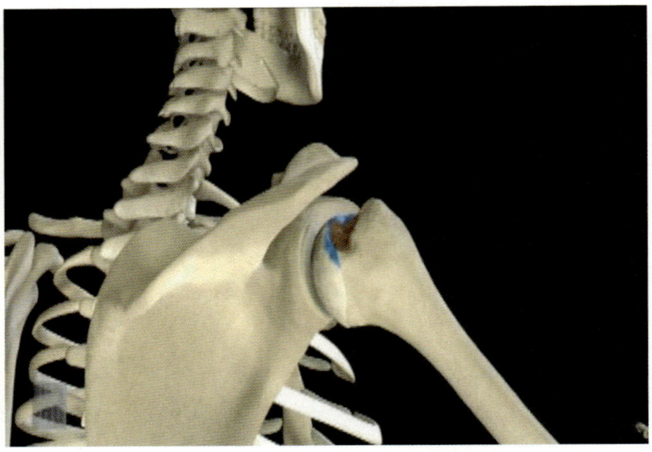

Fig. 3.21 *Phase 4* → reduction time

3.5 Recurrent Traumatic Anteroinferior Instability: Algorithm of Treatment and Rehab

The values which we obtained for the H-S angle after the first dislocation episode correlate closely with whether the lesion mechanism occurred in the ABD or ADD position, as reported by Burkhart [31].

Data obtained during an FTAD show that the humerus and scapula are orientated at specific angles when the Hill-Sachs lesion is formed, depending on the lesion mechanism.

When the dislocation occurs in the ADD position, the H-S angle is smaller (16.1° ± 2.9°), and the longitudinal axis of the Hill-Sachs is not parallel but, with the joint in the functional position of external rotation and abduction, passes diagonally across the anterior glenoid. It is improbable that the glenoid rim will be engaged; these *non-engaging* lesions are therefore not as likely to contribute to recurrent instability.

In cases of dislocations in ABD, the H-S angle is larger (32.4° ± 4.7°), and the longitudinal axis of the Hill-Sachs lesion is more oblique with respect to that of the humerus and parallel to the glenoid. These lesions are termed *engaging* and are more likely to result in symptomatic shoulder subluxation or dislocation.

It is also interesting to note that all the Hill-Sachs lesions were on track, not only because they were lateral to the *glenoid track* but also because in no case was glenoid bone loss sufficiently pronounced as to transform an "on-track" lesion into one which was "off track."

The movement associated with lesion mechanisms in FTASD is often, but not always, one of abduction, external rotation, or extension. In this case the Hill-Sachs lesion in the ABD position is orientated parallel to the glenoid (*engaging* lesion); if the lesion mechanisms of subsequent episodes are also in the ABD position, the morphology, location, and orientation of the humeral bony lesion will be repeated.

However, after an FTASD with the arm at side, the orientation of the Hill-Sachs lesion in the ABD position is *non-engaging*, but the joint is unstable in the anteroinferior direction because of the capsule-ligamentous lesion, and further episodes may result in a lesion with a different orientation and location with respect to the previous one, creating an overlap that forms a confluent Hill-Sachs lesion.

The application of these observations to the clinical context, particularly after a first episode of anteroinferior glenohumeral dislocation, involves, where possible, studying the mechanism of formation of the Hill-Sachs lesion (ABD mechanism of lesion Hill-Sachs lesion is more engaging versus ADD mechanism) and confirming its morphological and structural characteristics by means of CT imaging.

With correct interpretation, this information, together with other predictive factors (age, sex, sport, glenoid bone loss, soft tissue quality, associated lesions, etc.), may be used to orient the patient more precisely toward either conservative treatment or tailored surgical intervention. Bearing in mind that subsequent dislocation episodes may lead to enlargement of the Hill-Sachs lesion or keep it confluent, in some cases surgery is indicated after an initial episode in order to prevent an on-track Hill-Sachs lesion from becoming off track.

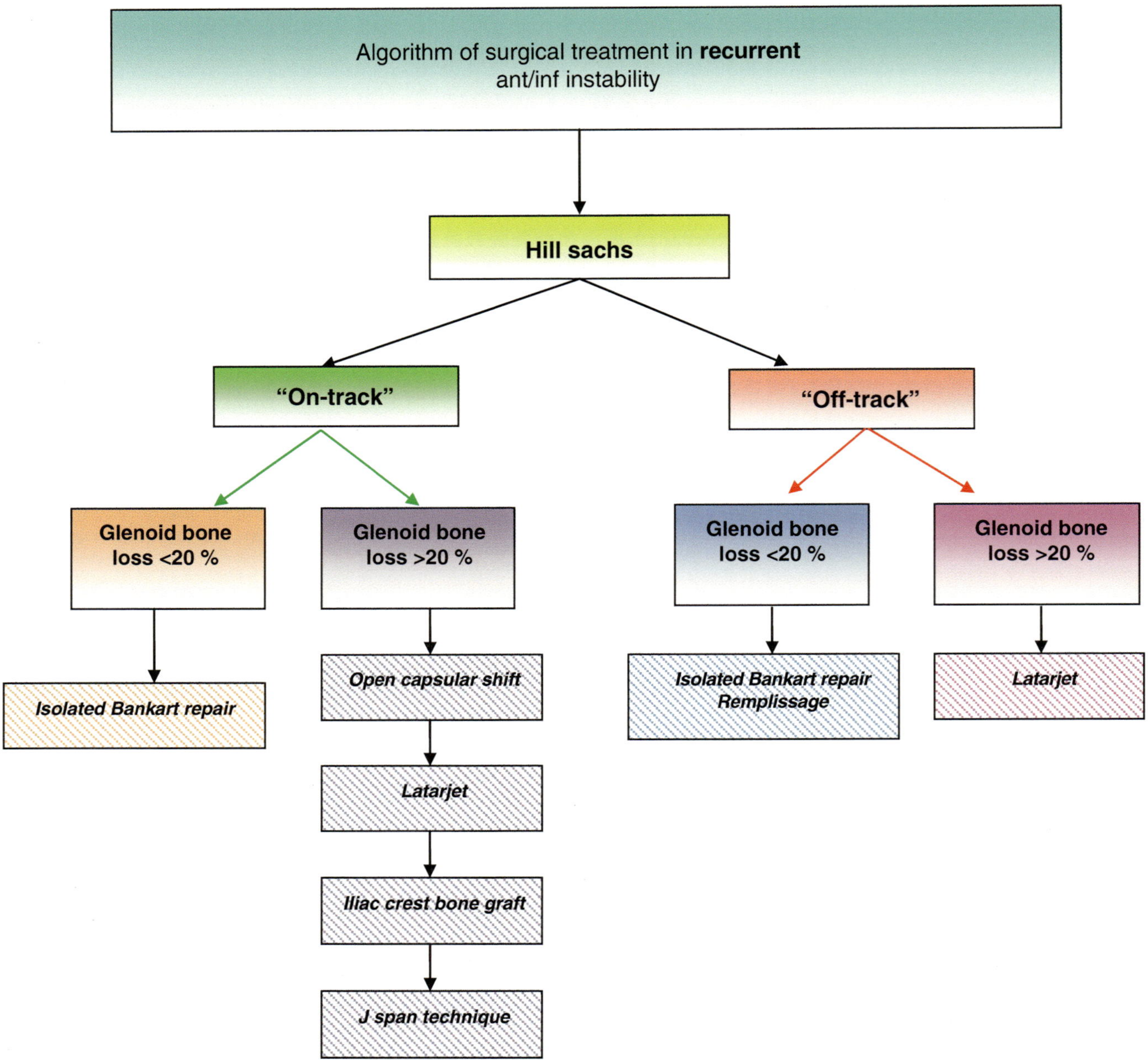

Take-Home Message

- The "cutting edge" of the glenoid bone loss in international literature is described to be around 20/21 %, even if in recent reports it seems to be lower around 13/14 %.
- Of course, in the same anatomical pathological conditions, different surgical techniques can lead to excellent clinical results. Further studies will focus attention to improve the indication, patient selection, timing of surgery, surgical techniques, and biological issue.

Surgical Treatments: Algorithm

- *Hill-Sachs lesion is on track, and glenoid bone loss ranges from 0 to 20 %*; the treatment is arthroscopic Bankart repair.
- *Hill-Sachs lesion is on track, and glenoid bone loss is over 20 %*; there are different treatments that are internationally recognized: open capsular shift, Latarjet, iliac crest bone graft, and J span technique.
- *Hill-Sachs lesion is off track, and glenoid bone loss ranges <20 %*; the treatment is isolated Bankart repair and remplissage (infraspinatus tenodesis to fill the humeral head defect avoiding the engaging of the Hill-Sachs with the anterior glenoid).

The increased recognition of the HSL in recurrent instability highlights the need to better address the bone deficiency of the humeral head in addition to the arthroscopic Bankart repair (repair of the torn anterior glenoid labrum and capsule). In 2008 Wolf and colleagues [69] described an arthroscopic method of filling the HSL by infraspinatus tenodesis and posterior capsulodesis, currently known as "remplissage" (Fig. 3.22).

This technique has rapidly gained popularity as an arthroscopic technique to manage large HSLs and although most clinical studies on the procedure have found it to be successful [69–76].

The primary stabilization feature of the remplissage procedure is that the infraspinatus and joint capsule form a mechanical block that contacts the glenoid rim at the "glenoid track," limiting the humeral head's lateral translation. This impediment to translation, however, may also lead to a restriction of ROM in the apprehension position.

- *Hill-Sachs lesion is "off track," and glenoid bone loss ranges >20 %*; the treatment is Latarjet (Fig. 3.23) because of its triple effect due to:
  1. *The bone support of the coracoid graft, that enlarge the platform of the inverted pear glenoid*
  2. *The sling effect, because the common tendon and inferior part of the subscapularis that stabilize the anteroinferior glenohumeral joint in ABER position*
  3. *If fixed, the capsular repair with the coracoacromial ligament attached to the graft*

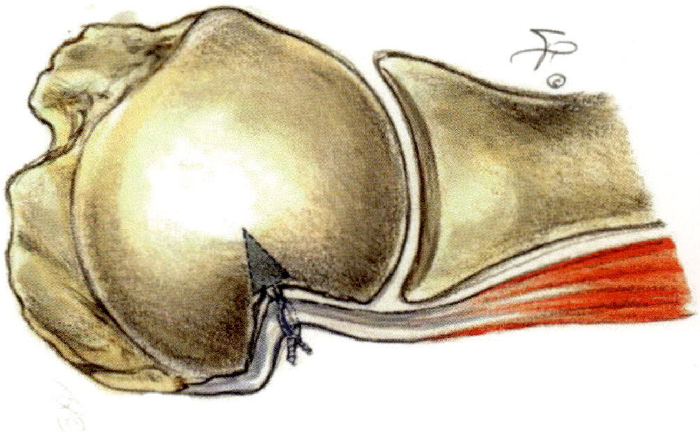

Fig. 3.22 Remplissage

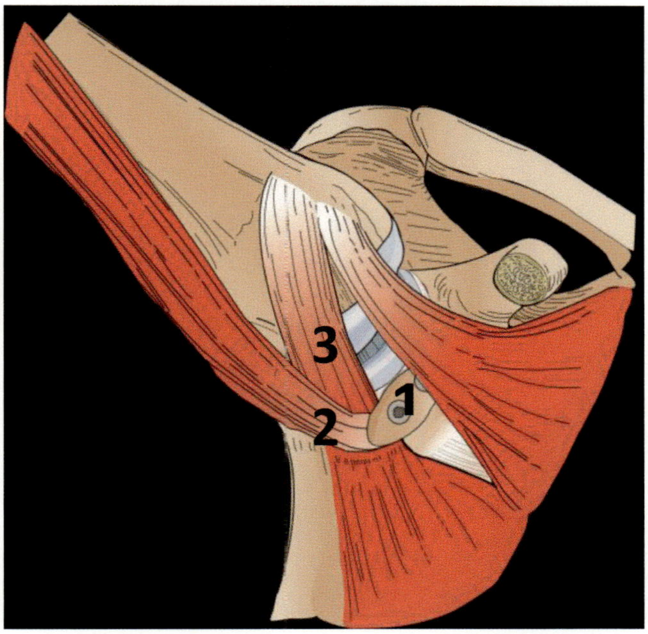

Fig. 3.23 Triple effect of the Latarjet technique. (*1*) Coracoid. (*2*) Common tendon. (*3*) Subscapularis and capsula

3.5.1 Arthroscopic Bankart Repair

The essential pathoanatomic lesion of a traumatic dislocation is the capsulolabral avulsion of the anteroinferior glenohumeral ligament complex (Bankart lesion); this lesion typically worsen with repeated injuries as previously described.

Anatomical reconstruction procedures have been aimed at reconstructing the anterior labrum using suture anchors.

It is well documented that restoration of stability can be reliably obtained by Bankart repair; if this is successful, however, there is some morbidity associated with it.

The following description of the arthroscopic Bankart repair procedure indicates in "SMALL CAPS" *the elements that take about 15 days to heal and in* "bold small caps" *the elements that take more than 6 weeks to heal.*

In an effort to restore stability to the shoulder while avoiding this morbidities, arthroscopic shoulder stabilization procedures have been developed and offer a number of advantages over traditional open techniques:

- Smaller incisions (ARTHROSCOPIC PORTALS) (Fig. 3.24)
- Less muscle dissection (*avoiding the iatrogenic lesion of the subscapularis is one of the main advantages of this technique*)
- Excellent visualization of the entire joint (*allowing clear surgical management of the pathology and of all the procedure's steps*)
- Less postoperative pain

The key point in this surgery is to repair with a shift from south to north the soft tissue lesion (Bankart lesion) to the subequatorial glenoid (soft tissue to bone healing) (Fig. 3.25).

The goal is reached through suture anchors that have to be able to withstand the forces required for rehabilitation until the normal bone to tissue interface is restored (Fig. 3.26).

Post-surgery rehabilitation must take the following into account:

1. ***Biological-specific healing rates of the surgical procedure:*** *skin incision (arthroscopic portals); in this case the healing process of the soft tissue (Bankart lesion) to the glenoid rim is crucial* (Fig. 3.27) *and of the infraspinatus to the Hill-Sachs if remplissage is performed* (Fig. 3.22).
2. ***Neuromuscolar and proprioceptive recovery:*** *must be gradual in the case of the affected body part and consistent with biological heeling timeframe, but can be faster for the kinetic chain links outside the involved shoulder.*
3. ***Return to working and/or sports activity.***

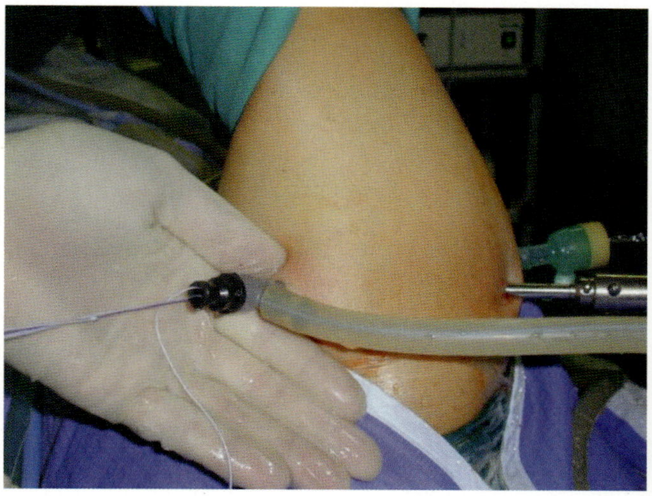

Fig. 3.24 Arthroscopic portals

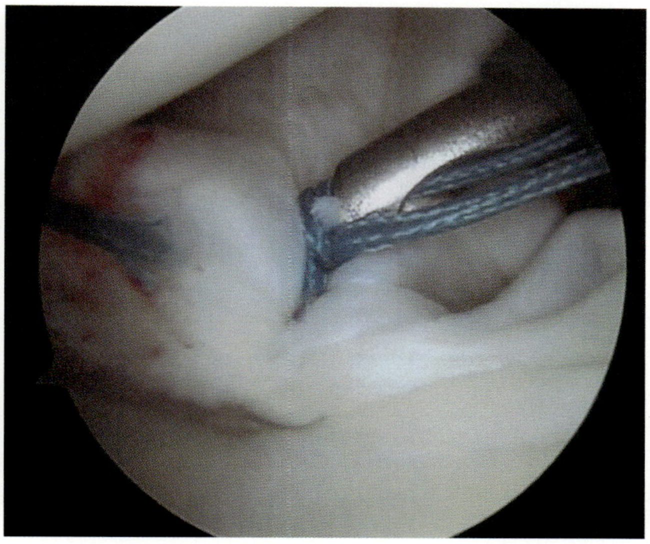

Fig. 3.26 Restoration of the ligaments to the bone

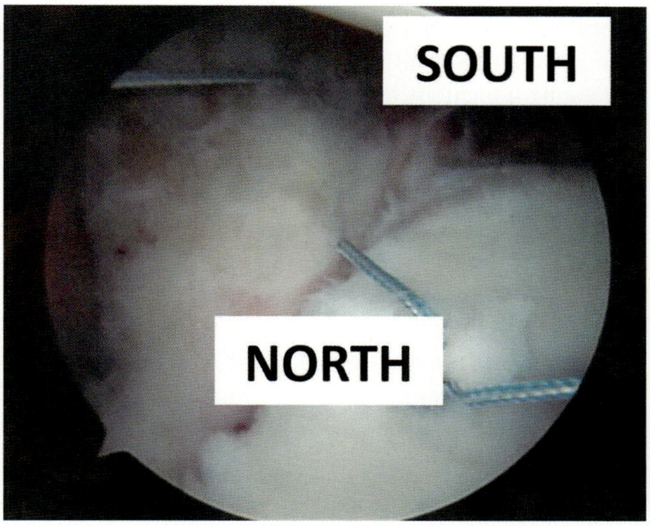

Fig. 3.25 Shift from south to north of the inferior capsule-ligamentous complex

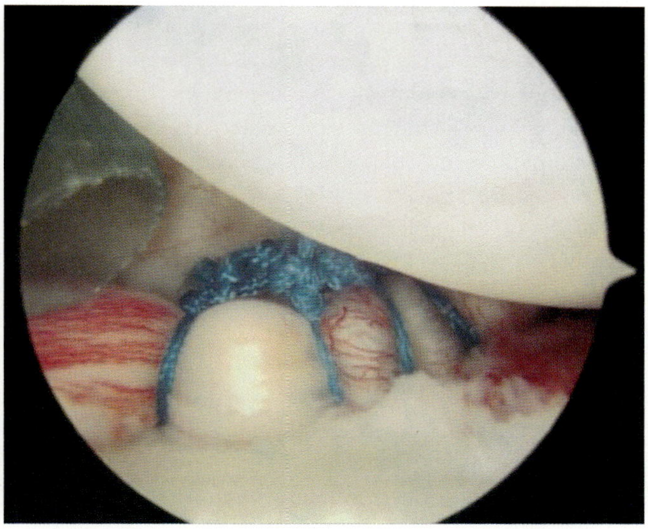

Fig. 3.27 Final view of the Bankart repair

3.5.2 Evaluation of the Shoulder following Arthroscopic Bankart Reconstruction

While it is beyond the scope of this chapter to completely review the comprehensive evaluation procedures applied in shoulder rehabilitation, it is however very important to discuss the most important portions of the objective evaluation applied following surgery.

Evaluation of the patient's static posture provides important information on scapular function and is one of the primary areas of initial focus in the initial evaluation postoperatively. Research has shown that the dominant shoulder is often lower than the non-dominant, not only in normal populations but can be significantly lower in the overhead athlete [77]. Understanding this typical relationship is important for the clinician as patients presenting after dominant shoulder surgery who hold their shoulder in a position higher than the non-dominant shoulder may be guarding and or have upper trapezius hypertonicity and may require rehabilitative interventions to address this compensatory condition. Additionally, observation of the patient in the resting position with the arms at the side and viewing the shoulder girdle and scapular region posteriorly will allow for inspection of the muscular structure and bulk in the periscapular region. Specific focus is given to the rotator cuff and scapular musculature for visual observation. Indentation over the infraspinous fossa of the scapula is common in overhead athletes [78, 79] and can be particular evident after dislocation and chronic instability indicating rotator cuff weakness and focused rehabilitation on the rotator cuff. Prominence of the scapular spine coupled with indentation within the infraspinous fossa is key indicator of infraspinatus atrophy [78, 79]. The use of the hands on hips position if the patient can assume this position (gently resting the hands on the hips with the thumbs pointing posteriorly) can accentuate the visual appearance of the atrophy if present in this region (Fig. 3.28). Patients with more severe atrophy may have suprascapular nerve involvement [78, 79]. Impingement of the suprascapular nerve can occur at the suprascapular notch and the spinoglenoid notch and form paralabral cyst formation commonly found in patients with superior labral lesions [80]. Particular attention is focused on this part of the visual observation in the evaluation process.

Additionally, prominence of the scapular borders both at rest and in the hands on hips position can indicate scapular dysfunction [81] and alert the clinician to the need for additional early focus and attention on the scapular stabilizers in the rehabilitation program. This visual observation technique with the arms at rest and in the hands on hips position constitute a static scapular evaluation and can indicate the need for the inclusion of early scapular exercise in the rehabilitation program. McMahon et al. [82] has shown that patients with glenohumeral joint instability have decreased muscular activity in the serratus anterior during active elevation than normal control subjects. The common association of scapular dysfunction and shoulder instability has been reported in several clinical investigations [83].

Dynamic scapular evaluation is also very important but is often not possible in the immediate postoperative evaluation due to patient's inability to perform large arcs of active movement. Kibler et al. [83] has provided a clinically useful classification of scapular dysfunction identifying three distinct types or patterns of scapular dysfunction. Table 3.1 lists the three types in their classification. Patients in the immediate postoperative phase often present with type III superior scapular dysfunction due to force couple imbalance and the characteristic "shrug" sign during attempts at arm elevation (Fig. 3.29). Additionally, increases in medial (internal) rotation are also common with instability as well [83] (Fig. 3.30).

Despite limitations in the ability to perform large arcs of active elevation in the initial postoperative evaluation of the patient following arthroscopic Bankart, revisiting the full evaluation of the scapula complete with dynamic assessment of scapulothoracic motion and further classification using the Kibler system is indicated later in the rehabilitation process.

In addition to scapular evaluation, careful assessment of range of motion provides an indication of joint capsular status and identifies potential areas of motion restriction. The physiotherapists evaluation of range of motion should include objective documentation of movement most often involves the use of a goniometer or inclinometer and specific standardized movement techniques to enhance accuracy and reliability. The motions of primary importance in the evaluation following arthroscopic Bankart are forward flexion, coronal plane and scapular plane abduction, and internal and external rotation. Measurement of humeral rotation should include the use of scapular stabilization to prevent scapular compensation and dilution of the glenohumeral measurement [84, 85]. Initial measurement of the postoperative extremity most often includes passive range of motion in all planes and measurement of humeral rotation with 45° of abduction (Fig. 3.31). Baseline measures on the dominant extremity can include active flexion and abduction, as well as humeral rotation passively without overpressure in 45° and 90° of abduction.

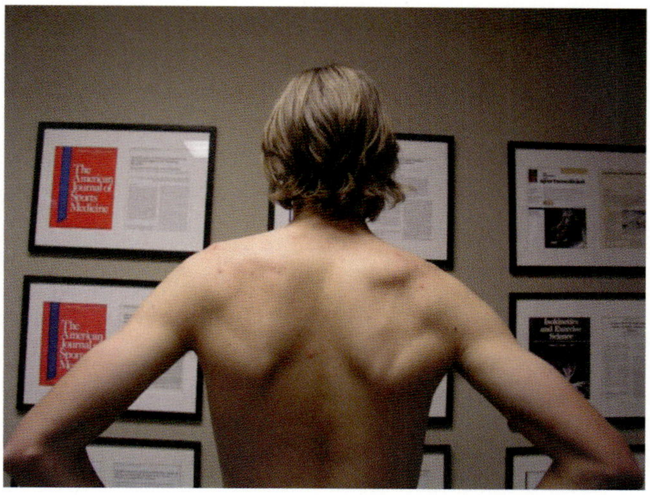

Fig. 3.28 Visual identification of Infraspinatus atrophy with the patient in the hands on hips position

Table 3.1 Kibler scapular classification

Type	Plane of dysfunction	Summary of visually observed dysfunction
I	Sagittal	Inferior angle of the scapula prominent
		Increase anterior tilting of the scapula
II	Transverse	Medial border of the scapula prominent
		Increased internal rotation of the scapula
III	Coronal	Increased superior translation of the scapula excessive superior movement of the scapula during active arm elevation, superior border prominent

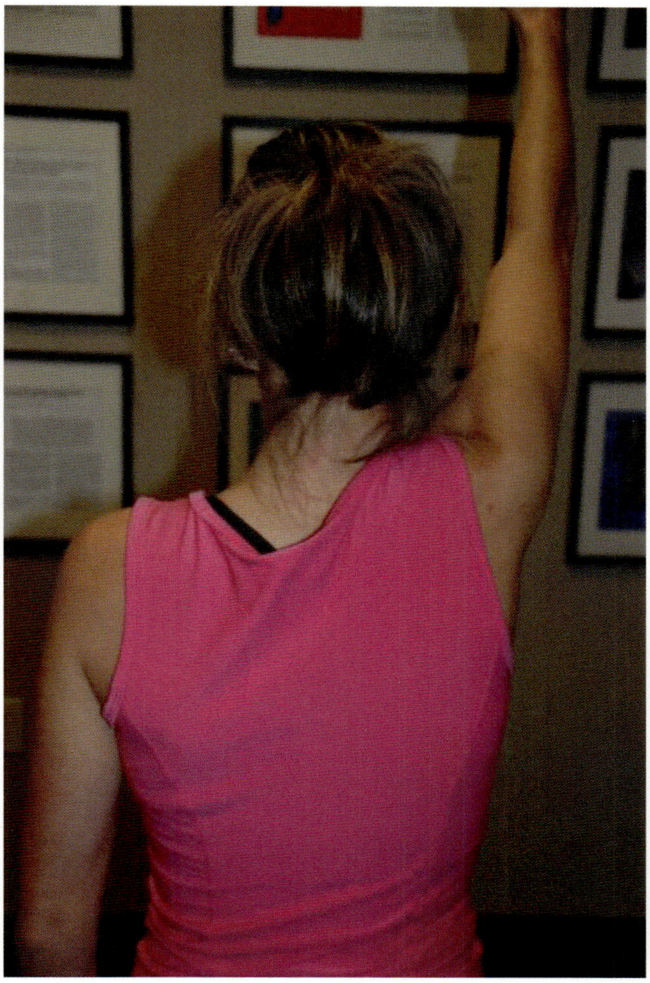

Fig. 3.29 Superior (type III) Kibler scapular pathology

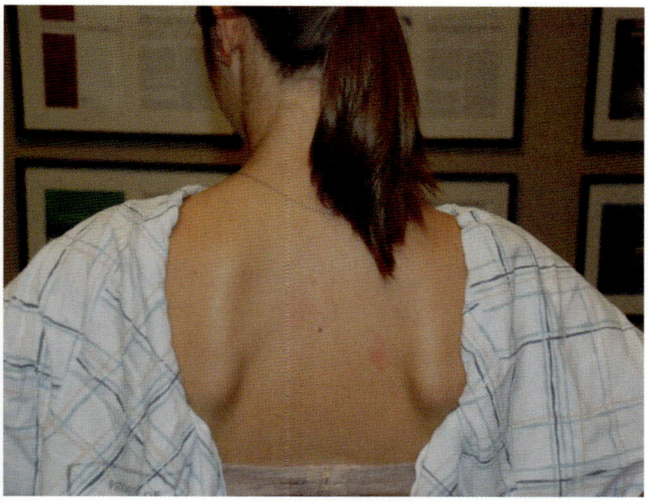

Fig. 3.30 Medial (type II) Kibler scapular pathology

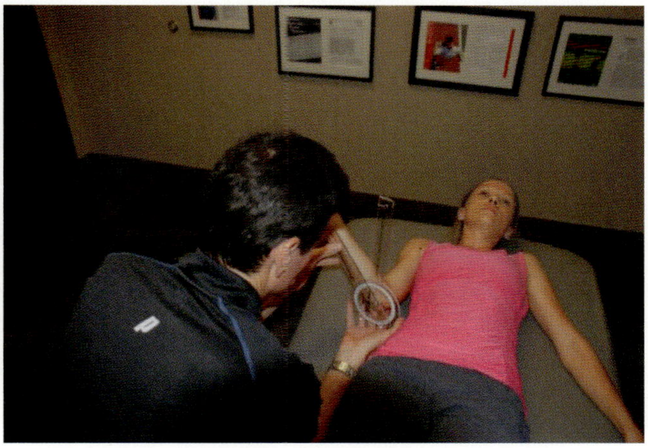

Fig. 3.31 Measurement of humeral external rotation in 45° of abduction in the early postoperative evaluation

Special Tests Used in the Postoperative Evaluation

Several special tests can be applied in the initial evaluation that can provide useful information on the baseline status of the shoulder following stabilization surgery. These include the dis-association test, the sulcus sign, and anterior posterior humeral head translation tests. Additionally, applying the Beighton Hypermobility Index can provide an estimate of the patient's systemic mobility status.

- *Dis-Association Test:* This maneuver involves performing a very simple circumduction movement of the humerus and assessing the patient's ability to dis-associate the humerus from the scapula. Patients with significant glenohumeral joint hypomobility and early apprehension toward movement will simply move their entire body and scapula along with the examiner's movement of the humerus and also exhibit much apprehension with this early movement. Patients with less restricted capsular status and no apprehension toward subtle movement will simply allow the examiner to perform the circumduction maneuver while maintaining a normal posture (Fig. 3.32).
- *Multidirectional Instability (MDI) Sulcus Test:* A very important test used to evaluate the stability of the shoulder is the MDI sulcus test (Fig. 3.33). This test is the primary test used to identify the patient with MDI of the GH joint. Excessive translation in the inferior direction during this test most often indicates a forthcoming pattern of excessive translation in an anterior or posterior direction or in both anterior and posterior directions [86]. This test, when performed in the neutral adducted position, directly assesses the integrity of the superior glenohumeral ligament and the coracohumeral ligament [87]. These ligaments are the primary stabilizing structures against inferior humeral head translation in the adducted GH position [88]. To perform this test, it is recommended that the patient be examined in the seated position with the arms in neutral adduction and resting gently in the patient's lap. The examiner grasps the distal aspect of the humerus using a firm but unassuming grip with one hand, while several brief, relatively rapid downward pulls are exerted to the humerus in an inferior (vertical) direction. A visible "sulcus sign" (tethering of the skin between the lateral acromion and the humerus from the increase in inferior translation of the humeral head and the widening subacromial space) is usually present in patients with MDI [89]. The presence of a positive MDI test postoperatively would indicate the need for a slower progression of range of motion interventions postoperatively and even help dictate the amount of immobilization needed. Early aggressive rehabilitation in a patient who presents with a sulcus sign would be contraindicated.

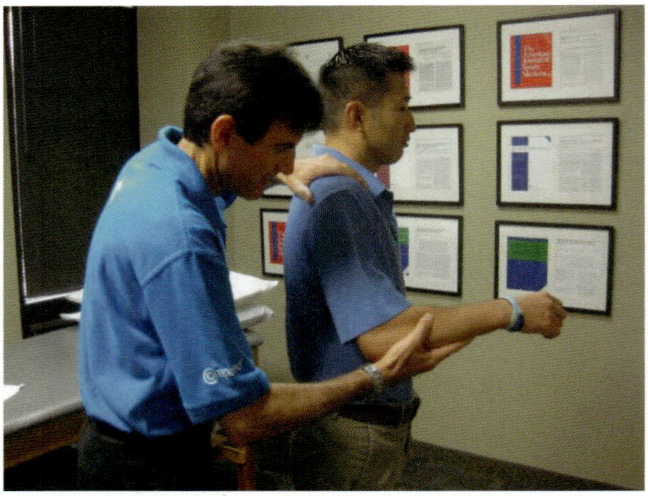

Fig. 3.32 Shoulder dis-association test

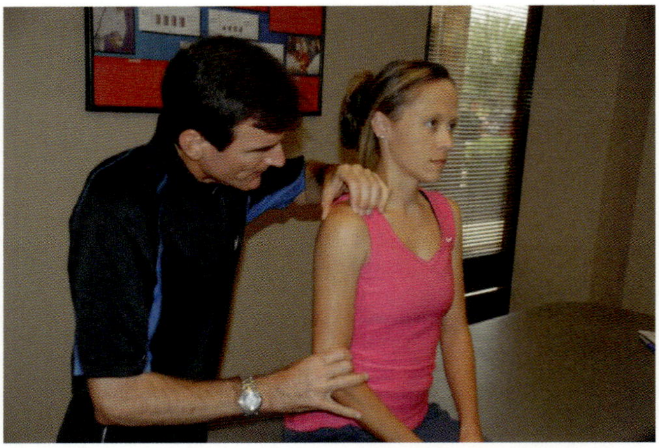

Fig. 3.33 Multidirectional instability (MDI) sulcus test

- *Anterior and Posterior Translation (Drawer) Tests:* Gerber and Ganz [90] and McFarland et al. [86] have reported on the anterior and posterior translation tests and recommend their use in the supine position due to greater inherent relaxation of the patient. The use of the supine position also allows the patient's extremity to be tested in multiple positions of GH joint abduction, thus selectively stressing specific portions of the GH joint anterior capsule and capsular ligaments. Figure 3.34 shows the supine translation technique for assessing and grading the translation of the humeral head in the anterior direction. It is important to note that the direction of translation must be along the line of the GH joint, with an anteromedial and posterolateral direction used because of the 30° version of the glenoid [1]. This is accomplished by ensuring that the examiner places the patient's GH joint in the scapular plane as pictured. Testing for anterior translation is performed in the range between 0° and 30° of abduction, between 30° and 60° of abduction, and at 90° of abduction to test the integrity of the superior, middle, and inferior GH ligaments, respectively [87, 88]. Posterior translation testing typically is performed at 90° of abduction because no distinct thickenings of the capsule are noted, with the exception of the posterior band of the inferior GH ligament complex [88]. Grading (assessing the translation) for this test is performed using the classification of Altchek and Dines [91]. This classification system defines grade I translation as humeral translation within the glenoid without edge loading or translation of the humerus over the glenoid rim. Grade II represents translation of the humeral head up over the glenoid rim with spontaneous return on removal of the stress. The presence of grade II translation in an anterior or posterior direction without symptoms does not indicate instability but instead merely represents laxity of the GH joint. Unilateral increases in GH translation in the presence of shoulder pain and disability can ultimately lead to the diagnosis of GH joint instability [4, 92]. Grade III translation, which is not seen clinically in orthopedic and sports physical therapy, involves translation of the humeral head over the glenoid rim without relocation upon removal of stress. Ellenbecker et al. [93] tested the intrarater reliability of humeral head translation tests and found improved reliability when using the main criterion of whether the humeral head traverses the glenoid rim. Similar to the findings of the MDI sulcus test, increases in humeral head translation identified postoperatively would again indicate the need for less emphasis on early postoperative range of motion and greater immobilization of the extremity. This will be discussed later in this chapter.

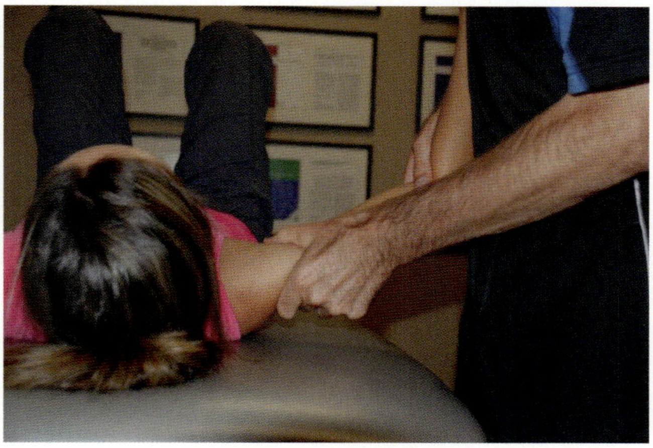

Fig. 3.34 Anterior humeral head translation test

- *Beighton Hypermobility Index:* In addition to the previously mentioned translation and provocation tests used for instability testing of the patient with shoulder dysfunction, a series of tests to assess the overall mobility or presence of generalized hypermobility are valuable during clinical evaluation of the shoulder in the overhead athlete [92]. The Beighton Hypermobility scale or index was originally introduced by Carter and Wilkinson [94] and modified by Beighton and Horan [95]. This scale is comprised of nine individual tests each assessed bilaterally (except for trunk flexion) which are used to assess the generalized hypermobility of the individual. These tests include: passive hyperextension of the 5th MCP joint; passive thumb opposition to the forearm; bilateral elbow, and knee hyperextension; and standing trunk flexion with knees fully extended (Fig. 3.35a–c). Several authors have documented the psychometric properties of the Beighton scale with reliability estimates ranging from 0.74 to 0.84 [96]. Several cutoff criterion have been used to determine how many of the individual tests must be positive to rate an individual as hypermobile with no overwhelming consensus [97]. Some studies have used 2 of the 9 measures as positive to grade the individual as hypermobile with other research using 4/9 to achieve this hypermobile rating [4, 97]. This scale can be used as an important classification for patients with GH joint instability or in patients where an understanding of underlying mobility status is important to determine progression rates for ROM or mobilization [4]. Patients with a positive Beighton Hypermobility Index would again be progressed more slowly with their range of motion and stretching following surgery in the initial postoperative phase of the rehabilitation protocol. This summary provides only a small portion of the key parts of the complete evaluation of the patient following arthroscopic Bankart reconstruction. The evaluation of neurological status including extremity light touch sensation, proprioception, distal grip strength, and vascular (capillary) refilling is and additional important component.

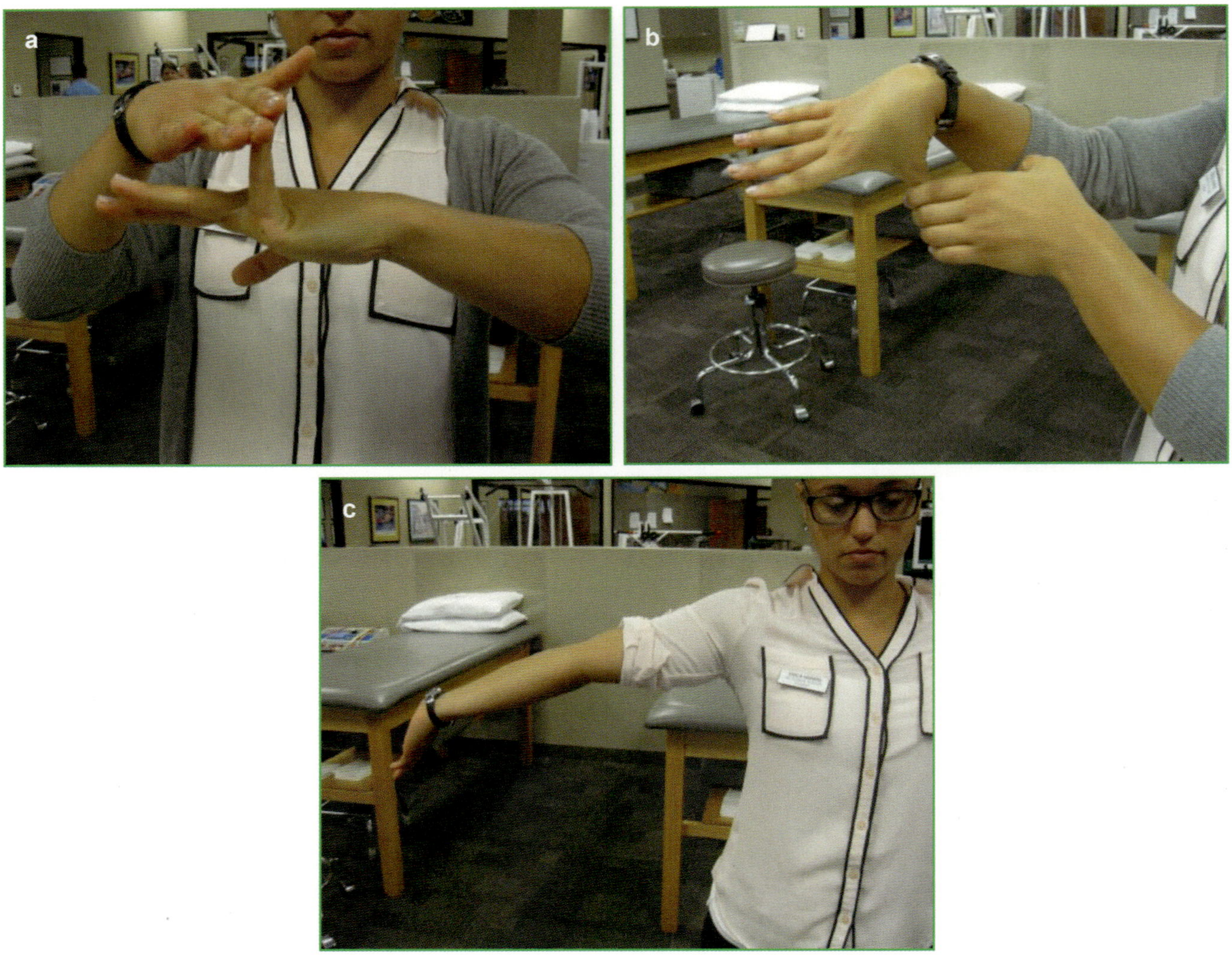

Fig. 3.35 (**a–c**) Several positive components of the Beighton Hypermobility Index

3.5.3 Rehabilitation following Arthroscopic Bankart

Individual patient progression following surgical repair of a Bankart lesion is applied during all stages of the rehabilitation process; however, for the purposes of this chapter and also prevalent in many clinical and research applications, a protocol-based presentation of the critically important steps will be outlined in this section of the chapter. Knowledge of and close communication of the specific surgical procedures performed between the orthopedic surgeon and the physiotherapist are of critical importance [98]. This allows for a complete understanding of the structures involved and also alerts the physio of any concomitant surgical procedures and anatomical structures that were addressed. Examples of concomitant surgical procedures that have a significant effect on postoperative rehabilitation procedures are: superior labrum anterior posterior (SLAP) repair, acromioplasty, distal clavicular excision, rotator cuff debridement and/or repair, capsular plication/shifting, biceps tenodesis, or tenotomy.

Goals of Rehabilitation following Arthroscopic Bankart

- The surgical repair of the Bankart lesion coupled with the concomitant capsular shortening to address redundancy when applicable creates several challenges to the rehabilitation specialist. These are outlined in Table 3.2.

Initial Rehabilitation Phase: (Weeks 2–6)

Patients are initially immobilized in a sling for the first 4–6 weeks following surgery and often are instructed to perform gentle active assisted exercises such as Codman's (Pendulums) and elbow range of motion. The use of a sling with abduction pillow is now commonplace to more optimally position the extremity in the scapular plane with approximately 30° of abduction. Patients are commonly referred to physical therapy at 10 days to 2 weeks postoperatively to begin their rehabilitation progressions.

Following the initial evaluation as outlined earlier in this chapter, the patient initiates their rehabilitation with a primary focus on the following specific activities (Table 3.3).

The application of modalities to increase local blood flow and decrease postoperative pain is indicated and applied in rehabilitation protocols [99]. The use of electrical stimulation and moist heat to prepare the joint and the soft tissues for both range of motion and muscular activation interventions is recommended by several authors [99]. While not a major focus, these modalities can be utilized to enhance patient comfort and improve soft tissue extensibility [99].

- *Range of Motion Progression:* Early protected ROM is one of the most specific progressions followed during the initial 4–6-week period after surgery. Specifically, this protected ROM progression involves the limitation of external rotation ROM to minimize tensile stress to the anteroinferior aspect of the labrum, which was repaired during the Bankart reconstruction as well as minimize tensile loading and stress to the anteroinferior capsule, specifically the inferior glenohumeral ligament, which has often been plicated or shifted during the surgical reconstruction to address redundancy of patency. Typically there are little or no restrictions placed upon forward flexion and scapular plane abduction as well as internal rotation. Research guides the use of a specific ROM of external rotation and the performance of that external rotation in positions of abduction that specifically limit stress to the anteroinferior joint capsule and labrum. In addition to the actual amount of

Table 3.2 Goals of rehabilitation following arthroscopic Bankart

Goals
Gradually progress glenohumeral joint range of motion to address postoperative limitations in functional movement
Enhance scapular stabilization to ensure proper glenoid positioning during functional humeral ranges of motion
Significantly improve rotator cuff strength to provide primary dynamic stabilization of the glenohumeral joint to protect the repaired structures and safely minimize unwanted humeral translations
Progress the patient through evidence-based rehabilitation progressions that allow for transition to an interval functional sports and activity return program

Table 3.3 Interventions emphasized in the initial phase of rehabilitation

Modalities to decrease pain and postoperative inflammation
Manual scapular stabilization and scapular exercise progression
Protected range of glenohumeral joint range of motion
Initiation of rotator cuff strengthening using protected movement patterns and positions

external rotation used in the initial rehabilitation, the position of abduction used during external rotation ROM is also important, with basic science research providing guidance from the literature. Both Pagnani et al. [87] and O'Brien et al. [88] have eloquently performed basic science research that identifies which portions of the anterior glenohumeral capsule are under tension based on the position of glenohumeral abduction. During 90° of abduction, these studies have identified the inferior glenohumeral ligament as the primary restraint to anterior translation. This directly stresses the capsule where the Bankart repair has occurred. External rotation in the first 30° of abduction at the patient's side places more specific tensile loading near the superior glenohumeral ligament and superior capsular structures. These basic science studies provide much of the specific information applicable to rehabilitation of the patient following Bankart reconstruction.

Black et al. [100] studied capsular tension in Bankart repairs in cadavers at 0° of abduction in the coronal plane. They identified a "low-tension zone," which occurred in the first 46.5° of external rotation in this position. After 45° of external rotation, researchers found a significant rise in tension in the anterior capsule. Additionally, research by Penna et al. [101] provides additional support for the limitation of external rotation following Bankart reconstruction. Their study provided additional insight by testing cadaveric specimens in multiple positions of abduction as well as following Bankart reconstruction and Bankart reconstruction with capsular shortening. Specifically, stress on the anteroinferior capsulolabral complex following Bankart repair along versus Bankart repair with capsular shortening was significantly different with external rotation (1.1 N versus 5.3).

Additionally, when comparing the effects of Bankart repair alone to Bankart repair with capsular shortening in the position of external rotation and abduction, it produced significant differences (4.6 versus 17.7). Therefore, knowledge of whether capsular shortening (plication or shifting) was performed during surgery does have an effect on the anatomical stress applied during both abduction and abduction with external rotation following surgery.

The progression of external rotation following surgery follows a progression from occurring in approximately 30–45° of abduction while the humerus is placed in the scapular plane (Fig. 3.36) during the first 2–6 weeks post-op to occurring in 90° of abduction after week 6–8 based on mobility status of the patient (Fig. 3.37). The study by Penna et al. [101] objectively supports this gradual progression as the values generated representing anteroinferior capsulolabral stress with Bankart reconstruction with capsular shortening increase from 5.3 N with no abduction to 17.7 N with abduction. These studies help the clinician to understand the internal capsular ramifications of limited external rotation ROM and provide rationale for the safe progression of external rotation ROM in the patient with anterior instability. Using this initial range of external rotation allows the patient to perform a functional ROM without jeopardizing the labral repair by exposing it to increased tensile loading.

The use of accessory joint mobilization during the initial rehabilitation consists of grade I oscillations to modulate pain, with particular avoidance of accessory mobilizations in anterior directions to protect the capsulolabral repair. Other directions of joint mobilization in progressive grades can be applied (i.e., posterior glide, caudal glide) if the patient presents with significant range of motion limitation from the initial period of immobilization postoperatively. Typically only lower grades of mobilization (Maitland grades I, II) are

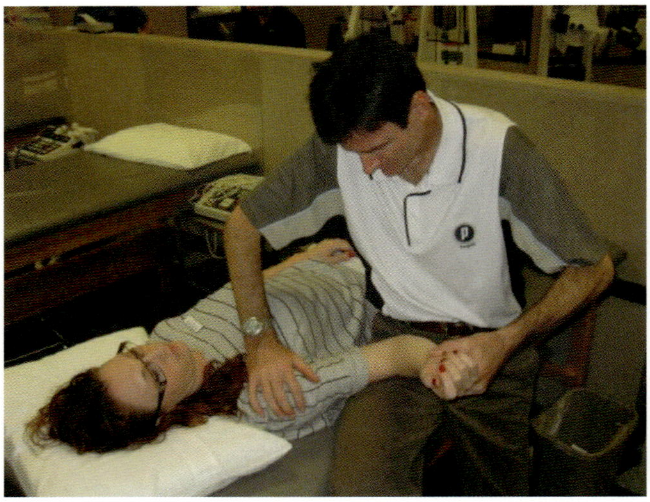

Fig. 3.36 External rotation ROM in the scapular plane with 30° of abduction used in the early postoperative rehabilitation

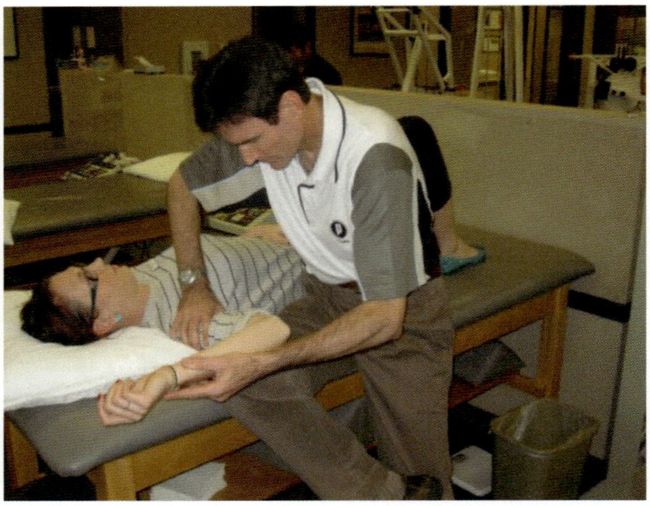

Fig. 3.37 External rotation ROM progression performed in 90° of abduction in the scapular plane performed after 6–8 weeks

applied unless significant capsular hypomobility has developed. An important concept to emphasize during the early phase of rehabilitation of the previously unstable shoulder that has undergone arthroscopic Bankart reconstruction is the distinction between range of motion and stretching. In the early phase of rehabilitation, many patients simply require range of motion of the shoulder, without aggressive end-range overpressure to protect the capsular tissue and repaired labrum. Early stretching is not necessarily a common practice again unless the patient does present with significant range of motion limitations. Careful objective monitoring of glenohumeral joint range of motion with comparison to the contralateral extremity is warranted to ensure that postoperative rehabilitation is not re-creating a hypermobile environment and is instead restoring optimal range of motion and capsular tension.

- *Scapular Stabilization and Early Rotator Cuff Activation:* In the initial phase of rehabilitation, specific procedures can be used to activate the stabilizing musculature of the glenohumeral joint and scapular articulation. These occur with very controlled, low loading schemes, and higher repetition bases to improve local muscular endurance [102].

Manual techniques are initially recommended to directly interface the clinician with the patient's scapula, to bypass the GH joint and allow for repetitive scapular exercise without undue stress to the rotator cuff in the early phase. Figure 3.38 shows a specific technique recommended and used by this author to manually resist scapular retraction. Activation of the serratus anterior and lower trapezius force couple is imperative to enable scapular upward rotation and stabilization during arm elevation [83]. Rhythmic stabilization applied to the proximal aspect of the extremity, progressing to distal with the GH joint in 80–90° of elevation in the scapular plane, can be initiated to provide muscular co-contraction in a functional position. Additionally, with this technique, a protracted scapular position can be utilized to enhance the activation of the serratus anterior [103, 104], due to research identifying decreased muscular activation of this muscle in patients with glenohumeral joint instability [82].

Kibler et al. [105] have published several key exercise movements that recruit the serratus anterior and lower trapezius and can be used early in rehabilitation due to the lower levels of elevation and external rotation inherent in these movements. This minimizes subacromial impingement and capsulolabral stress and makes the exercises well tolerated by patients early in rehabilitation. Figures 3.39 (Robbery)

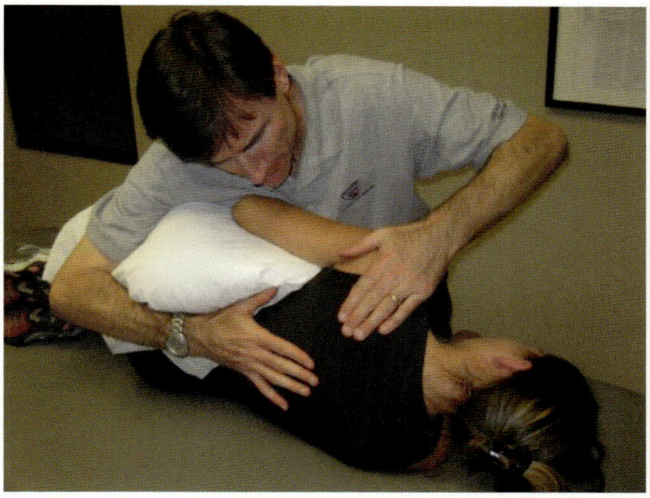

Fig. 3.38 Manual scapular resistive exercise performed by the physio to illicit early force couple activation for scapular stabilization

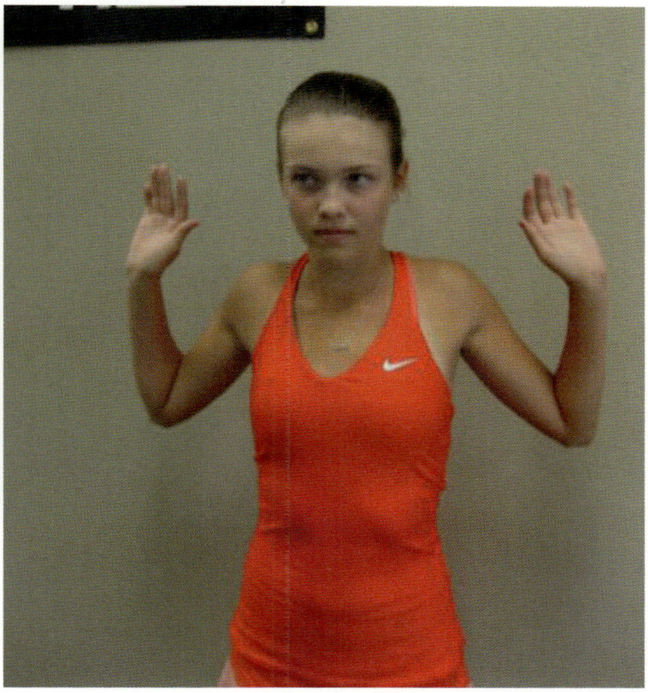

Fig. 3.39 Robbery

and 3.40 (lawnmower) exercises have extensive EMG verification by Kibler et al. [105] and Tsurike and Ellenbecker [106]. The lawnmower exercise can even be applied with the patient's arm in a sling to provide early scapular stabilization exercise with minimal capsulolabral stress. The serratus punch performed in supine (Fig. 3.41) is utilized and found to elicit 60 % or greater MVIC levels in the serratus anterior musculature [107].

According to Davies [108], an initial resistive exercise progression for the rotator cuff often commences with isometric exercise followed by isotonic exercise and then finally more functional plyometric and isokinetic resistance applications. This allows for increased challenge and specificity in the exercise progression. This progression is particularly useful in postoperative rehabilitation following arthroscopic Bankart.

One study highlights the importance of early submaximal exercise in increasing local blood flow. Jensen et al. [109] studied the effects of submaximal (5–50 %) maximum voluntary isometric contraction (*MVIC*) contractions in the supraspinatus tendon measured with laser Doppler flowmetry).

Results showed that even submaximal contractions increased perfusion during all 1-min contractions but produced a post-contraction latent hyperemia following the

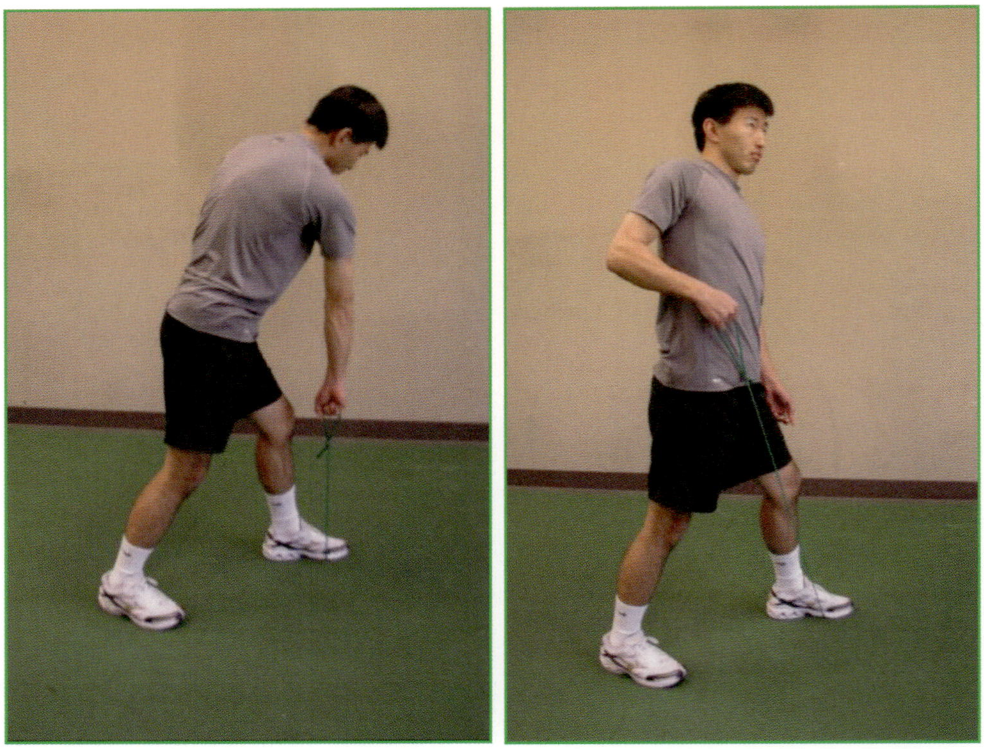

Fig. 3.40 Lawnmower exercise

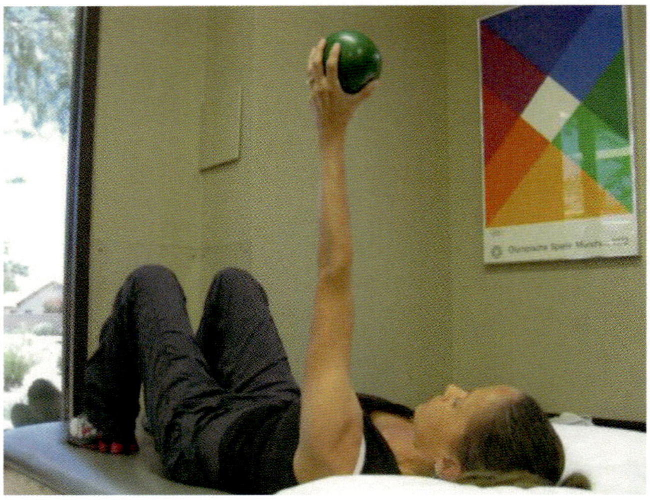

Fig. 3.41 Serratus punch exercise

muscular contraction. These findings have provided a rationale for the early use of IR and ER isometrics or submaximal manual resistance in the scapular plane with low levels of elevation to prevent any subacromial contact and capsular stress early in the rehabilitation process. Figure 3.43 shows an early application of isometric exercise for the posterior rotator cuff called "dynamic isometrics" where elastic resistance is used to provide known loading in an isometric format as a step is taken by the patient away from the attachment point of the band/tubing to increase resistance accordingly. The use of elastic resistance with known, calibrated elongation resistance values allows the clinician to safely prescribe isometric exercise dosing appropriately for the patient. A towel roll is used under the axilla to most appropriately position the patient's shoulder for rotator cuff exercise [110–112].

An initial isotonic rotator cuff exercise progression recommended to increase rotator cuff strength is shown in Fig. 3.42. These exercises are based on electromyographic (EMG) research, showing high levels of posterior rotator cuff activation [113–117], and they place the shoulder in positions well tolerated by patients in the initial stage of rehabilitation. Resistance is not initially applied performing only active range of motion and based on patient tolerance resistance levels are progressed in ½ pound increments (0.25 KG). In patients following arthroscopic Bankart, side-lying ER and prone extension with an externally rotated (thumb out) position are utilized first, with progressions to prone horizontal abduction occurring at 6–8 weeks following surgery. The use of the exercise prone ER with scapular retraction can only be added later in the rehab progression once the patient has regained the abduction/external rotation motion inherent in

Fig. 3.42 Rotator cuff isotonic exercise program

1. SIDELYING EXTERNAL ROTATION:
Lie on uninvolved side, with involved arm at side, with a small pillow between arm and body. Keeping elbow of involved arm bent and fixed to side, raise arm into external rotation. Slowly lower to starting position and repeat.

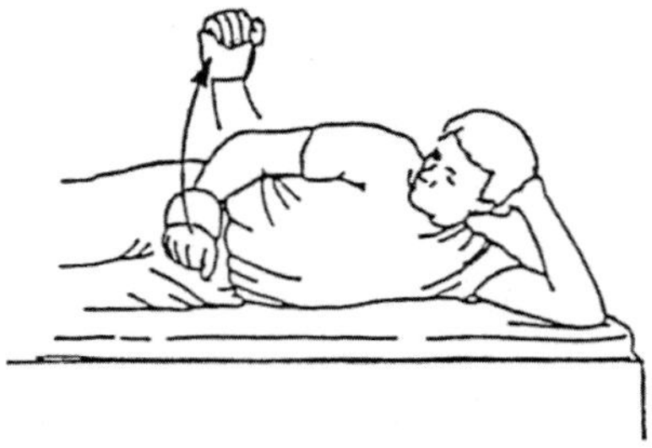

2. SHOULDER EXTENSION:
Lie on table on stomach, with involved arm hanging straight to the floor. With thumb pointed outward, raise arm straight back into extension toward your hip. Slowly lower arm and repeat.

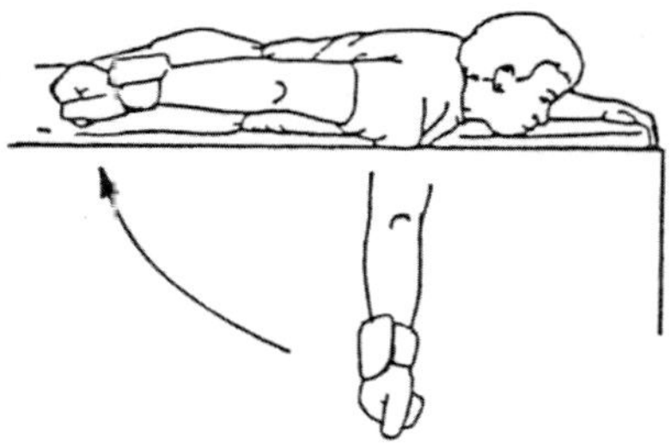

3. PRONE HORIZONTAL ABDUCTION:
Lie on table on stomach, with involved arm hanging straight to the floor. With thumb pointed outward, raise arm out to the side, parallel to the floor. Slowly lower arm, and repeat.

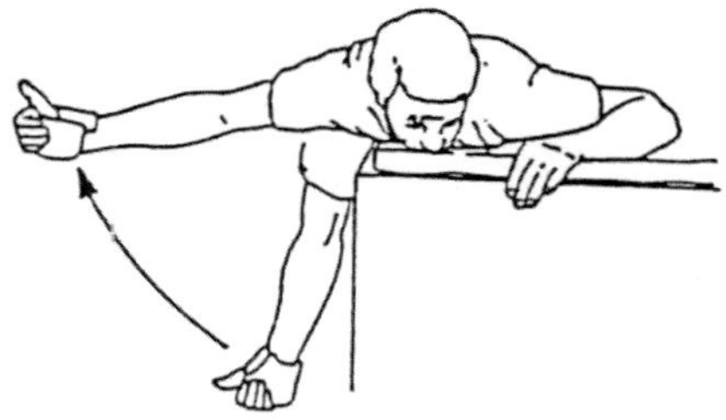

4. 90/90 EXTERNAL ROTATION:
Lie on table on stomach, with shoulder abducted to 90 degrees and arm supported on table, with elbow bent at 90 degrees. Keeping the shoulder and elbow fixed, rotate arm into external rotation, slowly lower to start position, and repeat.

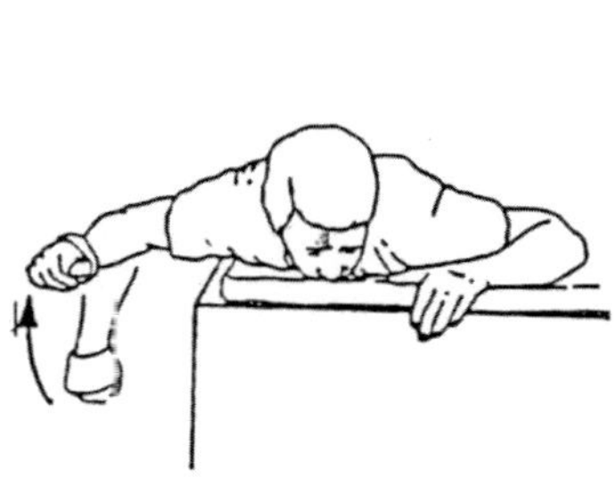

this exercise and higher levels of rotator cuff and scapular strength are present. Prone horizontal abduction is used at 90° of abduction to minimize the effects resulting from subacromial contact [118]. Research has shown that this position creates high levels of supraspinatus muscular activation [115, 116], making it an alternative to the widely used empty can exercise, which often can cause impingement through the combined inherent movements of IR and elevation. Three sets of 15–20 repetitions are recommended to create a fatigue response and improve local muscular endurance [102].

It is important to point out the importance of emphasizing proper scapular positioning during rotator cuff exercises such as side-lying external rotation, prone extension, and prone horizontal abduction. Cools and colleagues [111] have shown enhanced activation of the rotator cuff during exercise conditions where emphasis was placed on proper scapular positioning. The author of this chapter recommends careful monitoring of naturally occurring scapular motion during rotator cuff exercise as opposed to attempts to lock the scapula in a retracted position during humeral motion (rotator cuff exercise patterning).

The efficacy of these rotator cuff exercises in a 4-week training paradigm has been demonstrated, and 8–10 % increases have been noted in IR and ER strength measured isokinetically in healthy subjects [119–121]. Training of the rotator cuff and scapular musculature has resulted in modification and improvement of the ER to IR ratio, improved strength, and endurance of the rotator cuff and performance enhancement [119–122].

All exercises for ER strengthening in standing and side-lying are performed with the addition of a small towel roll placed in the axilla as pictured (Fig. 3.43). In addition to assisting in isolation of the exercise and controlling unwanted movements, this towel roll application has been shown to elevate muscular activity by 10 % in the infraspinatus muscle when compared with identical exercises performed without towel placement [116]. Another theoretical advantage of the use of a towel roll to place the shoulder in approximately 20–30° of abduction is that it prevents the "wringing out" phenomena shown in cadaver research investigating shoulder microvascularity. Rathburn and MacNab [110] showed enhanced blood flow in the supraspinatus tendon when the arm was placed in slight abduction as compared with complete adduction. Finally, another research study has further supported the use of a towel roll or pillow between the humerus and the torso under the axilla during a humeral rotational training exercise.

Graichen et al. [123] studied 12 healthy shoulders using MRI at 30°, 60°, 90°, 120°, and 150° of abduction. A 15 N force was performed, which resulted in an abduction isometric contraction or an adduction isometric contraction. Adduction isometric muscle contraction produced a significant opening or increase in the subacromial space in all positions of GH joint abduction. No change in scapular tilting or

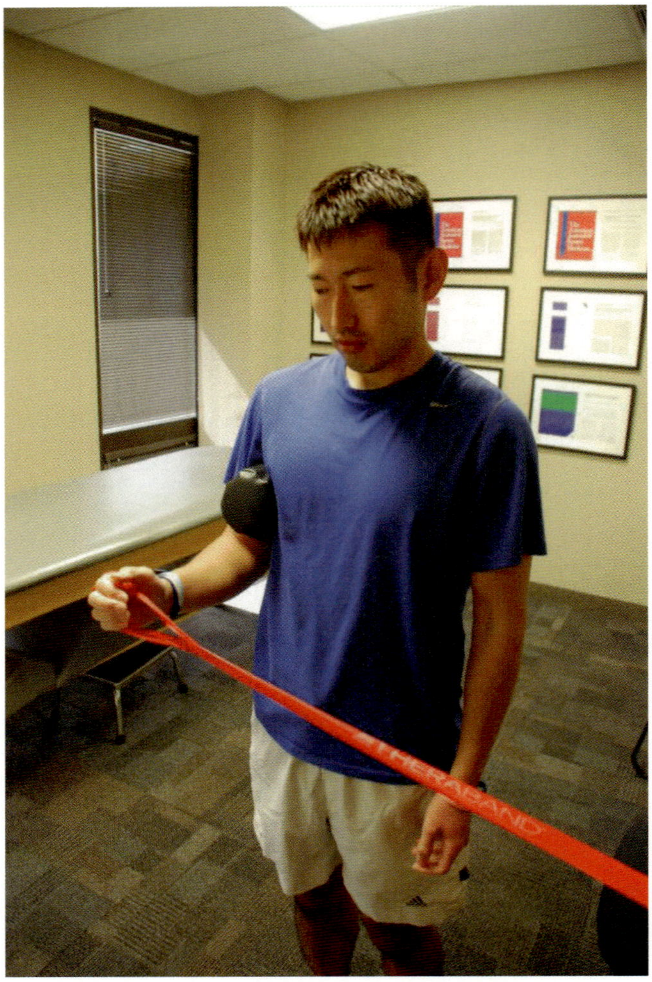

Fig. 3.43 External rotation at the side with elastic resistance

scapulohumeral rhythm was encountered during abduction or adduction isometric contractions. Results from this research can be applied for the patient with impingement during humeral rotation exercise. The use of the towel roll can facilitate an adduction isometric contraction in patients who may need enhanced subacromial positioning due to impingement during the humeral rotation exercise [123].

Research by Bitter et al. [124] has provided guidance regarding the use of resistive exercise in shoulder rehabilitation. They measured EMG activity of the infraspinatus and middle and posterior deltoid during ER exercise in healthy subjects. Muscular activity was monitored during ER exercise at 10, 40, and 70 % activation levels (percentage of maximal). This important study found increased relative infraspinatus activity when the resistive exercise level was at 40 % of maximal effort, indicating more focused activity from the infraspinatus and less compensatory activation of the deltoid. This study supports the use of lower-intensity strengthening exercise to optimize activation from the rotator cuff and to de-emphasize input from the deltoid and other prime movers, which often occurs with higher-intensity resistive loading.

Ramifications of Concomitant Surgical Procedures

Patients who undergo arthroscopic Bankart reconstruction often have other surgical procedures that have specific implications in the rehabilitation protocol. Patients who in addition to anteroinferior labral detachment also have superior labral detachment and subsequent *SLAP repair* have specific guidelines and limitations in their immediate postoperative care. Active contraction and resistance to the bicep are indicated in patients who have concomitant superior labral repair. This includes holding all elbow flexion resistance exercises including rowing, upper body ergometry, and forearm supination exercise to limit bicep activation. This is deferred for the first 6–8 weeks following surgery [122]. Progression to external rotation with 90° of glenohumeral joint abduction is also delayed until after 6–8 weeks following surgery to minimize the effects of the peel back mechanism and ultimately protect the repair of the superior labrum [125].

Patients who also had rotator *cuff repair* have limitations in early strengthening of the rotator cuff based on tear size and degree of tendon involvement. Additionally, patients who also undergo subacromial decompression and or distal clavicular excision may have greater pain and a delayed return of pain-free elevation and horizontal adduction, respectively, due to the osseous reaction to the surgical procedure and need for additional healing time for these structures. While these concomitant procedures do not preclude the patients' ability to progress and follow the protocol for arthroscopic Bankart reconstruction, they do require modification and altered progression rates due to the involvement of additional anatomical structures in the surgical procedure.

When *remplissage* is performed because a medial Hill-Sachs that is off track, we have to consider that the infraspinatus tendon is repaired into the humeral head bone loss; some precautions need to be underlined:

- Restriction of the *internal rotation* and *horizontal adduction, pushing movements*, and *bench press,* etc.
- Immediate motion for external rotation at 45° abduction and flexion PROM to 90° for 4 weeks
- Initiate internal rotation ROM at 6–8 weeks post-op
- *Full ROM* at 8–12 weeks (loss of external rotation expected)

Intermediate Phase (Weeks 6–12)

Objective characteristics of patients capable of progressing the intermediate phase of rehabilitation are outlined in Table 3.4. Typical timeframes for this transition occur between 6 and 8 weeks based on the degree of initial range of motion loss, concomitant surgical procedures, and the patients' tolerance to the initial phase of postoperative rehabilitation.

Progression of range of motion to terminal ranges occurs during this phase of rehabilitation in all planes. Range of motion is particularly progressed for external rotation now in 90° of functional abduction in the scapular and eventually coronal plane. Clinicians are guided by the baseline range of motion in the contralateral extremity for goal setting as well as the patient's preoperative instability history, presence of bone loss, and arm dominance. These factors may indicate through collegial consultation with the referring surgeon, setting range of motion limitations less than the contralateral extremity to further protect and provide a more stable and limiting capsular component following surgery. For example, patients with extensive preoperative dislocation histories, presence of glenoid or humeral bone loss, and decreased abduction external rotation functional ergonomic or athletic demands may be considered for less complete range of motion return. Care must be taken however not to leave the patient with range of motion limitations that could lead to obligate translations [126] and predispose the patient for future capsulorraphy arthropathy [127].

Table 3.4 Objective characteristics of patients progressing to the intermediate phase

Achievement of 45–60° of external rotation ROM in 45–60° of abduction
Ability to functionally elevate the shoulder to 90°
Tolerance of initial rotator cuff and scapular exercise progression (>3+/5 grade MMT)
Ability to tolerate basic ADL's outside the sling with minimal to no pain

Progression of Rotator Cuff and Scapular Stabilization

Additional scapular stabilization exercises in this phase of rehabilitation include ER with retraction (Fig. 3.44), an exercise shown to recruit the lower trapezius at a rate 3.3 times greater than the upper trapezius and to utilize the important position of scapular retraction [128]. Once non-guarded, external rotation is present, this exercise can be applied with scapular retraction being emphasized during execution. Multiple seated rowing variations, continued manual scapular protraction/retraction resistance exercise performed by the therapist with hand placements directly on the scapula as well as the use of the 90° elevated closed-chain exercise (Fig. 3.1) consisting of the patient's hand over a small Swiss ball with perturbations applied to add proprioceptive feedback and stimulate co-contraction in this functional position, are all used during this rehabilitation phase. For patients who perform a significant amount of work or sports activity in a closed-chain upper extremity environment, rhythmic stabilization progressions are applied starting in quadruped (Fig. 3.45) to enhance proximal stabilization.

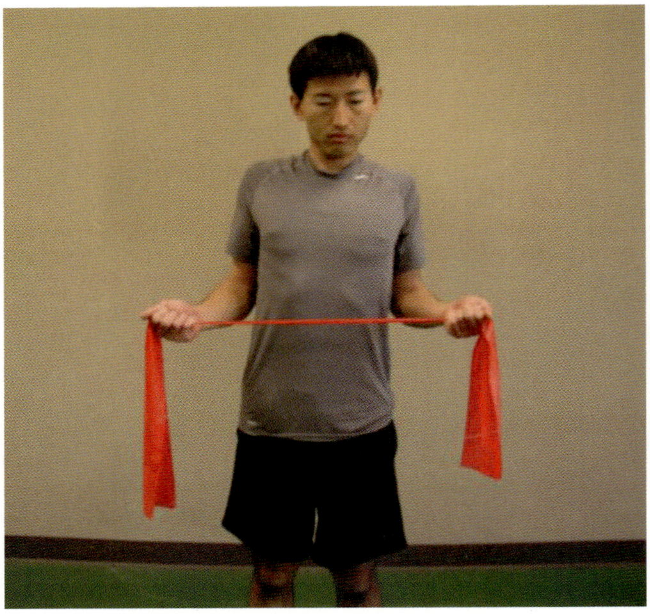

Fig. 3.44 External rotation with scapular retraction bilateral with elastic resistance

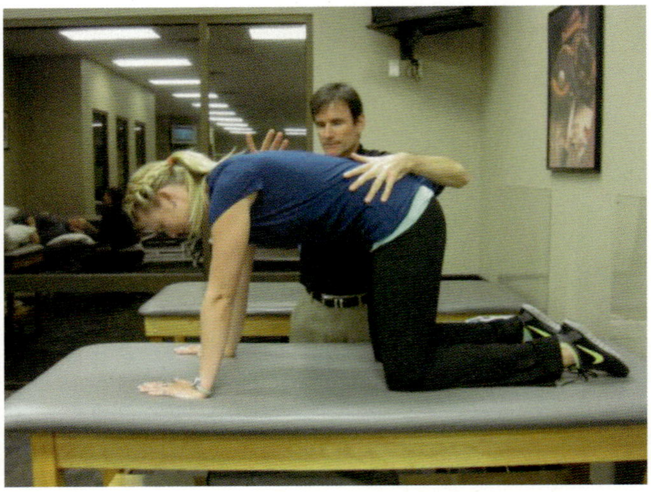

Fig. 3.45 Quadruped rhythmic stabilization exercise for closed-chain co-contraction of the shoulder musculature

Rotator cuff exercise is progressed to include oscillation-based interventions such as external rotation oscillation (Fig. 3.46) and side-lying body blade (Fig. 3.47). These exercises are time based, starting with sets of 30 s to improve endurance. Chen et al. [129], Ebaugh et al. [130] have both shown the negative effects on scapular positioning and humeral head translational control with rotator cuff fatigue. In addition to the more challenging exercises added during this phase of rehabilitation, the position of humeral elevation is now increased during rotator cuff and scapular exercise. Figure 3.48 shows the initial exercise applied for external rotation strengthening in 90° of abduction with elastic resistance. Pertubations can be applied by the physio in the 90/90 position to further invoke muscular activity and co-contraction in the functional 90/90 position. This 90/90 exercise with elastic resistance is also accompanied by the prone 90° abducted ER exercise (see Fig. 3.42) to facilitate the rotator cuff and lower trapezius and other scapular stabilizers during rehabilitation [107, 114–116]. The external rotation focus in strengthening of the rotator cuff is based on basic science research showing how the

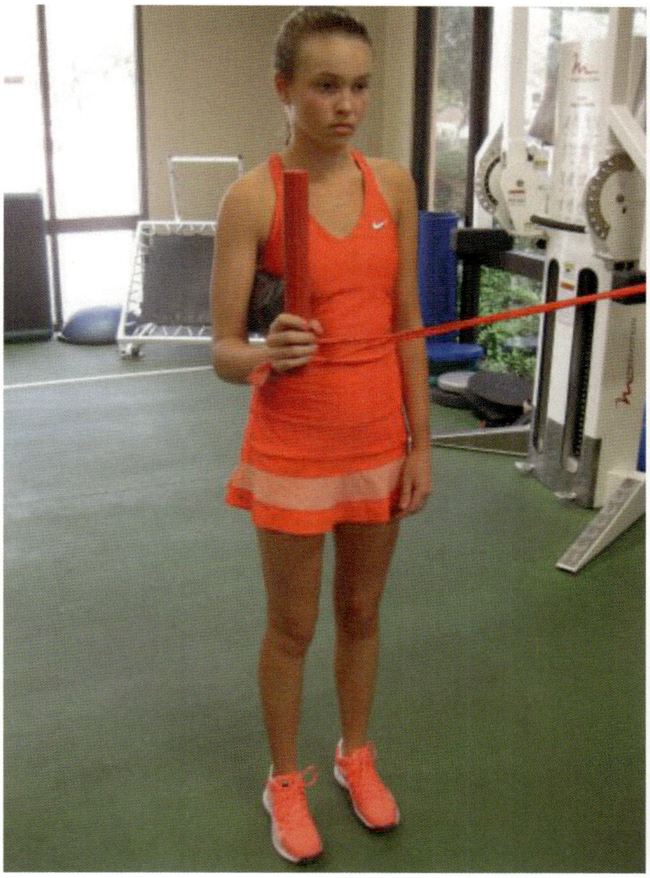

Fig. 3.46 External rotation oscillation

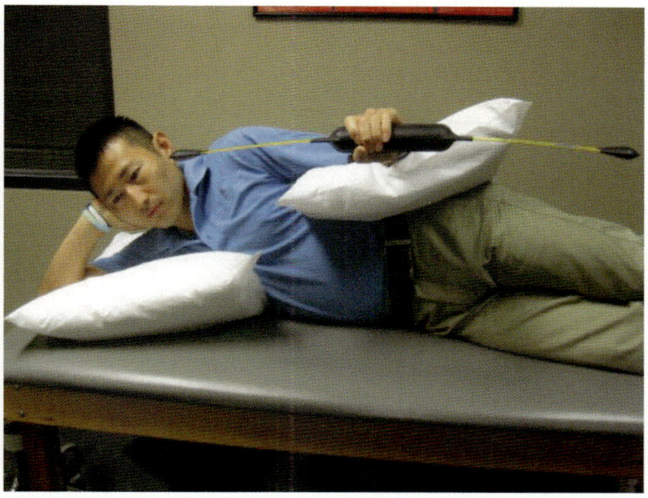

Fig. 3.47 Side-lying body blade oscillation exercise

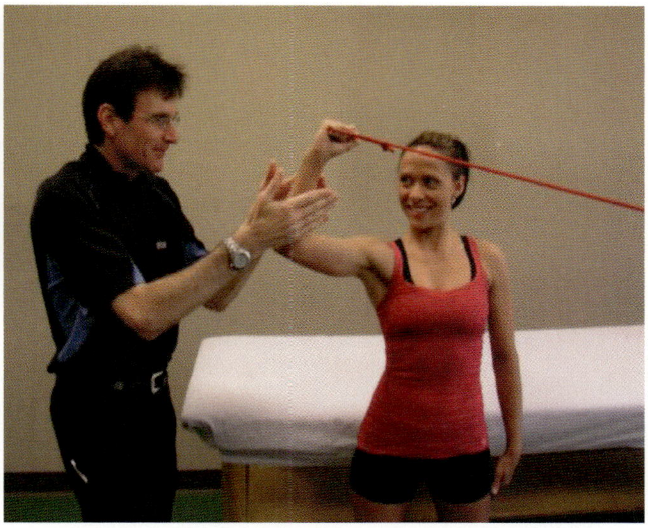

Fig. 3.48 External rotation at 90° of abduction in the scapular plane with physio applied perturbation

posterior rotator cuff is active in preventing anterior translation during glenohumeral motion. The posteriorly directed force supplied by the posterior rotator cuff can provide key stabilization to limit anterior translation and limit stress to the repaired labrum and capsulolabral complex [131]. Internal rotation strengthening is also added during this phase of the rehabilitation. Exercises for internal rotation include elastic resistance internal rotation with the arm in neutral adduction with a towel roll under the shoulder, as well 90° abducted internal rotation. An exercise application to stimulate contraction of the internal rotators in a functionally rapid way can be achieved by ball dribbling at 90° of elevation with 90° of elbow flexion (Fig. 3.49). The addition of rhythmic stabilization by the physio is also indicated and applied during rest periods with this exercise. Close monitoring occurs of the ER/IR muscular strength ratio for patients with glenohumeral joint instability and rotator cuff pathology.

Ellenbecker and Davies [122] have provided a significant review of this topic, and the literature has established a key ratio of 2:3 for the ER/IR ratio with the external rotators being 66 % as strong as the internal rotators in a normal healthy shoulder. Byram et al. [132] have shown this ER/IR ratio to be predictive of serious shoulder injury in elite overhead athletes further reinforcing the guidance of this key ratio in strength programming during rehabilitation. Biasing the ratio to include values greater than 66 % has been recommended [122] to ensure that posterior rotator cuff strength can off-set the larger internal rotational stresses during functional activities. A range between 2:3 and 3:4 has been recommended for this ratio, and thus the 66–75 % ER/ Ratio has become a dynamic stabilizing reference to guide the amount of internal rotation strengthening and optimal muscle balance during shoulder rehabilitation by many clinicians [120–122].

Return to Function Phase (12–16 Weeks)

Objective characteristics for patients making the important transition to the final "return to functional phase" are listed in Table 3.5. This phase emphasizes the continued restoration of functional range of motion as well as extensive higher level rotator cuff and scapular exercise focused to return the patient to their full functional level. Some of the key resistive exercise additions during this phase of rehabilitation are the functional plyometric exercise progression and isokinetic resistance application for shoulder internal and external rotation. The addition of isokinetic exercise (if available) not only provides optimal accommodating resistance throughout the range of motion but allows for detailed testing and muscular balance measurement (ER/IR ratio) not possible with manual muscle testing. The use of a handheld dynamometer can also provide critically important objective strength data [133] to direct ER/IR normalization and guide exercise administration and end stage program development.

Plyometric exercise progression is initiated at this time in the rehabilitation progression. Several studies reported in the literature show increases in upper extremity function with plyometric exercise variations [119–134]. The functional application of the eccentric pre-stretch, followed by a powerful concentric muscular contraction, closely parallels many upper extremity sports activities and serves as an excellent exercise modality for transitioning the active patient to the interval sports return programs. Figures 3.50 and 3.51 show two plyometric side-lying external rotation

Table 3.5 Objective characteristics of patient's transitioning to the return to activity phase

No apprehension with end range of motion all planes
ROM levels within approximately 10 % of contralateral side
Tolerance of 90/90 functional position with resistive exercise and perturbations
Muscle strength at 4/5 all planes without pain provocation

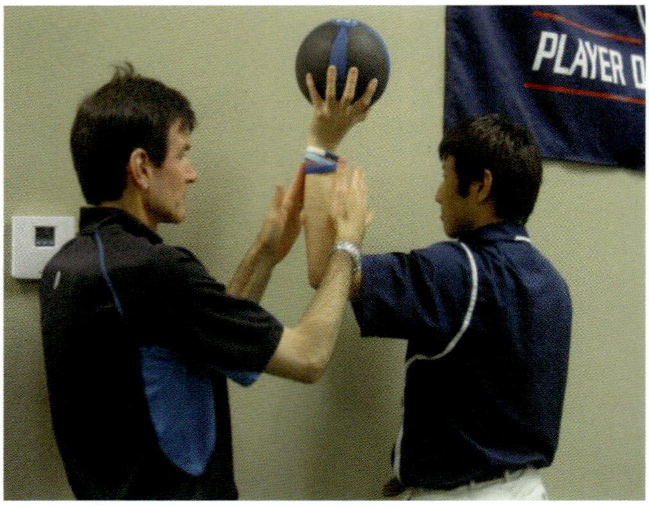

Fig. 3.49 Internal rotation plyometric ball dribbles with rhythmic stabilization

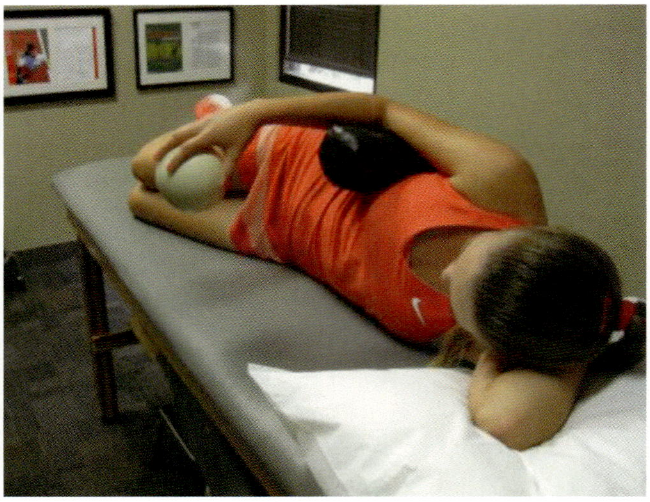

Fig. 3.50 Side-lying plyometric ball drops

exercises used to develop posterior rotator cuff strength with Figs. 3.52 and 3.53 showing similar versions of plyometric exercise in the 90/90 position. These exercises have been studied by Ellenbecker et al. [134], who demonstrated high levels of peak EMG activity of the lower trapezius (118–131 % MVIC) and infraspinatus (85–103 %) during these important exercises. Carter et al. [119] studied the effects of an 8-week training program of plyometric upper extremity exercise and ER strengthening with elastic resistance performed at 90° of glenohumeral joint abduction. They found increased eccentric ER strength and concentric IR strength and improved throwing velocity in collegiate baseball players, thus showing the positive effects of plyometric and elastic resistance training in overhead athletes.

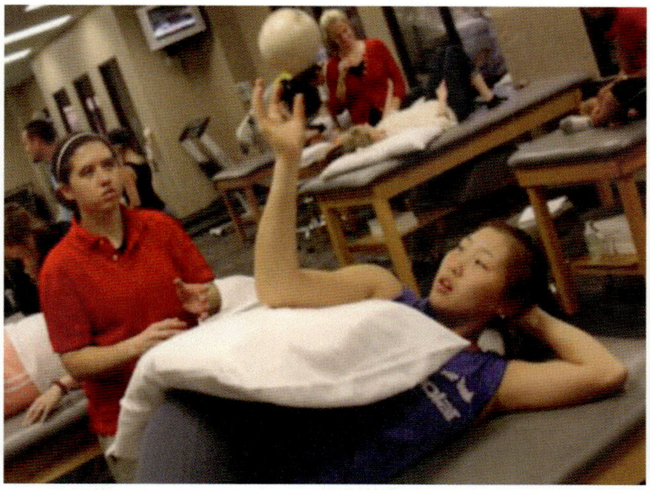

Fig. 3.51 Side-lying plyometric reverse catches

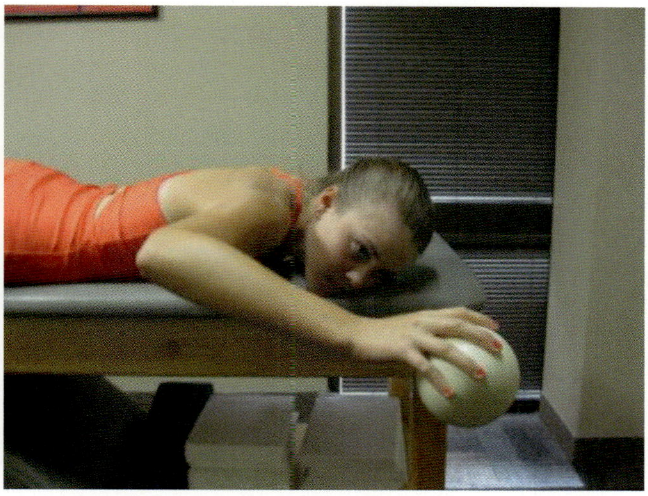

Fig. 3.52 90/90 prone plyometric ball drops

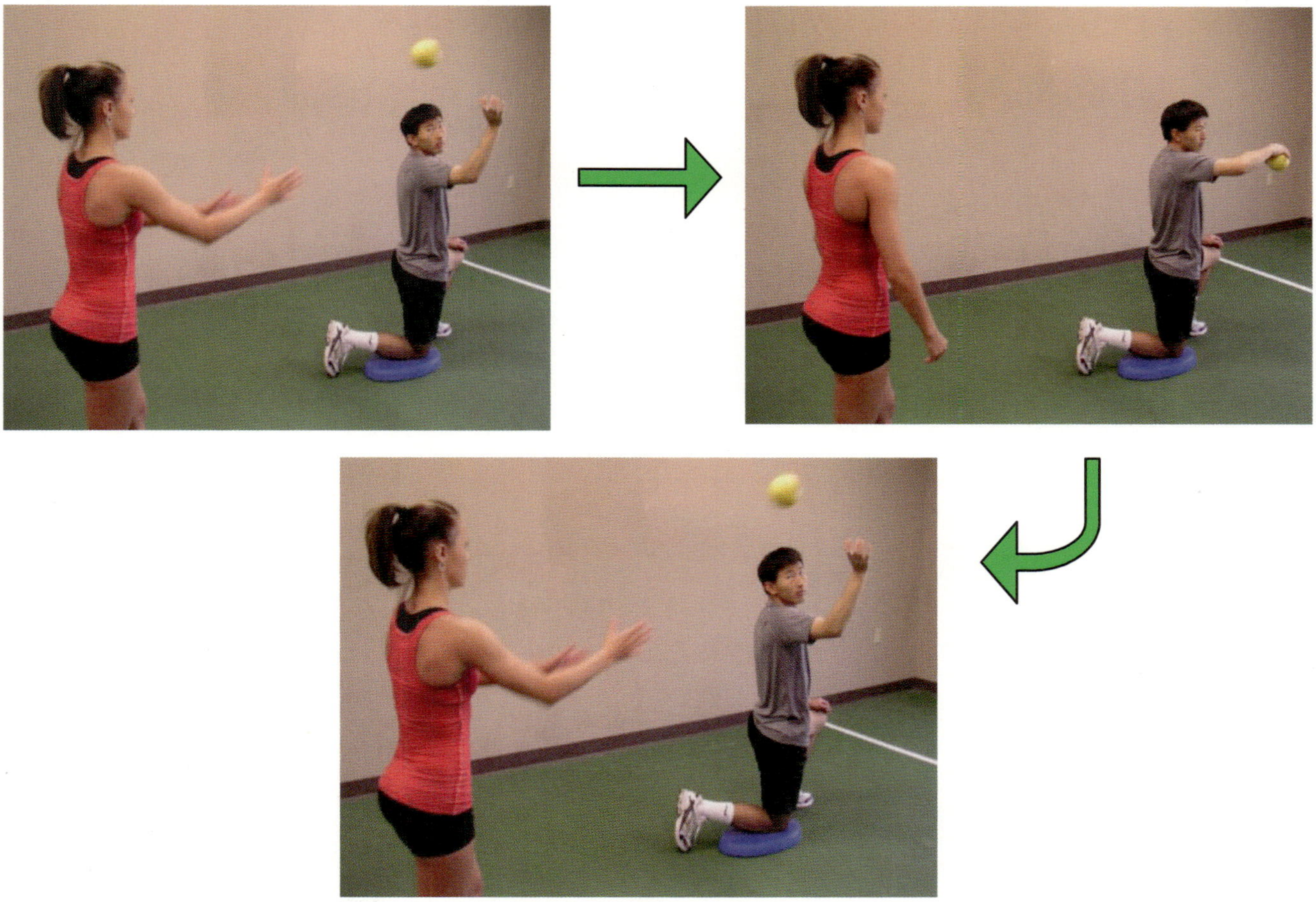

Fig. 3.53 90/90 prone plyometric reverse catches

For the athlete returning to contact sports such as basketball and football, internal rotation plyometrics can also be used to provide an abduction external rotation stress requiring muscular recruitment and stabilization to counter the negative potential effects of the abduction external rotation stress. Figure 3.54 shows the initial application of this type of provocational plyometric performed at 45–60° of abduction in the supine position with support provided by the floor or additional padding to limit the external rotation range of motion during the acceptance phase of the exercise with a medicine ball. Figures 3.55 and 3.56 show standing variations of plyometric exercises for internal rotation strength development that assist with the return to functional activities such as throwing. Functional activity or sports simulation drills are added during this phase as well for golf (Fig. 3.57a, b) and tennis (Fig. 3.58) using the controlled progression of medicine balls and a plyoback machine or partner.

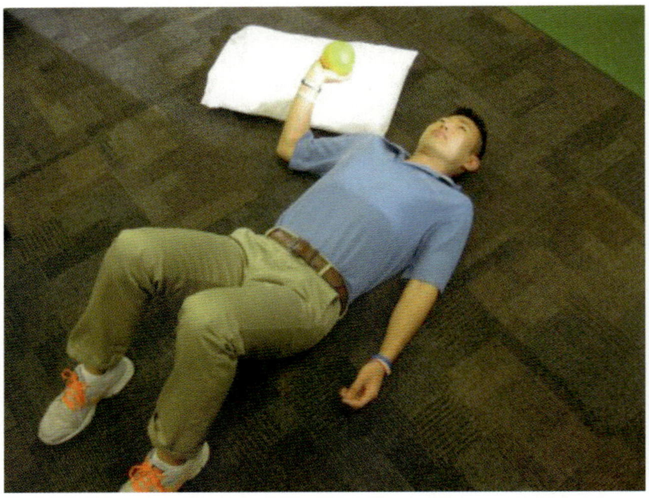

Fig. 3.54 Supine internal rotation provocational plyometric ball tosses

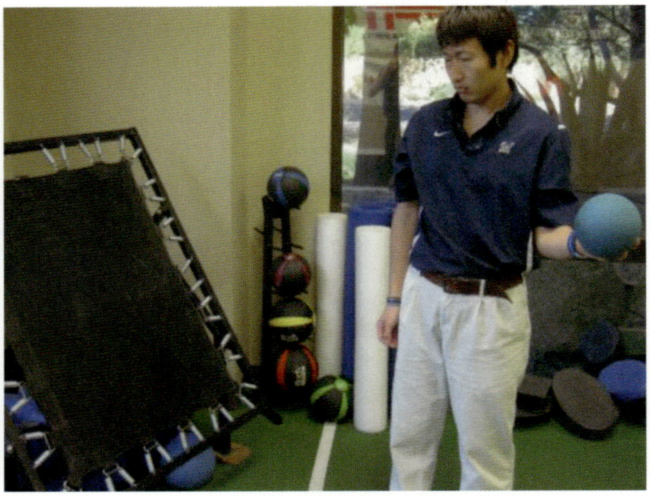

Fig. 3.55 Internal rotation standing plyometrics in neutral ab/adduction position

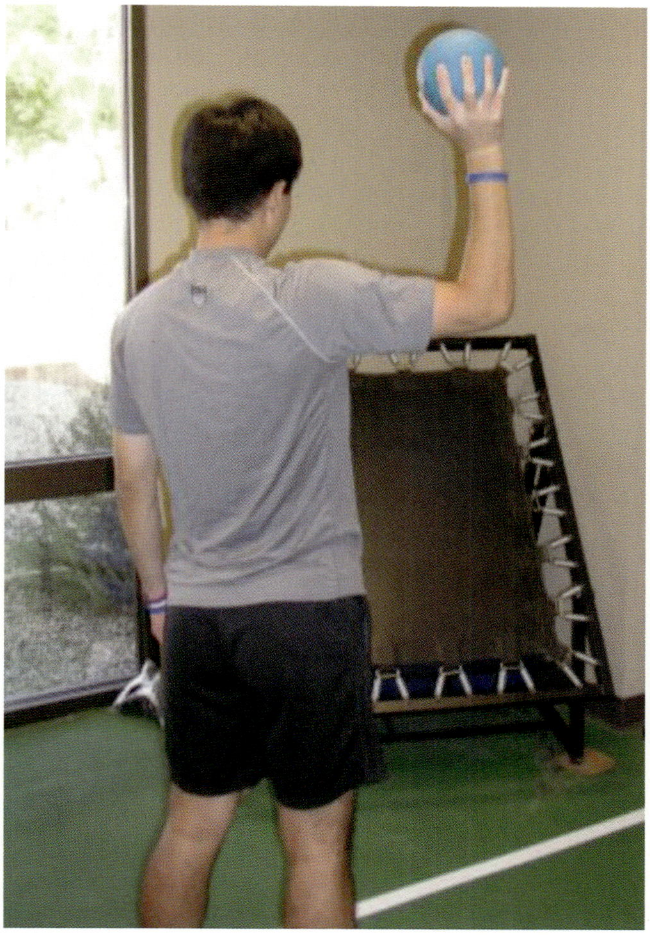

Fig. 3.56 Internal rotation standing plyometrics with 90° of abduction

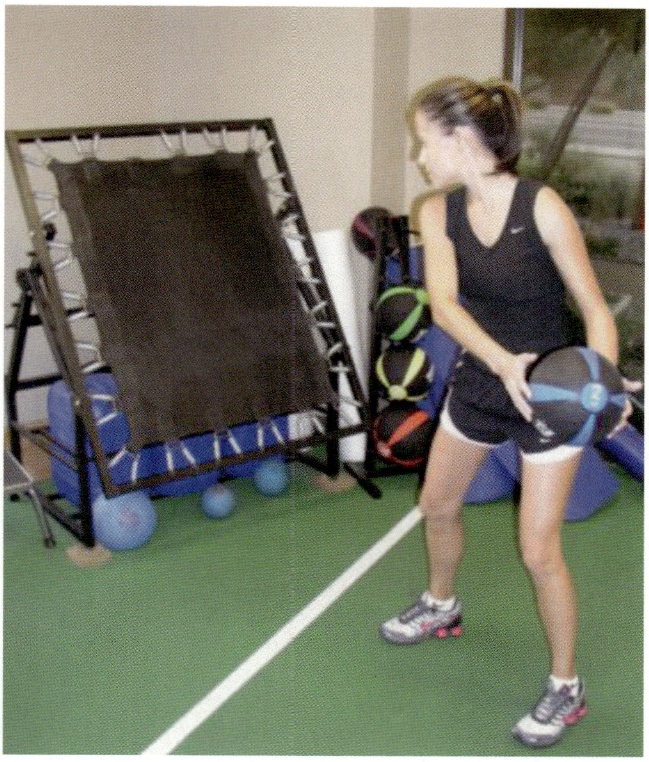

Fig. 3.58 Sports-specific tennis groundstroke plyometric

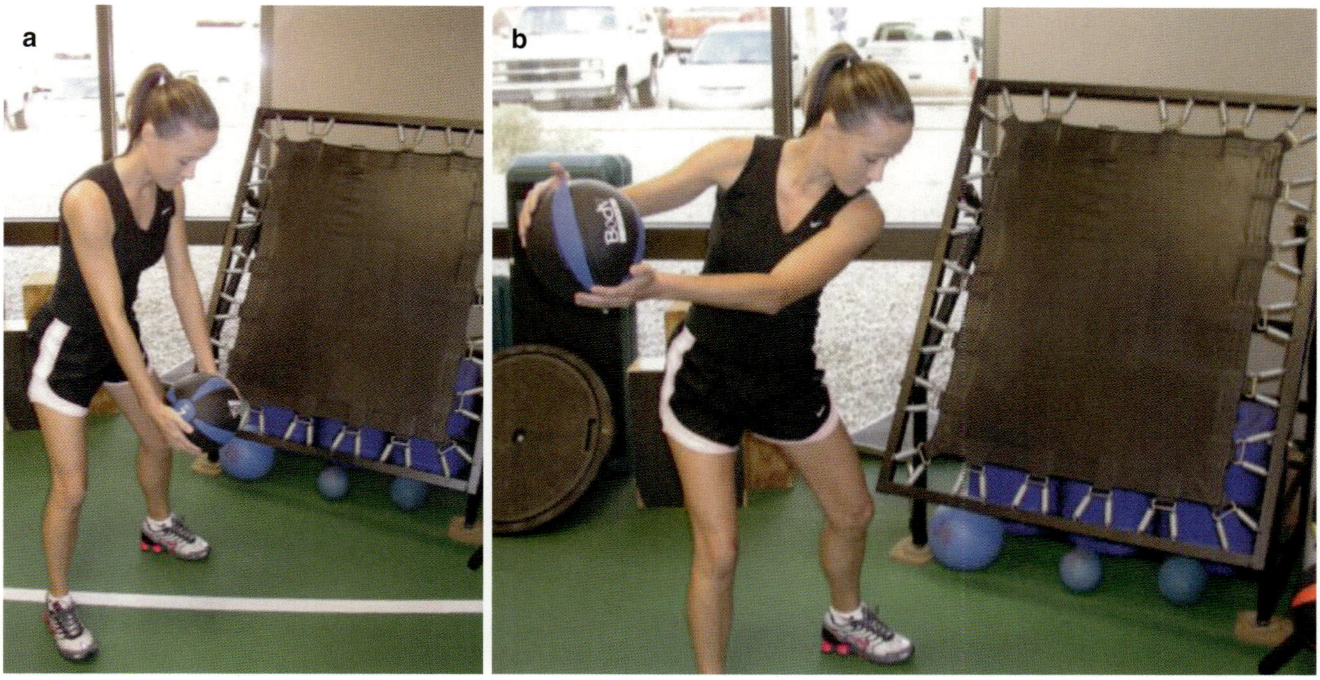

Fig. 3.57 (**a**, **b**) Sports-specific golf plyometric

As the patient tolerates isotonic exercise with 2–3 lb (Fig. 3.45) and also can perform rotational training without pain using medium-level elastic resistance, isokinetic rotational exercise is initiated in the modified base position. This position places the GH joint in 30° of flexion and 30° of abduction, and it uses a 30° tilt of the dynamometer relative to the horizontal (Fig. 3.59) [108, 135]. This position is well tolerated and allows the patient to progress from submaximal to more maximal levels of resistance at velocities ranging between 120° and 210° per second for nonathletic patient populations and between 210° and 360° per second during later stages of rehabilitation in more athletic patients. The use of the isokinetic dynamometer is also important to quantify objectively muscular strength levels and, most critically, muscular balance between the internal and external rotators [108, 135]. Achieving a level of IR and ER strength equal to that of the contralateral extremity is an acceptable initial goal for many patients; however, unilateral increases in IR strength of 15–30 % have been reported in many descriptive studies of overhead athletes [108, 136–138]; thus, greater rehabilitative emphasis may be required to achieve this level of documented "dominance." Progression of the patient to the 90/90 position for isoinertial exercise (Impulse, Inc, Noonan Georgia) (Fig. 3.60) as well as on an isokinetic dynamometer (Fig. 3.61) with the shoulder elevated 90° in the scapular plane further provides an optimal training stimulus to increase rotator cuff strength in sports and activity-specific positions [122–139].

A predominance of IR/ER patterning is used during isokinetic training. This focus IR/ER exercise is based on an isokinetic training study by Quincy et al. [140], who showed that IR/ER training for a period of 6 weeks not only can produce statistically significant gains in IR and ER strength but can improve shoulder extension/flexion and abduction/adduction strength as well. Training in the patterns of flexion/extension and abduction/adduction over the same 6 weeks produced only strength gains specific to the direction of training. This overflow of training allows for a more time-efficient and effective focus in the clinic during isokinetic training.

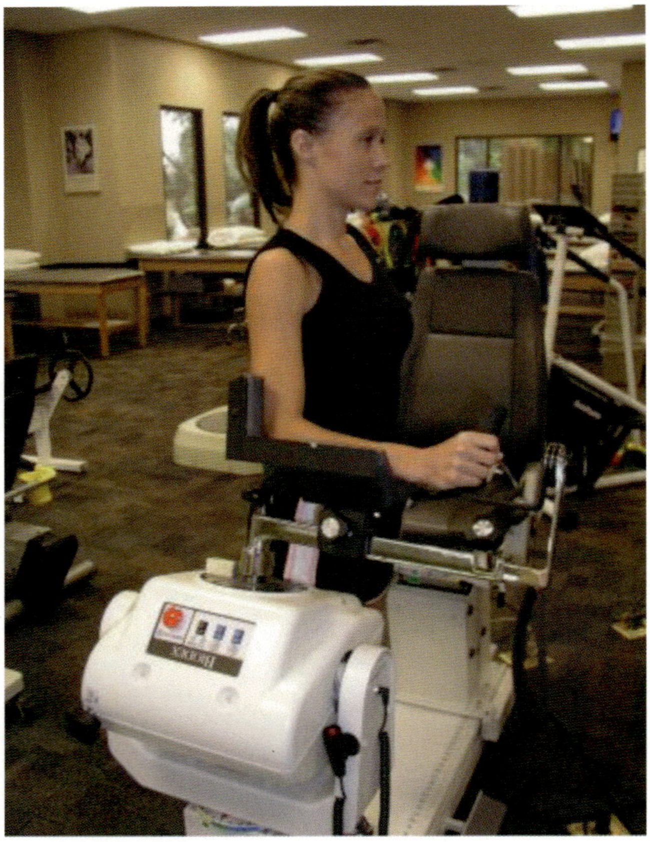

Fig. 3.59 Internal/external rotation in the modified base position on the Biodex Isokinetic Dynamometer

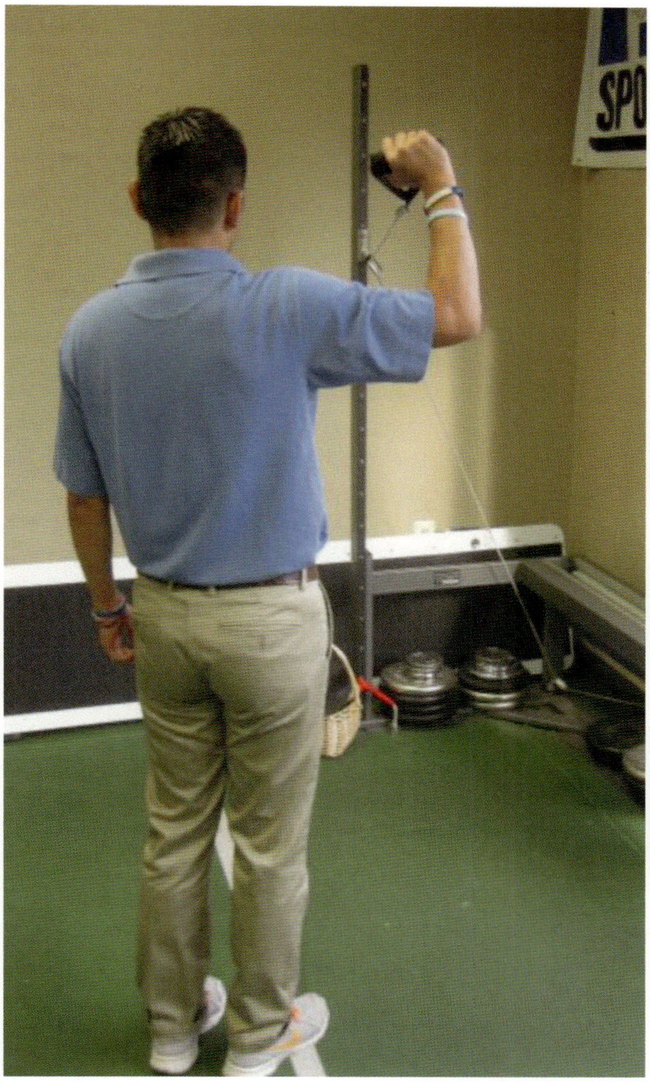

Fig. 3.60 Isoinertial external rotation exercise on the impulse trainer

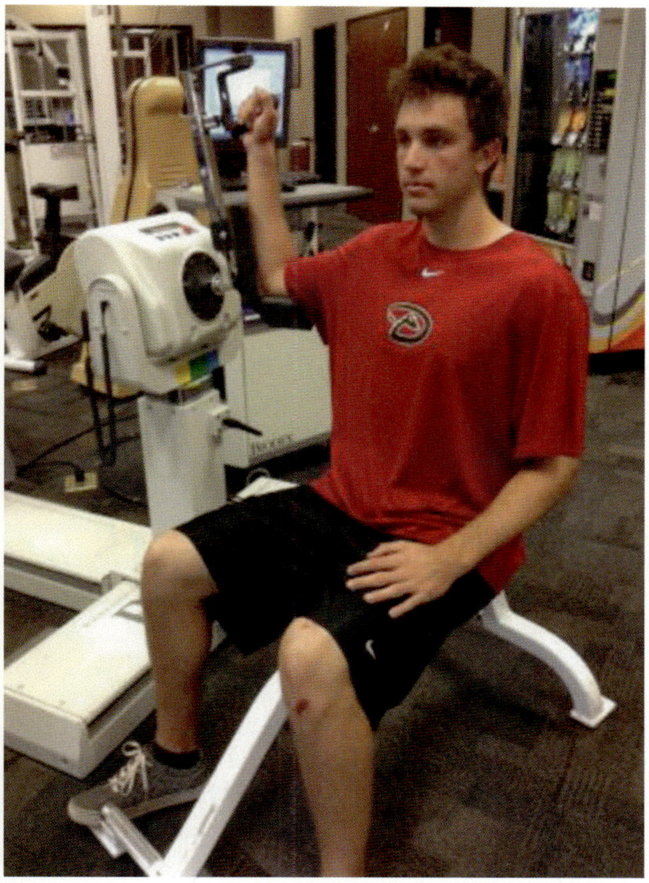

Fig. 3.61 Isokinetic internal/external rotation training position with 90° of elevation in the scapular plane

Objective Criterion to Progress to Sports and Functional Activities

One of the most challenging aspects of the rehabilitation of the patient following arthroscopic Bankart is the clinical decision-making that occurs prior to progressing the patient back to their sports or functional activity. The use of objective data is recommended to guide this decision. Table 3.6 outlines the important components and findings of a return to activity evaluation for patients following Bankart repair.

The use of objective testing outlined in Table 3.6 allows the clinician to base the individual's functional return on objective parameters that can be measured and re-assessed as needed during the later stages of rehabilitation. Future prospective studies will provide key evidence basis for the use of guidelines such as those listed and their ability to predict successful functional activity and sports performance following both non- and post-surgical shoulder injury and subsequent rehabilitation.

Interval Sports and Functional Activity Return Programs Following Arthroscopic Bankart

While it is beyond the scope of this chapter to review and provide all return to activity programs following stabilization surgery, several key concepts will be discussed and recommendations given for a return to traditional fitness weightlifting and tennis program to provide examples of the characteristic stepwise progressions applied to minimize re-injury risk and optimize success and functional performance ratios.

Returning a patient following arthroscopic Bankart to traditional weightlifting requires modification and education regarding increased stress from inherent glenohumeral positions which place the shoulder in excessive amounts of horizontal adduction and with some exercises excessive elevation. These exercises can increase anterior capsulolabral stress and impingement, respectively. Bleacher and Ellenbecker [141] and Gross et al. [142] have provided guidelines for patients with instability and rotator cuff disease regarding the return to traditional weightlifting. General concepts such as alternate-day performance (rest between strength training sessions), lower weight and higher repetitions, and most important exercise position and movement pattern modifications (Table 3.7). Limitation in range of motion with bench presses and removal of all behind the head exercises such as lat pull and military press with modified movement pattern recommendations are recommended for patients following Bankart reconstruction.

Also of key importance with the weightlifter is for them to continue with rotator cuff and scapular exercise training to maintain the ER/IR muscle balance and ensure key levels of rotator cuff stabilization forces remain following discharge from physical therapy.

Characteristics of an interval sports return program for tennis include alternate-day performance, as well as gradual progressions of intensity and repetitions tennis activities. For the interval tennis program, the initial use of a foam ball and progressing to a series of low compression tennis balls both used during the teaching process of tennis to young children are recommended and followed. These balls are recommended for use during the initial phase of the return to tennis program and are thought to result in a decrease in impact stress and increased patient tolerance to the early tennis specific activity. Additionally, performing the interval program under supervision, either during physical therapy sessions or with a knowledgeable tennis teaching professional or coach, allows for the biomechanical evaluation of technique and guards against over-zealous intensity levels, which can be a common mistake in well-intentioned, motivated patients, especially adolescents. Using the return program on alternate days, with rest between sessions, allows for recovery and decreases the risk re-injury.

This interval tennis program has been published previously [143], and a modified version is included (Table 3.9) in this chapter. It includes updated information on the use of the different tennis ball progressions and takes the player through a series progressing from groundstrokes to volleys and finally serves and overheads. Additionally, having the patient's racquet and string type/tension evaluated by a qualified tennis teaching professional is recommended as certain racquet and string characteristics may be indicated for patients when returning from shoulder injury.

Table 3.6 Objective guidelines for return to sports and functional activity

Pain-free range of motion without apprehension at end range of motion
Range of motion within 10 % of contralateral extremity unless anatomical factors supersede it
Muscular strength within 10 % of the contralateral extremity for IR and ER strength with isokinetic testing or hand held dynamometer
Manual muscle testing (MMT) great 5-/5 for all planes of motion without pain provocation
ER/IR muscular strength ratio >66 % with objective testing

Table 3.7 Modifications of traditional weight lifting for patients following anterior stabilization

Exercises	Shoulder pathology	Modification(s)
Flat bench press	Anterior instability	*Grip* <1.5 biacromial width
		ROM limitations <15° shoulder extension (towel on chest, to block motion, or use of physio ball, smith machine to limit ROM)
Cable Fly's	Anterior instability	*Hand spacing* (1–1.5 biacromial width)
		ROM limitation – shoulder extension, horizontal abduction anterior to coronal plane
		Glenohumeral abduction angles <90° maintaining
		Elbows below shoulder level
Pec deck	Anterior instability	*ROM* limitations – shoulder horizontal abduction anterior to coronal plane
		Glenohumeral abduction angles <90° adjusting seat level
Dumbbell Fly's	Anterior instability	*ROM* limitations – shoulder horizontal abduction, extension anterior to coronal plane (Swiss ball or wide bench limiting movement)
		Glenohumeral abduction angles between 45° and 70°
		Elbow flexion angles 70–90°
Traditional push-up	Anterior instability	*Hand spacing*: <1.5 xs biacromial width
		ROM limitations – shoulder horizontal abduction anterior to coronal plane (medicine ball, 45 cm Swiss ball at sternal level)
		Glenohumeral abduction 45–70°
		End range – "plus" position
Lat pull down	Anterior instability	Perform with bar in front of head, NOT behind the head
Front and lateral raise	Anterior instability	Humerus in external rotation (thumb up) position and block ROM to 0–90 only to minimize rotator cuff stress
Military press	Anterior instability	The use of dumbbells, not barbell, limits ROM to 90–120° of elevation maximum, always in front of head, never behind head

Outcomes Following Arthroscopic Bankart

One final concept to discuss in closing section of this chapter is outcomes following arthroscopic Bankart reconstruction. The rehabilitation concepts discussed throughout this chapter can return functional range of motion and rotator cuff and scapular strength to patients with unilateral glenohumeral instability for surgical stabilization. Our own outcomes research on patients following arthroscopic Bankart reconstruction obtained via a retrospective review shows an average return of 160° of forward flexion, 150° of abduction, and 78° of external rotation at 90° of abduction and 42° of internal rotation at 90° of abduction. These values compared to the baseline (contralateral extremity) show 5° greater forward flexion, 21° deficits in abduction, and 16 deficits in internal and external rotation with 90° of abduction. This ROM data shows nearly full elevation range of motion return and the largest deficits in abduction and rotational range of motion. Additional outcomes data published by Kim et al. [144] specifically deals with the comparison of early aggressive rehabilitation versus immobilization and delayed rehabilitation in 62 nonathletic patients who underwent arthroscopic Bankart for unidirectional glenohumeral joint instability in a 3-year follow-up study. The results of Kim et al. [144] show no significant difference in re-dislocation rate in patients who received more aggressive early rehabilitation and range of motion intervention. There were improved patient satisfaction in the immediate motion (aggressive rehabilitation) group as well as decreased postoperative pain ratings and faster return of range of motion. This study supports the application of immediate range of motion as compared to a group of patients with delayed ROM and longer immobilization times following arthroscopic Bankart.

Several meta-analyses have been published comparing the outcomes of open Bankart to arthroscopic Bankart. In a review of 2108 studies on shoulder instability in their meta-analysis, Lenters et al. [145] concluded that arthroscopic stabilization procedures did have significantly higher functional outcomes scores, but open stabilization procedures were superior at preventing recurrent instability and returning patients to work as compared to arthroscopic procedures. Petrera et al. [146] conducted a specific meta-analysis to compare arthroscopic to open Bankart results using suture anchors. They concluded that there was no significant difference in recurrent instability 6 versus 6.7 % between arthroscopic and open Bankart, but that there were superior functional results among the patients who had arthroscopic Bankart.

Finally, regarding long-term outcome, the association between anterior stabilization surgery and glenohumeral joint arthritis was studied by Castagna et al. [147]. They followed up patients after arthroscopic anterior stabilization surgery (10 year minimum follow-up) and found 29 % with mild arthritis and 10 % with moderate arthritis. There was no correlation with functional outcome and the presence of glenohumeral arthritis. The recurrence of instability following surgery in this long-term outcome study was 16 %. Further long-term outcomes research is necessary to best understand the sequela.

Take-Home Message

Summary

This material in this chapter was meant to provide a detailed description of an evidence-based protocol for rehabilitation following arthroscopic Bankart reconstruction. A thorough understanding of the surgical procedure for Bankart reconstruction with and without capsular shift as well as any concomitant surgical procedures will allow therapists to provide appropriate and optimal rehabilitation following surgery. Current outcomes evidence shows high-level functional results and lower recurrence of instability in follow-up studies. The goals of restoring a functional and stable range of motion platform coupled with highly fatigue-resistant scapular stabilization and rotator cuff strength and key are tenants of a comprehensive rehabilitation program for patients following this procedure.

3.6 Latarjet Technique

Latarjet technique is considered a non-anatomical surgical procedure; its goal is to stabilize the shoulder by compensating for the capsule-labral and osseous injury with an osseous and soft tissue check in that blocks excessive translation and restore stability.

Preoperative plain x-ray studies were performed in anteroposterior, internal and external rotation, and lateral, axillary, and Bernageau views. Preoperative CT scans are obtained for all patients to better evaluate the glenoid bone surface.

Anyway because the integrity of the glenoid is one of the elements that defines the surgical treatment, the reliability of plain radiographs is one of the key points.

According to Gerber [148], we look carefully at the anteroposterior (AP) radiographs of the shoulder where the anterior glenoid rim appears as a subchondral sclerotic line.

This sclerotic line can be interrupted for more than 5 mm (Fig. 3.62) in patients withanterior glenoid deficiencies; this absence is called loss of sclerotic glenoid line (LSGL) and have used it in clinical practice to document in a easy way bony lesion of the anterior glenoid rim that anyway if present need to be assessed with CT scan.

*The following description of the Latarjet surgical procedure indicates in "*SMALL CAPS*" the elements that take about 15 days to heal and in "*bold small caps*" the elements that take more than 6 weeks to heal.*

Our surgical technique is a modified Latarjet procedure using a mini plate developed by the authors.

THE SKIN (Fig. 3.63) is incised along the anterior axillary crease in a longitudinal fashion along the Langers line. The incision is placed lateral to the coracoid process. THE DELTOPECTORAL INTERVAL is identified, the cephalic vein is retracted laterally, and the interval is developed. The clavipectoral fascia is then incised at the lateral border of the conjoined tendon at its coracoid attachment, and the coracoacromial ligament is divided to facilitate exposure of the superior aspect of the capsule and, particularly, the rotator interval area. The bicipital groove and the lesser tuberosity are identified.

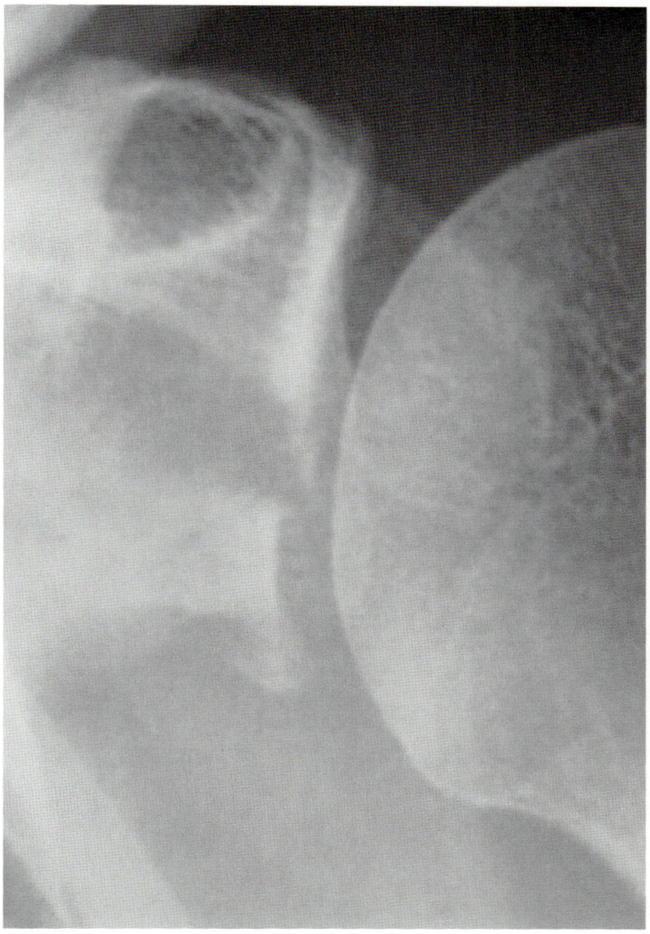

Fig. 3.62 (A-P view) note the breakage of the subchondral sclerotic line

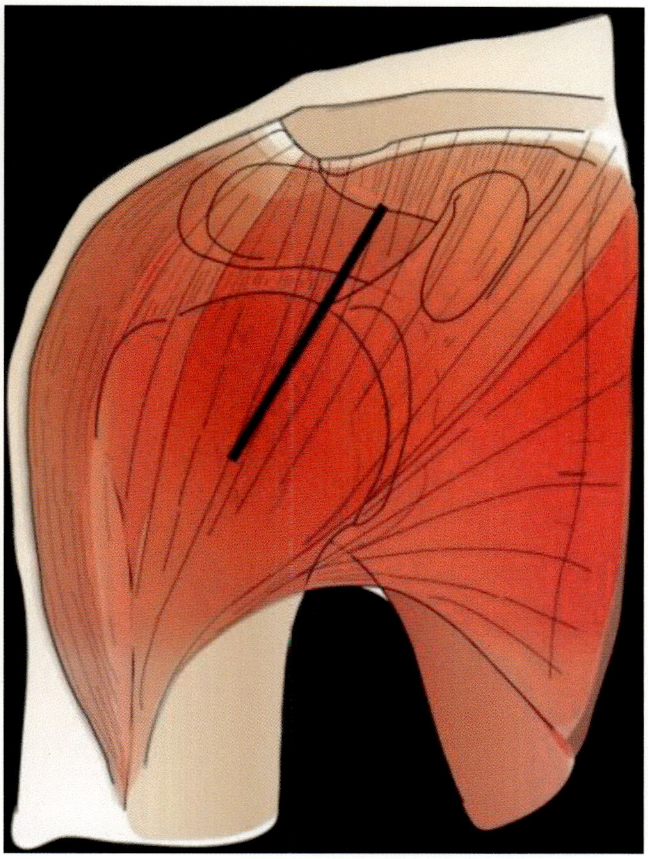

Fig. 3.63 Skin incision and deltopectoral approach

This procedure is performed using a local bone graft by the osteotomy of the terminal 2 cm of the coracoid process (Fig. 3.64), detaching the insertion of the pectoralis minor tendon. The coracoid bone graft is decorticated in the inferior surface until the cancellous bone. After the orizzontal split of the subscapularis tendon (Fig. 3.65) is performed, the coracoid bone graft is transplanted along with the conjoined tendon to the anteroinferior glenoid rim that is decorticated. The coracoid bone graft is positioned below the equator and no less than 2 mm from the glenoid cartilage (Fig. 3.66).

The coracoid bone graft is laid lengthwise and held in place with two bicortical partially treated (diameter 4 mm) cannulated screws and the eventually the mini wedged plate to improve compression (Fig. 3.67).

The mini wedged plate design has specific characteristics, each of which corresponds to a biomechanical function. It has a wedged profile. The wedge of the plate if placed medially under compression makes the coracoid bone graft rotate medially, thereby improving the bone match between the coracoid bone graft and the glenoid bone surface.

It has a figure of eight (8) configuration that allows a better torsional orientation of the plate on the dorsal-sloped coracoid surface. Four spikes for an improved stabilization of the plate-bone block and two screw holes for lag screws insertion. These features allow the plate to distribute the load evenly to the bone.

Post-surgery rehabilitation must take the following into account:

1. ***Biological-specific healing rates of the surgical procedure:*** *skin incision, cleavage plane, capsulotomy, tenotomy, or muscle-tendon split; in this case the bone-to-bone healing of the coracoid graft to the neck of the scapula is crucial.*
2. ***Neuromuscolar and proprioceptive recovery:*** *must be gradual in the case of the affected body part and consistent with biological heeling timeframes but can be faster for the kinetic chain links outside the involved shoulder.*
3. ***Return to working and/or sports activity.***

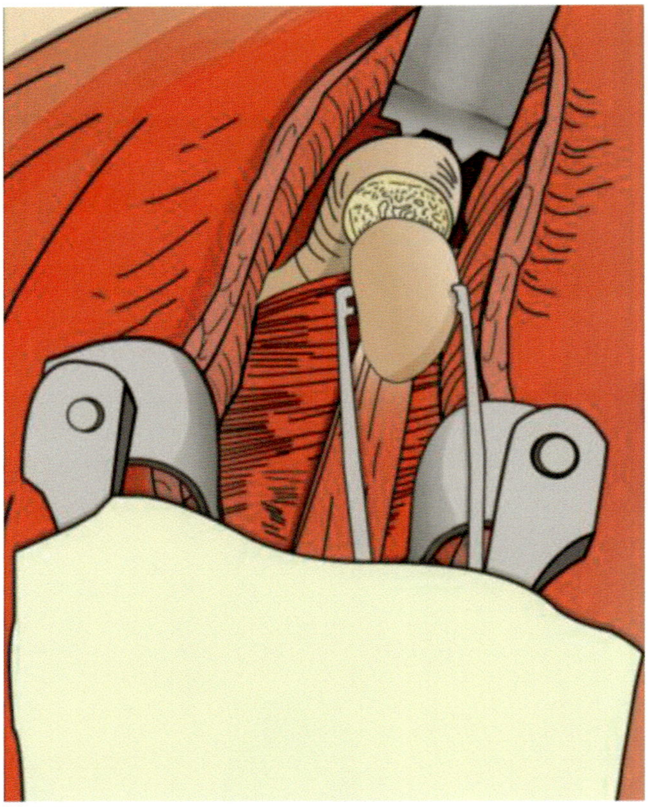

Fig. 3.64 Osteotomy of the coracoid at level of the "knee" in front of conoid and trapezoid

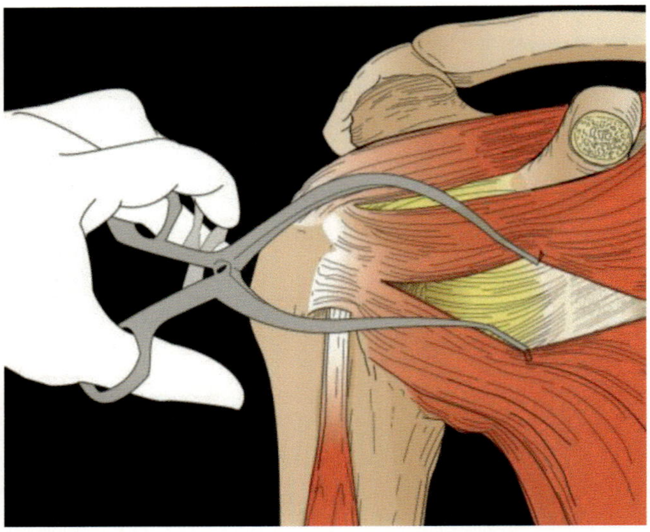

Fig. 3.65 Subscapular split

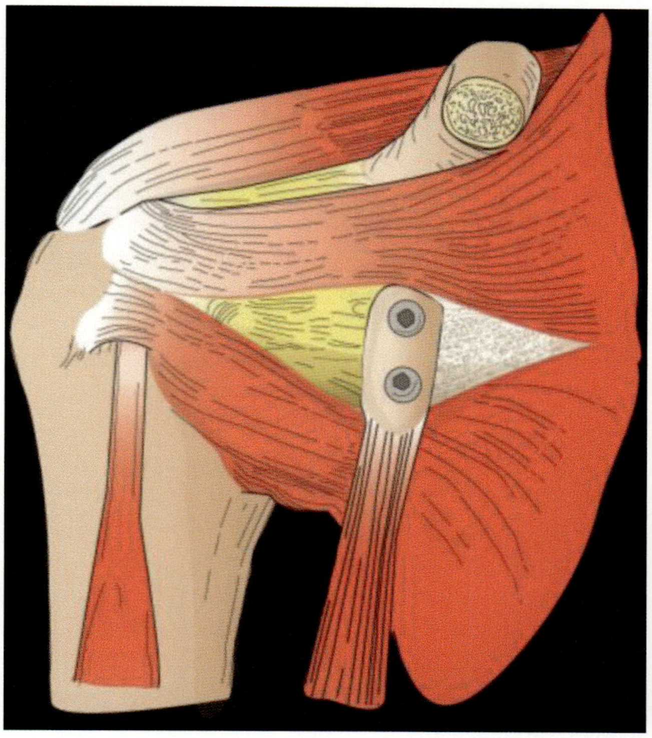

Fig. 3.66 Positioning of the coracoid between 3 and 6 o'clock

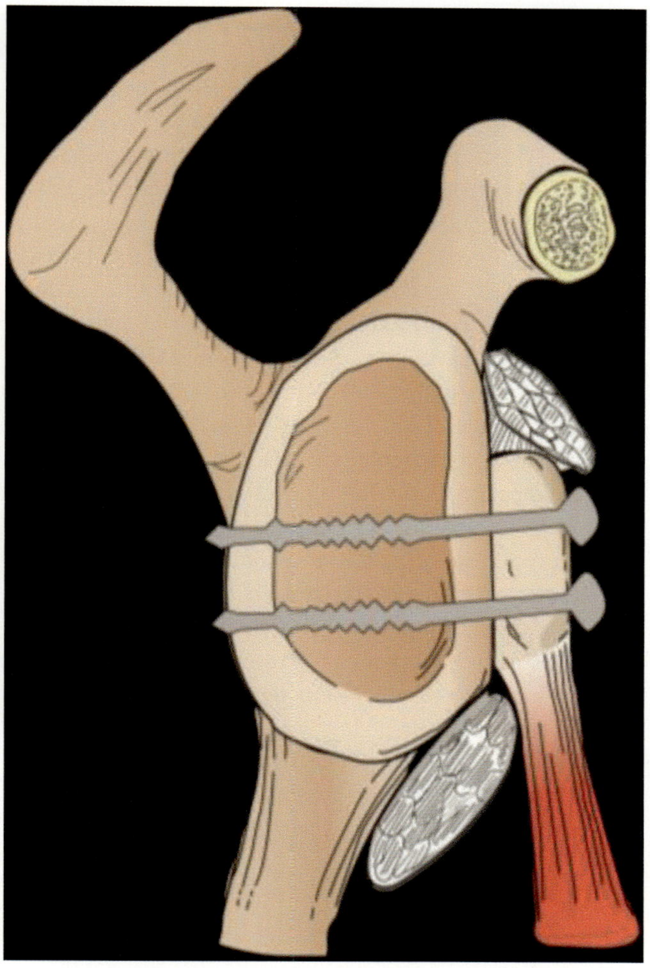

Fig. 3.67 Compression of the coracoid on the scapular neck

3.7 Rehabilitation following Latarjet Technique

Rehabilitation following reconstruction surgery using the Latarjet procedure plays a decisive role in reinstating musculoskeletal and proprioceptive functions. The following chapter looks at the methods and tools underpinning an appropriate rehabilitation protocol for this particular post-op situation.

As previously underlined, a good patient rehabilitation protocol must involve both orthopedic surgeon and physiotherapist.

Importantly, patients enrolled in any rehabilitation protocol must be approached as individuals in their own right with issues that range from the specifics of their post-surgical condition to their particular emotional state.

In fact experience advises against applying a standardized rehab protocol but rather the introduction of a series of exercises geared to restoring glenohumeral joint function within the framework of established goals, but implemented according to the pace of individual physical recovery and the subjective status of each patient. Hydrotherapy could have an important role in rehabilitation protocol if is managed by specialized equipe.

- *0–2 Weeks*: Following Laterjet surgery, the patient is requested to keep the involved limb in a sling (Fig. 3.68). At discharge from hospital, the patient is taught a gentle scapular retraction exercise (Fig. 3.69) to maintain correct periscapular posture and tropism. Since the surgical procedure involves transplanting the coracoid process that gives attachment to the short head of the biceps and the coracobrachialis – muscles that are involved in flexion and extension of the elbow and in pronation and supination of the forearm – any movements involving these must be carried out with care and in no way trigger a painful arc. In addition, the patient must be given clear instructions that any flexion/extension and pronation/supination are to be performed in a self-assisted fashion (Fig. 3.70).
- *15th Day*: Stitch removal and clinical control
  On removal of the stitches, it is possible to identify the patients among those with no subcutaneous hematoma or fever who are likely to develop fibrous adhesions in the glenohumeral joint – in our clinical practice defined as external rotation below 20 %. These adhesion-prone patients should start rehabilitation immediately under the supervision of a specialist team. Patients not presenting the warning signs of fibrous adhesions will generally begin physiotherapy on day 21 post-op.
- *21th Day*: On starting rehabilitation, the patient must be pain-free or with only minimum pain.

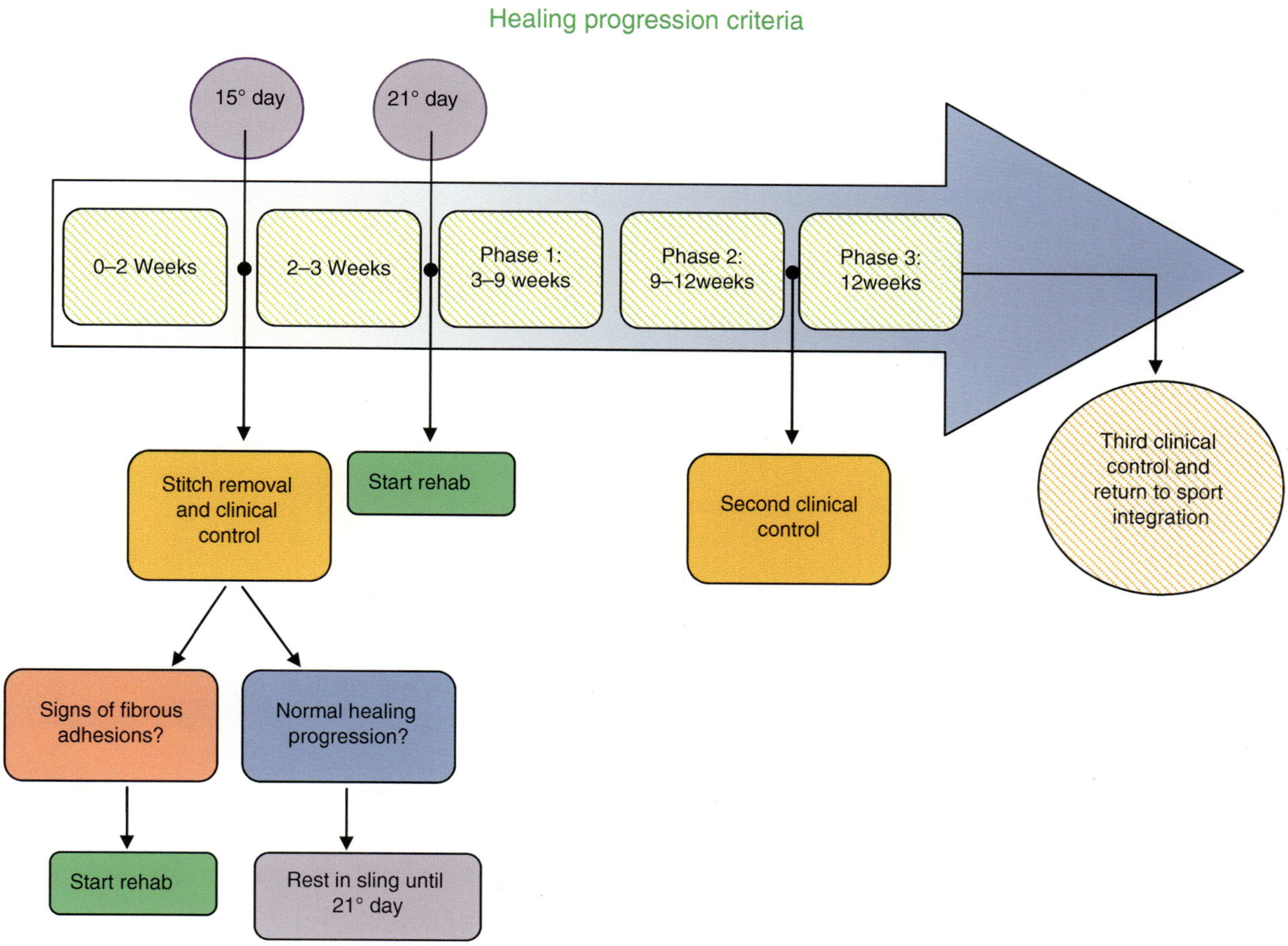

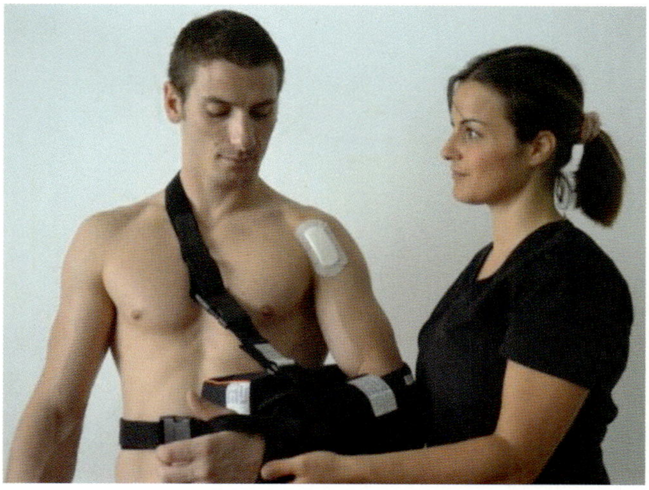

Fig. 3.68 Fitting arm sling before discharge

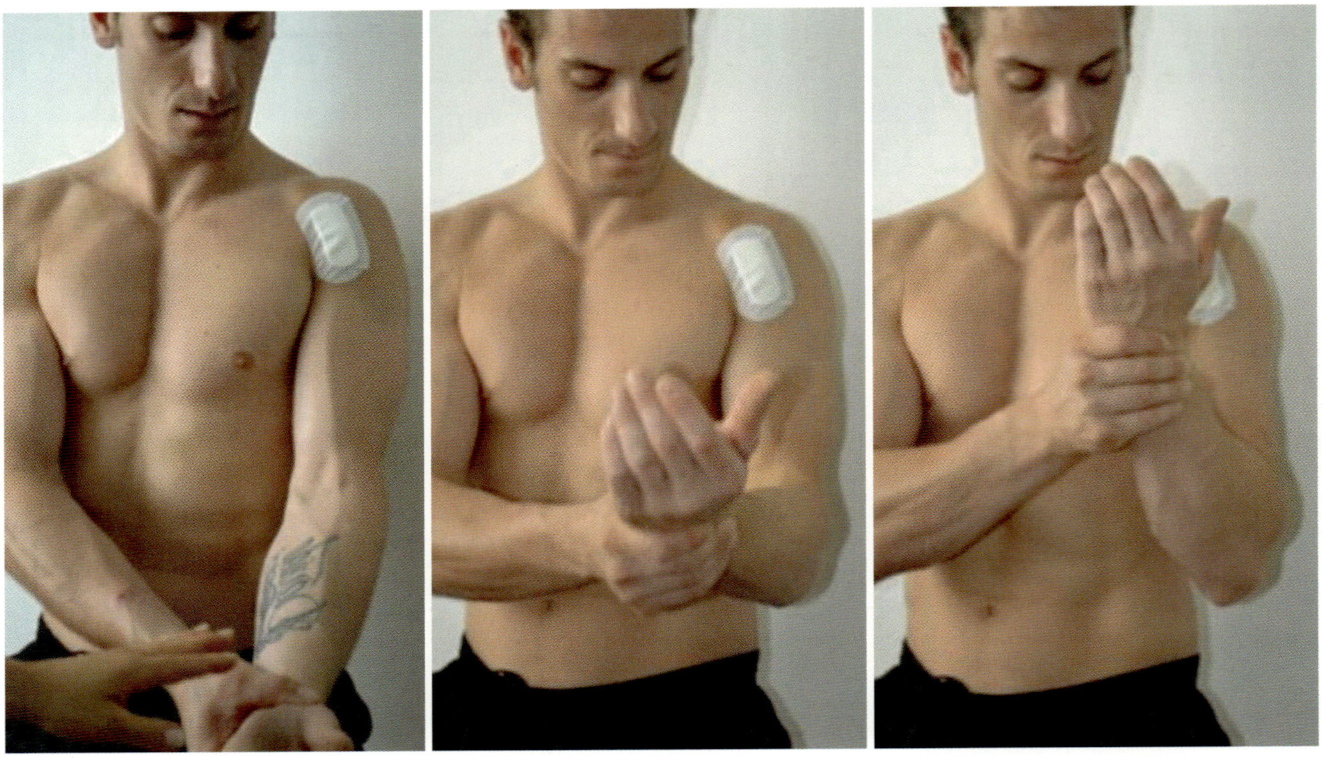

Fig. 3.69 Assisted elbow flexion-extension without sling

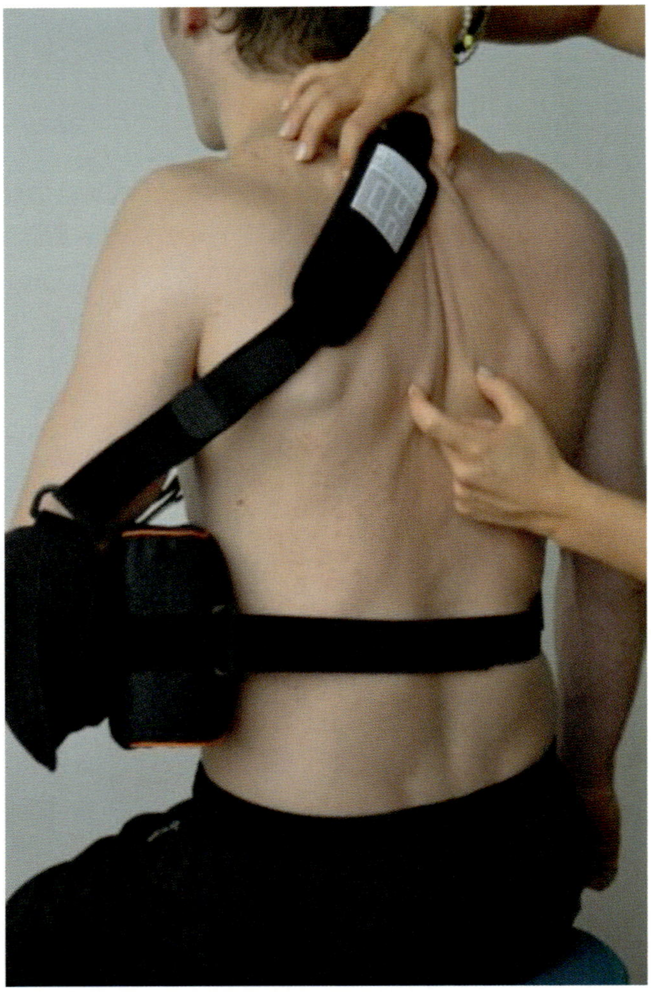

Fig. 3.70 Scapular retraction with sling

3.8 Physical Examination at Outset

- *Posture*:
  The patient's posture could be altered on account of the protraction induced by the sling (Fig. 3.71).

  Altered posture must be appropriately dealt with by the rehabilitation team. Restoring correct posture is decisive in this initial phase since it will facilitate subsequent movements, enhance muscle strengthening, and increase general exercise performance. Correct posture optimizes KINETIC CHAIN STRENGTH, reinforcing the proximal extremities and the DISTAL JOINT muscle structures (Fig. 3.72) [149].
- *Scapular Control*:
  The aim of physiotherapy in this phase is to maintain good scapular control with specific scapular closing exercises (Figs. 3.74 and 3.75) and allow gentle stretching of the anterior structures (Fig. 3.73) [150]. These are the first exercises initiating the physiotherapy procedure. They are to be performed, however, only if the patient feels no pain. Early muscle reactivation aims to prevent inhibition and loss of neuromuscular control [151].

  The exercise progression as proposed by Smith is the scapular clock, with the patient placing his hand on the wall with the arm elevated less than 90°.

  In this case the myoelectric activity of the deltoid and rotator cuff muscles is negligible, proving it to be a safe exercise geared specifically to recruiting the middle/lower trapezius and the serratus anterior.

  Propose scapular protraction and retraction and elevation-depression of the girdle [149, 150, 152].

  We prefer the first exercise (scapular protraction and retraction) (Fig. 3.75) since it has been shown to activate the lower adn middle trapezius and so is useful to avoid scapular girdle elevation and the possible compensation observed in scapular dyskinesia. However, the other movements proposed by the authors also appropriately reactivate the scapulothoracic muscles. In particular, active depression of the scapula triggers high electromyographic activity in the serratus anterior, while retraction activates the lower and middle trapezius.
- *ROM*: As a rule, residual passive range of motion following surgery should not be less than 50° passive and active elevation in the scapulothoracic plane. Starting progressive passive kinesis especially of the glenohumeral joint is essential if capsular contracture is to be avoided and joint ROM gradually restored.

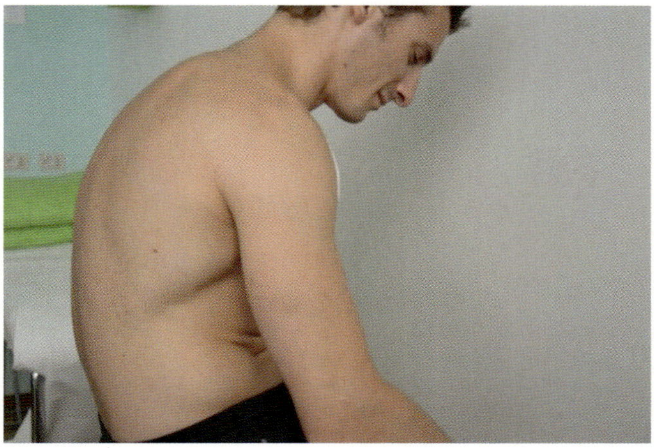

Fig. 3.71 Altered posture after wearing sling for approximately 3 weeks

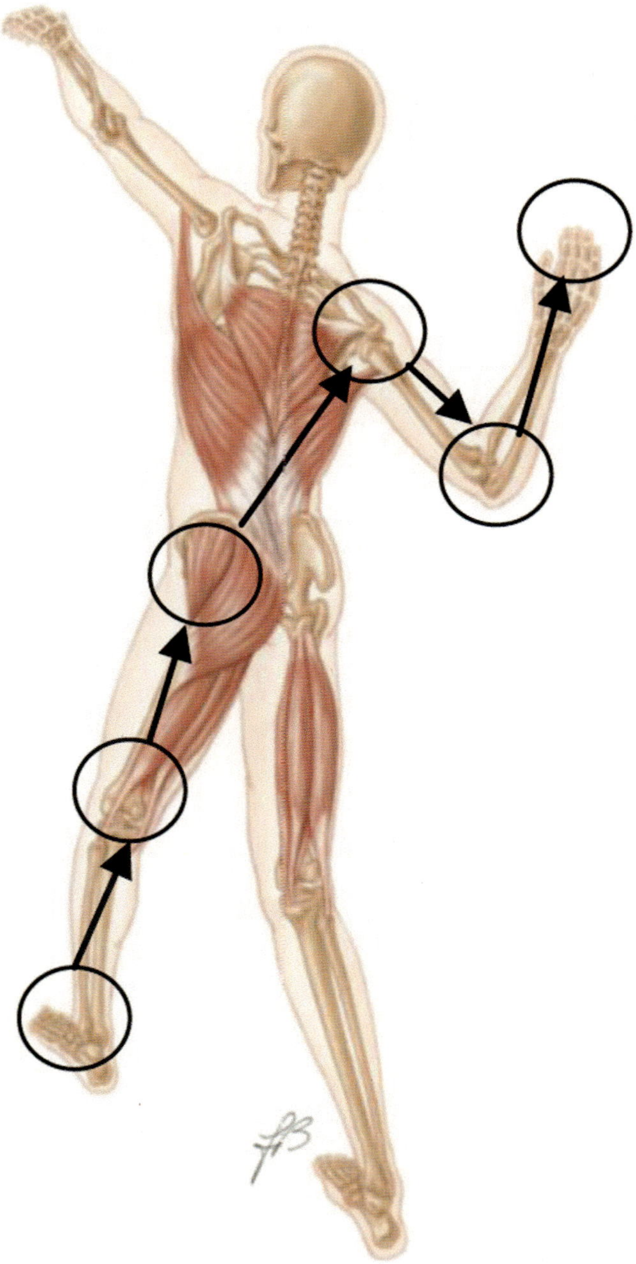

Fig. 3.72 Sequential kinetic chain activation

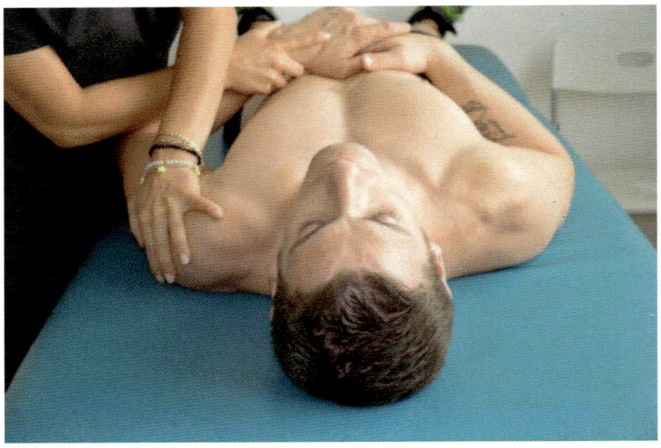

Fig. 3.73 Stretching of the anterior shoulder structure. *Often shortening or contracture of the pectoral muscle cause anterior scapula tilting*

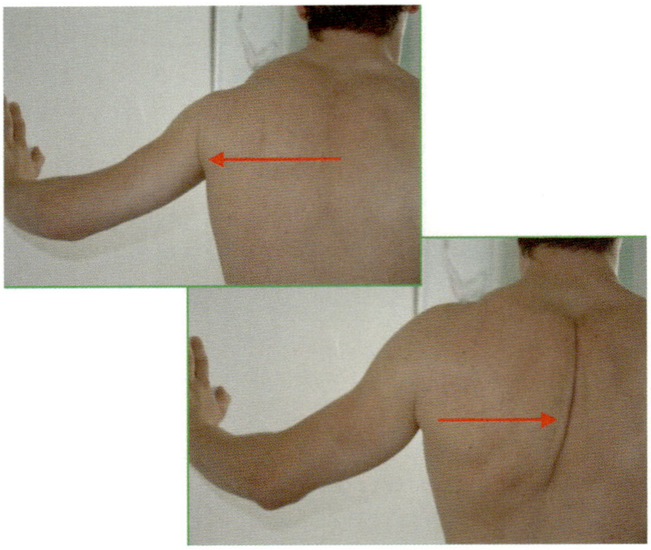

Fig. 3.75 Scapular clock: retraction and protraction

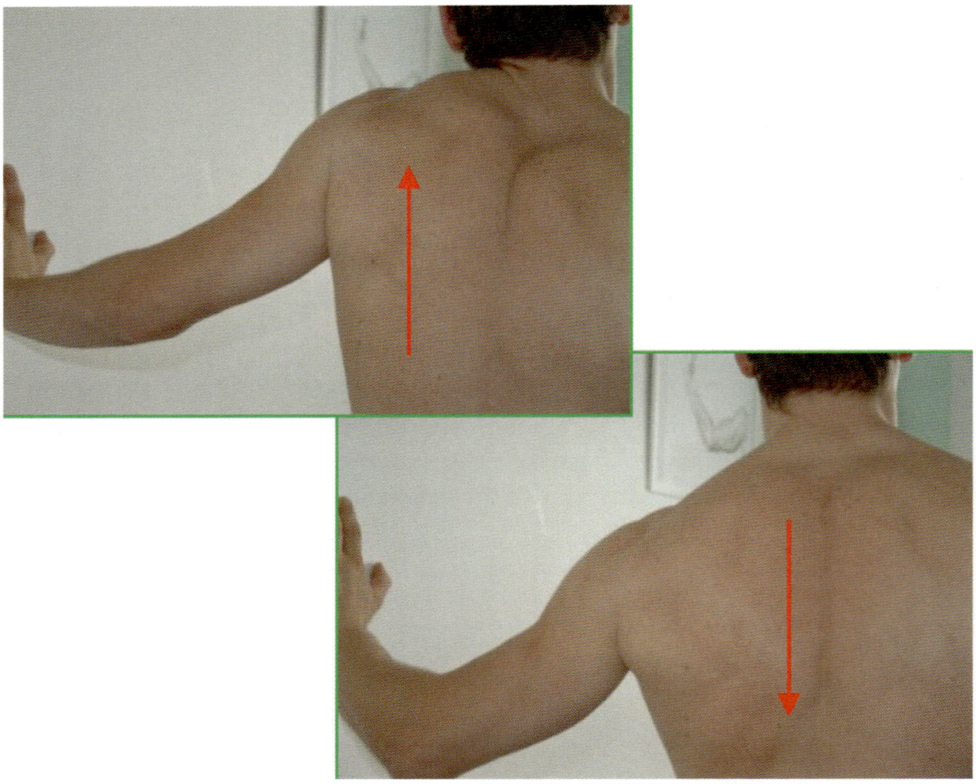

Fig. 3.74 Scapular clock: elevation and depression

Take-Home Message

Subscapular split versus *subscapular tenotomy* (Fig. 3.76a, b)

- Since the subscapular split procedure does not involve detachment of the subscapularis from the greater tuberosity, there is no tendon-bone healing period to be respected. As a result, internal rotation and external rotation exercises can be started earlier on. The subscapular tenotomy procedure, on the other hand, requires greater caution up to the 6th postoperative week, with active and passive external rotation and active internal rotation.

Take-Home Message

What is proprioception?

- Proprioception is a specialized sensory modality that gives information about extremity position and direction of movement. This kind of afferent sensory feedback is probably important in mediating muscular control of the shoulder joint [153–155].

- *Evaluate Core Stability:* In the first phase, it is important to assess patient posture and core stability so as to tailor the right sequence of goals to be obtained over the course of rehabilitation. As Kibler explains [156, 157], the various body segments play specific roles in the kinetic chain activation sequence. The muscles and joints of the hips, pelvis, and spine (known collectively as the core) are centrally located and can perform many of the stabilizing functions that the body requires if the distal segments are to perform their specific functions. Thus "core stability" provides proximal stability for distal limb mobility and function.

When assessing core stability and strength, it is important to evaluate the muscles working in an eccentric, load-absorbing function, the body segments in a closed-chain situation, and the resultant movements in the 3 planes of trunk motion. In the standing balance test, the patient is asked to stand on one leg and is given no further verbal cue. A positive test result, known as the Trendelenburg sign, is when the hip drops on the unsupported side (Fig. 3.77a, b). This indicates inability to control the posture and suggests proximal core weakness [156].

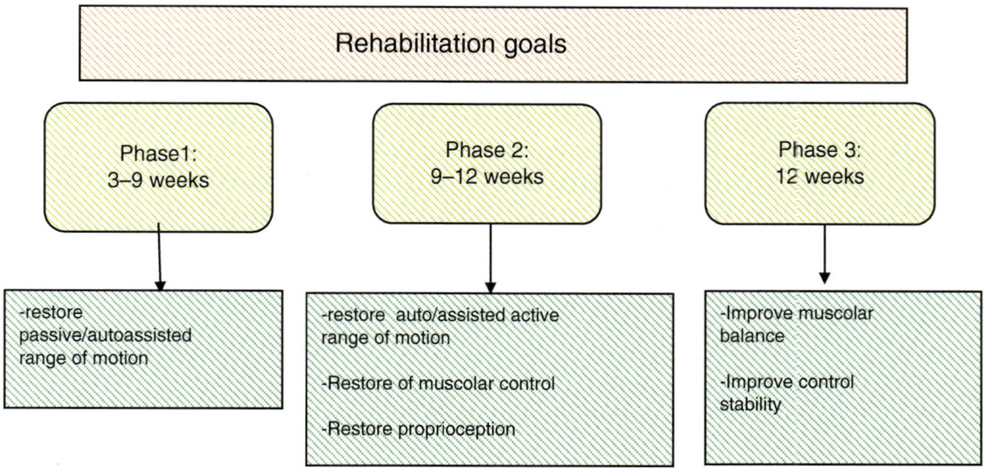

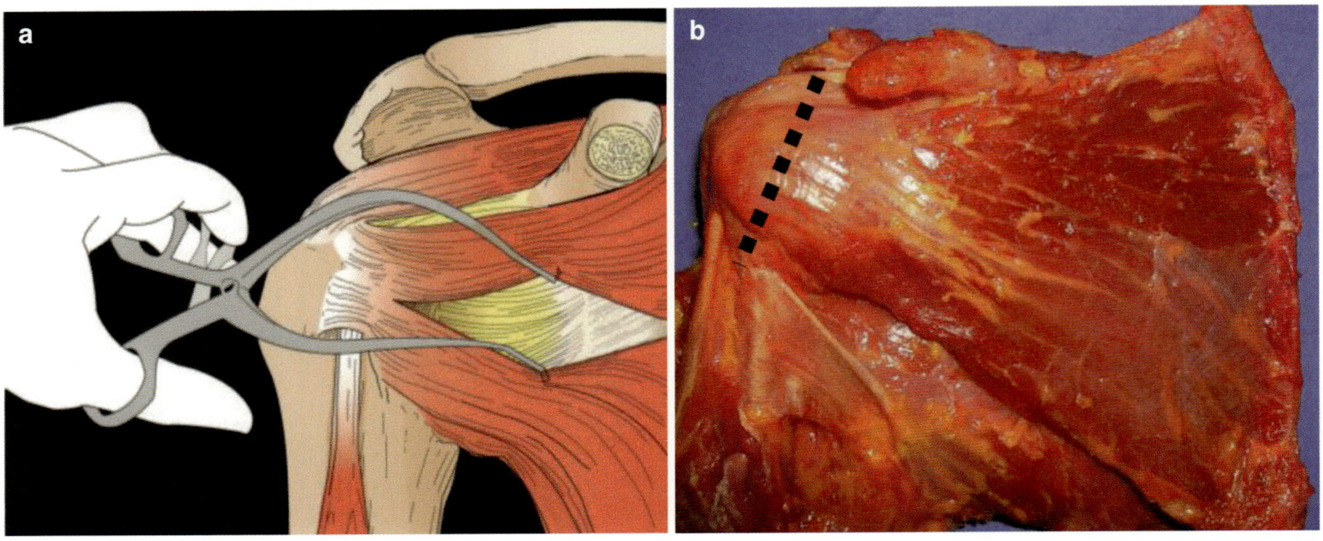

Fig. 3.76 (**a**) Subscapular split. (**b**) Subscapular tenotomy (*black dotted line*)

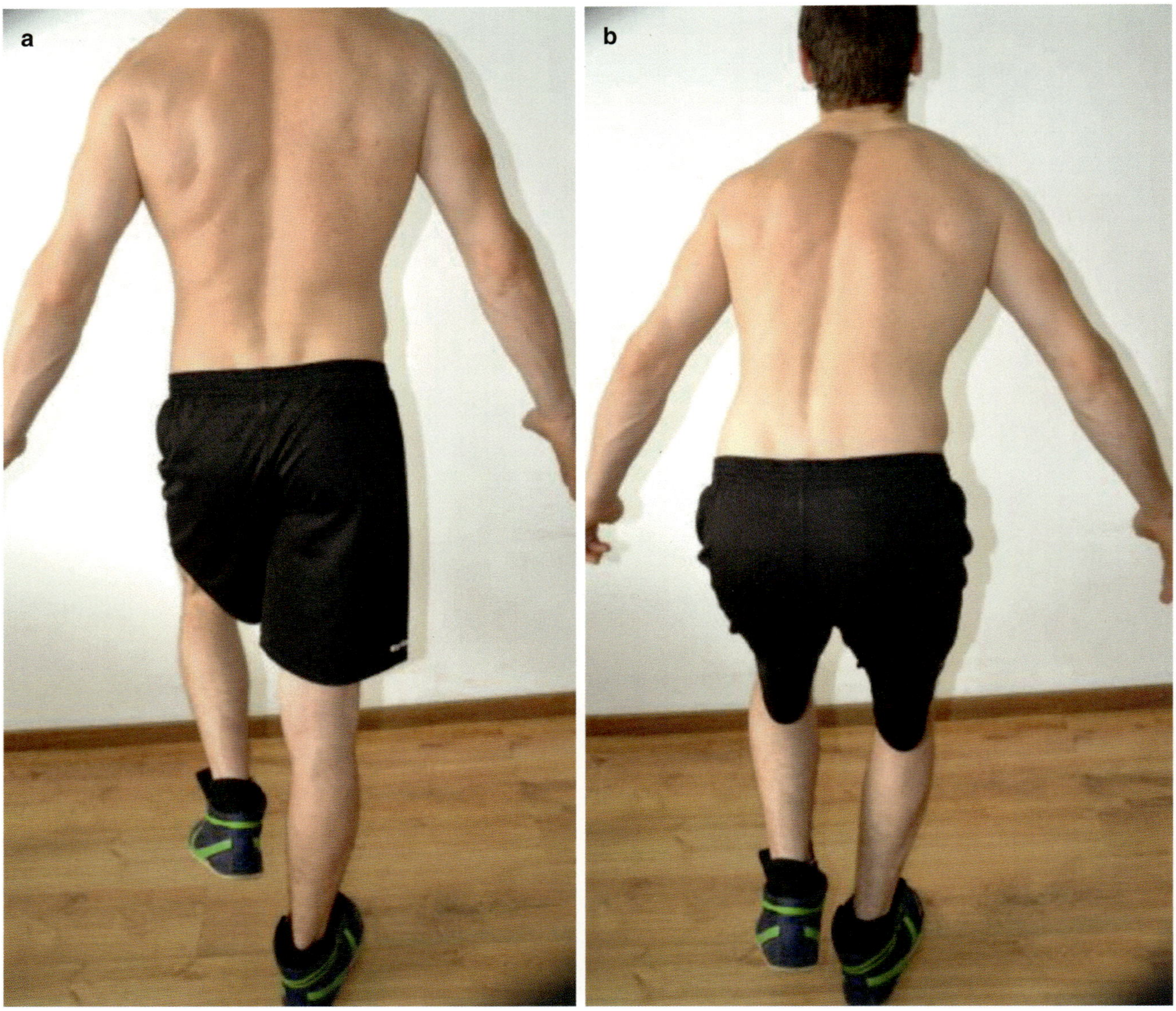

Fig. 3.77 (**a**, **b**) Trendelenburg sign

Phase I: 3–9 Weeks

The focus of rehabilitation is to restore normal joint arthrokinematics and reinstate the shoulder's physiologic range of motion, respecting biological post-op healing timeframes and patient pain thresholds, if any.

Goals	How to do
Protect and preserve the surgical repair	Comply with patient biological healing times after surgical reconstruction
	Sleep in supine position with a towel under the elbow to prevent shoulder hyperextension
	In side-lying sleep, put towel under the axilla to keep the shoulder in a neutral position
Reduction of inflammation and pain	Frequent cryotherapy for pain and inflammation
Achieve gradual restoration of passive range of motion (PROM)	Passive mobilization by physiotherapist and self-assisted exercises by patient keeping under 90° elevation in the scapulothoracic plane and 15°/20° external rotation (Fig. 3.78a)
	Supine passive arm elevation (Fig. 3.78b)
Enhance/ensure adequate scapular function	Scapular clock exercises (Figs. 3.74 and 3.75)
	Progress to scapular isometric exercises
	Ball squeezes (Fig. 3.85)
	Low row (Fig. 3.79) inferior glide (Fig. 3.80)
Restore proprioception	Proprioception ball exercise

- *Restore ROM*: ROM exercising is gradually increased as the connective tissues progressively heal and can successfully accommodate greater stress. Advancing pain-free ROM during this phase is essential to progressing toward full ROM by the next phase. Patients must be encouraged to complete the articular range with active assisted ROM exercises within a pain-free range and with passive mobilization (Fig. 3.78a, b).
- *Enhance/Ensure Adequate Scapular Function*: Kibler et al. [105] have demonstrated serratus anterior and lower trapezius activation in a closed kinetic chain (CKC) and in the absence of ROM with exercises like the low row, which increases external scapular rotation and posterior tilt, and the inferior glide, which induces scapular retraction (Figs. 3.79 and 3.80). Since muscle tone is likely to be reduced, special neuromuscular facilitation strategies must be adopted [150] to reinstate arthrokinematics and prevent compensation [149, 150, 152]. Kibler et al. [105] proposes open kinetic chain (OKC) exercises: the lawnmower (Fig. 3.81a, b), a diagonal exercise pattern going from the contralateral leg through the trunk up to the ipsilateral arm, which helps correct the position of the scapula in retraction thanks to the facilitation caused by the hip extension together with extension and rotation of the trunk.

The robbery exercise (Fig. 3.82a, b) is an OKC exercise, activating the periscapular district. Here too, the lower trapezius and the serratus anterior are recruited, but this time through hip and trunk extension and starting from a position of flexion with bilateral extension of the arms in adduction with the elbows flexed [158].

- *Proprioceptive Neuromuscular Control*:

The main goal of surgery is to restore not only the mechanical restraint lost with joint dislocation but also the proprioceptive deficits arising after joint injury [154].

Regaining proprioceptive and neuromuscular control must proceed in parallel with recovery of range of motion.

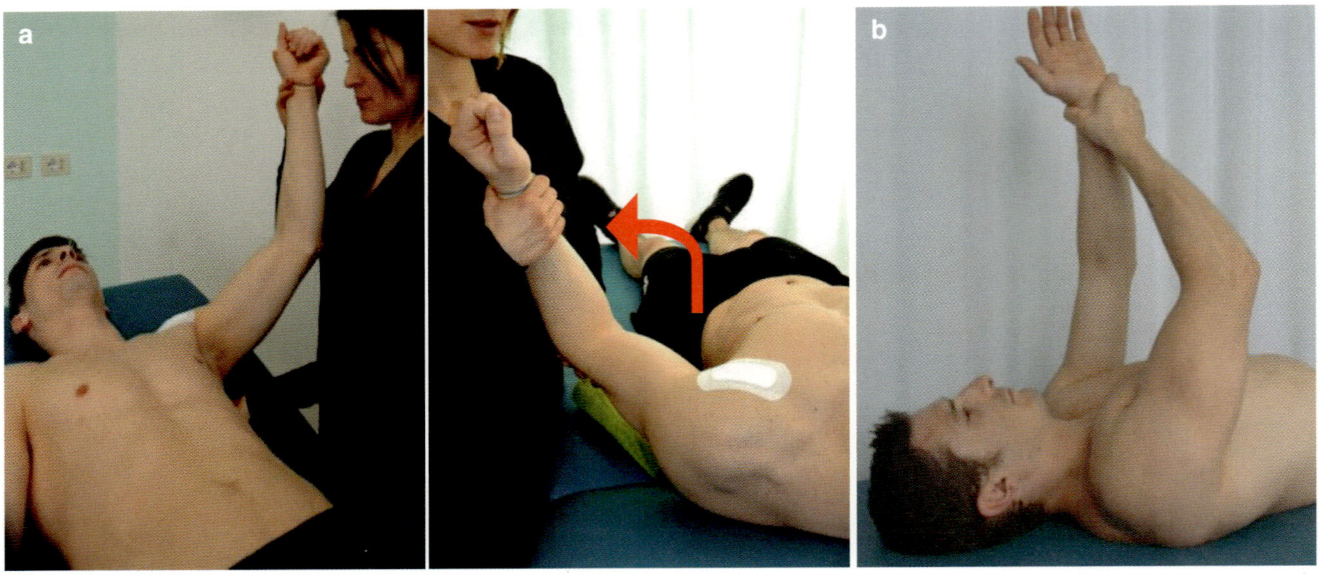

Fig. 3.78 (**a**) Passive mobilization in external rotation between 15° and 20°. (**b**) Lie on the back. Hold the affected arm at the elbow with the opposite hand. Using the strength of the opposite arm, lift the affected arm upward, as if to bring the arm until 90°, slowly lower the arm back to the bed

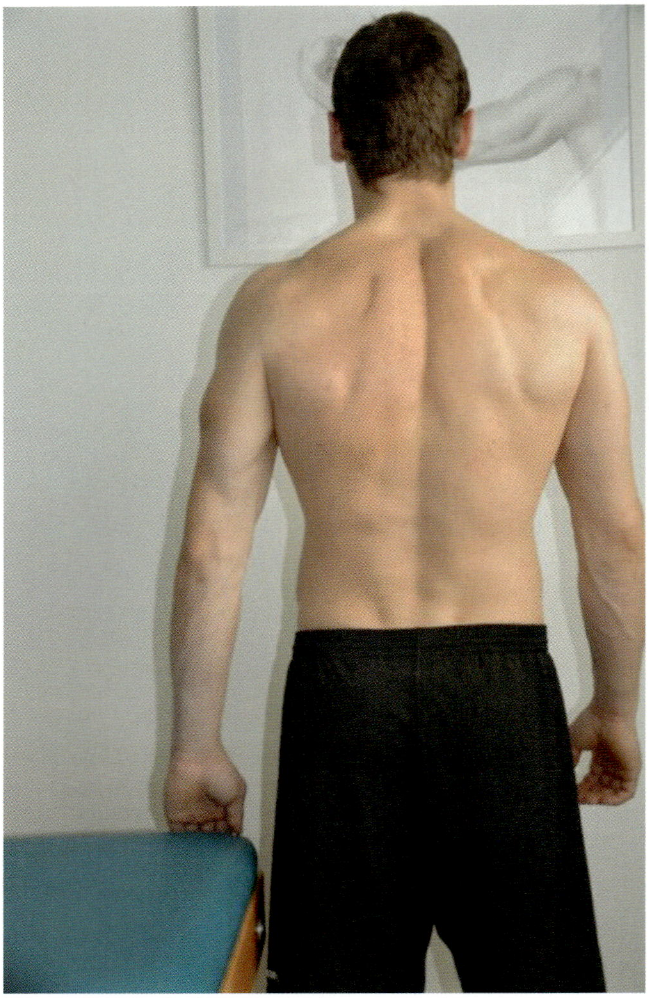

Fig. 3.79 Low row

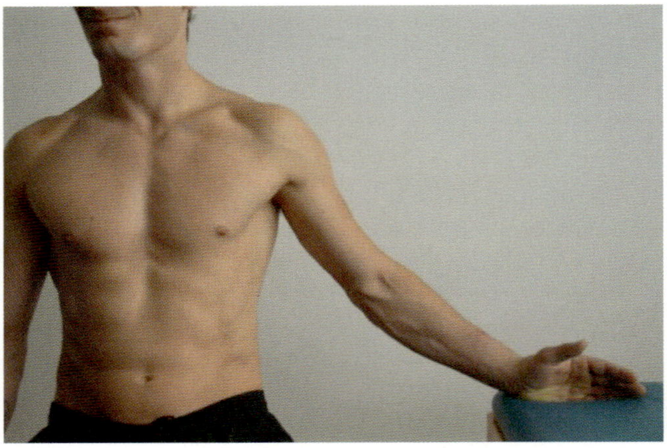

Fig. 3.80 Inferior glide

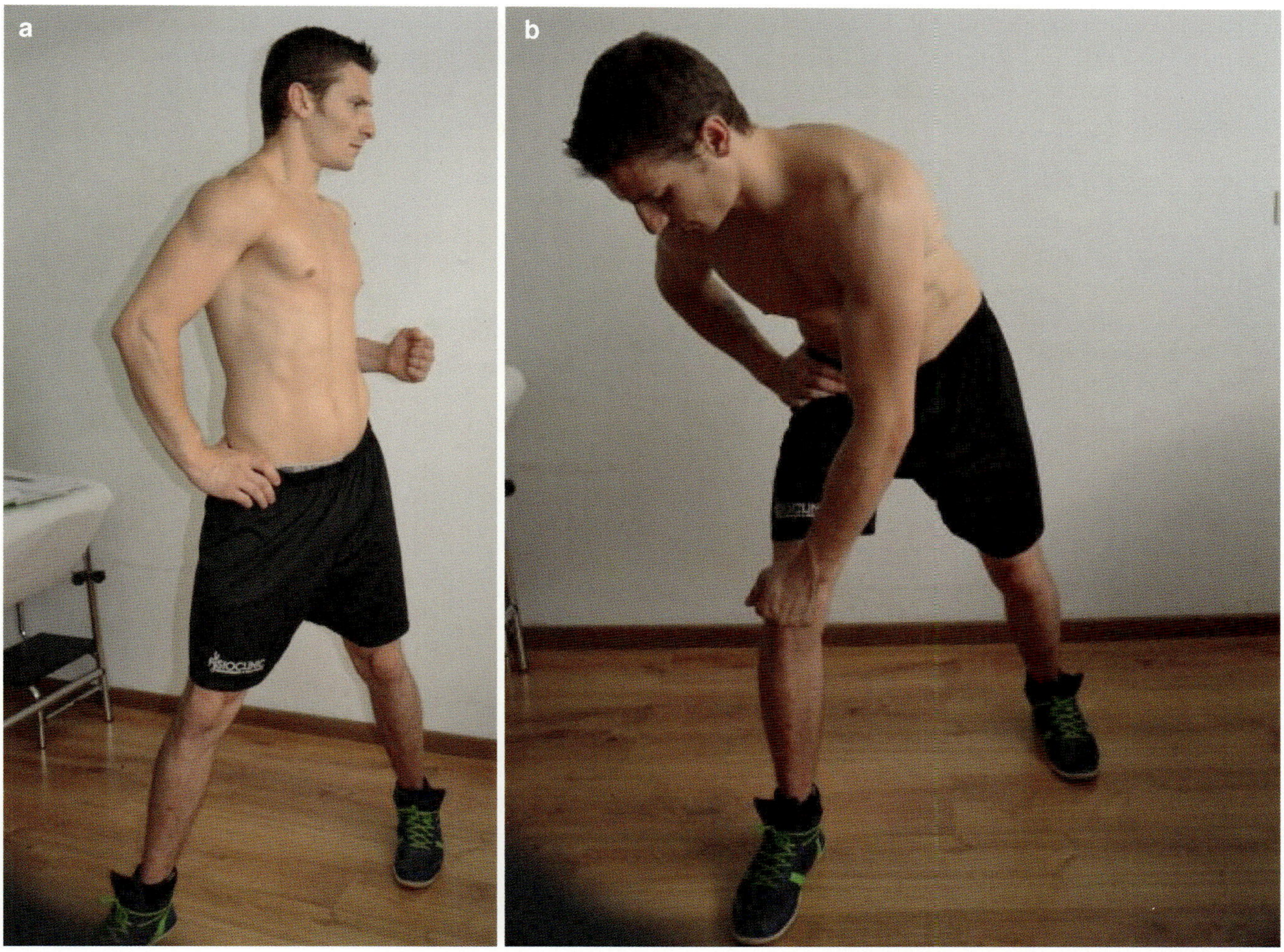

Fig. 3.81 (**a**) Initial position: scapular retraction exercise in closed kinetic chain. (**b**) Lawnmower final position

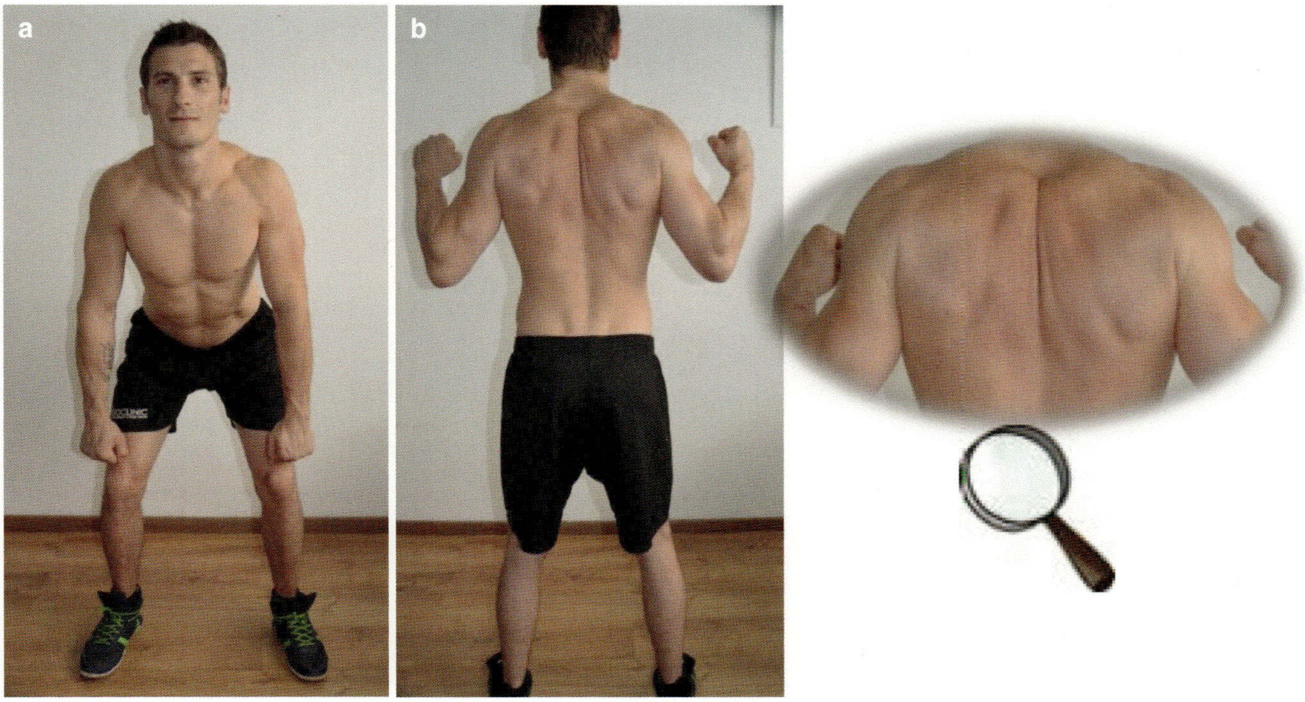

Fig. 3.82 (**a**) Robbery → Start position. (**b**) Robbery → Final position

To begin with, gentle but very useful neuromuscular control exercises can be implemented, starting from the supine position to avoid activation of the upper trapezius as explaned in chapter one.

- The involved limb must be supported by a small towel (Fig. 3.83a) so as to obtain the right glenohumeral mechanical position in the scapular plane.
  With the elbow at 90° and with the hand tightly closed, the patient is asked to push back against the force applied by the physiotherapist all along the forearm (Fig. 3.83b). Obviously, this exercise must be done under the patient's pain threshold.
  Exercise difficulty will be gradually increased. Based on the patient's improved response, the exercise will be increased in terms of resistance applied, proprioceptive response, and the adoption of different arm positions in different planes (Fig. 3.83c)
- Physioball isometric contraction to promote proprioceptive awareness. The exercise comprises a systematic movement management and control pattern that can be carried out eliminating visual feedback (with eyes closed) and flexing the knees to increase kinetic chain energy (Fig. 3.84).

Take-Home Message

- Between the 6th and 12th weeks, increasingly subscapular split and coracoid healing take place. From this moment, we can begin to strain these structures by biomechanical point of view.

Take-Home Message

It is important to perform the exercises with the arm abducted at around 20° to the scapular plane to ensure the best biomechanical alignment.

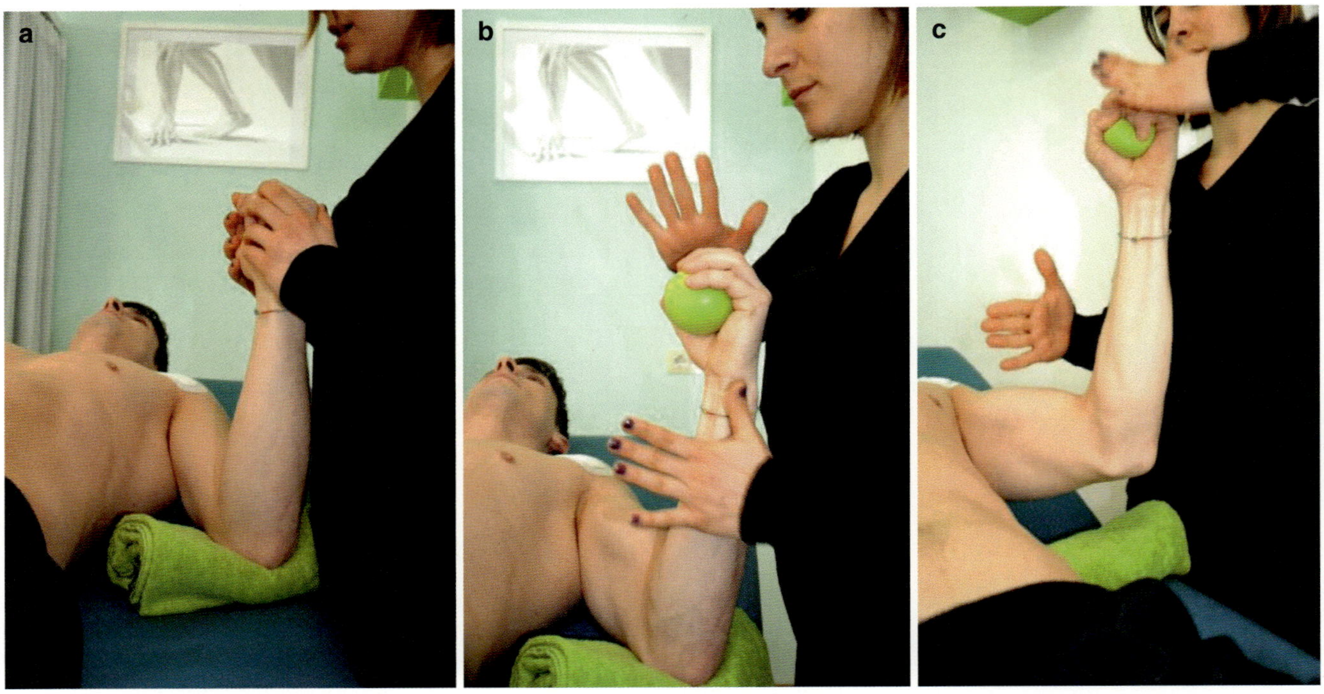

Fig. 3.83 (**a–c**) Progressively more difficult proprioceptive exercises with the arm unsupported in space

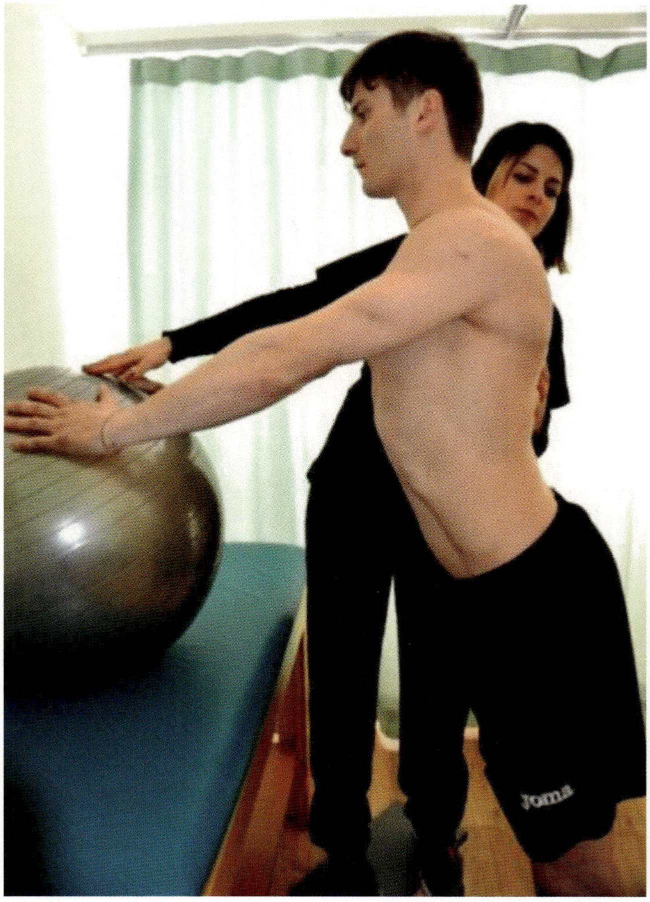

Fig. 3.84 Physioball isometric contraction

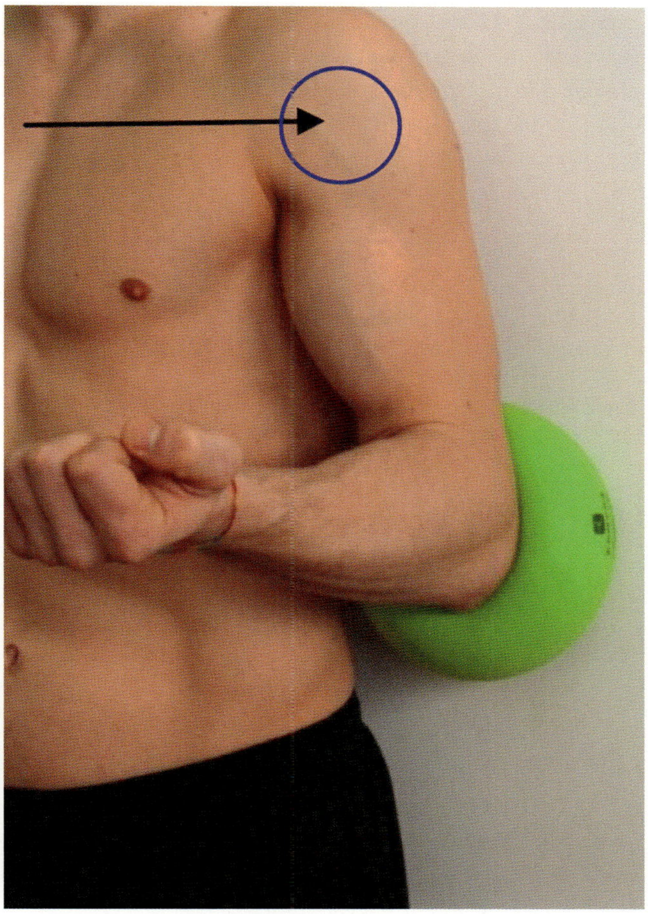

Fig. 3.85 Ball squeeze exercises

Phase II: 9–12 Weeks

After the 9th week, if the patient has acquired joint mobility of no less than 90° in passive-active elevation on the scapular plane, in the total absence of pain, he may pass to the next protocol phase.

Goals	How to do
Respect patient's biological healing rate	Continue cryotherapy as required
Progressively increase both active and passive ROM recovery	Passive, self-assisted and gradually active mobilization
Emphasize exercising the lower trapezius, the middle trapezius, and the serratus anterior to increase scapular retraction and establish muscular balance	Emphasize the scapulo thoracic muscles
	Exercises in side-lying position with and without external rotation to recruit middle and lower trapezius (Figs. 3.87 and 3.88)
	Isometric exercises with or without the application of force
	Prone exercises to improve lower and middle trapezius (Fig. 3.89)
Proprioceptive recovery	Flex bar

- *PROM and AROM Recovery*: Passive and active ROM must be continued throughout the second phase with self-assisted mobilization, stretching by the therapist and active exercises above 90° elevation (Fig. 3.86a, b).
- *Enhance/Ensure Adequate Scapular Function*: Equally important to strengthen the scapulothoracic muscles is the exercise of scapula closure, or pinch, shown in (Fig. 3.86a, b). The patient lies on his side with a towel support under the upper arm to maintain the correct shoulder joint position [159] and close the scapula. The patient is facilitated in his movements by the gravity-free side-lying position. In addition, De Mey et al. [160] have shown that this position inhibits the upper trapezius, instead specifically recruiting the middle and lower fibers of the muscle in order to maintain correct stabilization.

Ludewig et al. [161] further confirm the validity of these exercises, reporting the significantly different activation of the upper trapezius and the serratus anterior in the CKC push-up plus exercise (Fig. 3.90). In the plus phase – when the patient flexes his elbows to move toward the wall and in so doing pinches his scapulae – all the muscle fibers of the serratus anterior are maximally engaged.

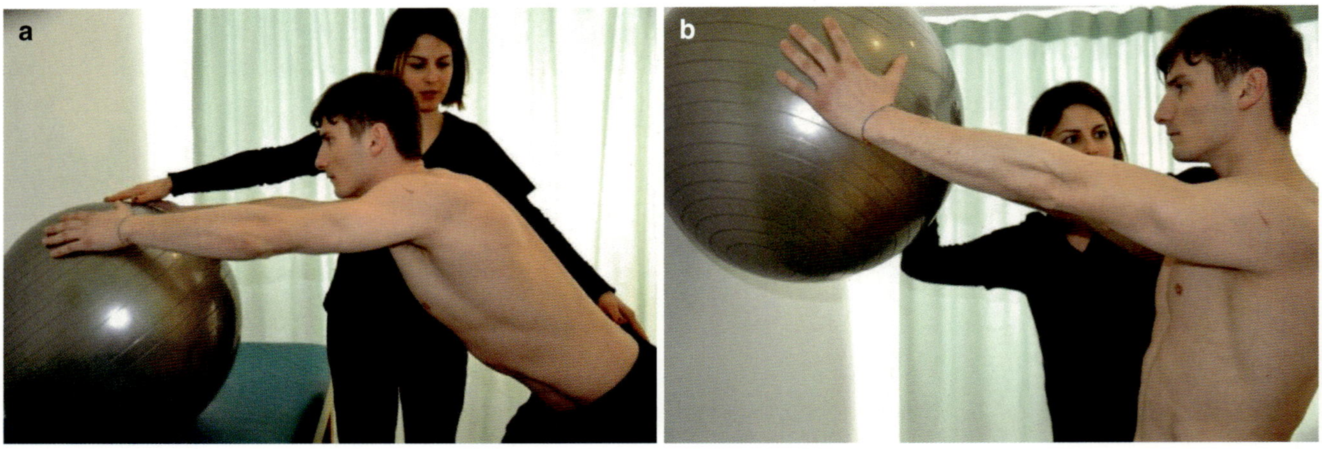

Fig. 3.86 (**a**, **b**) Gradual recovery of shoulder joint arc of motion

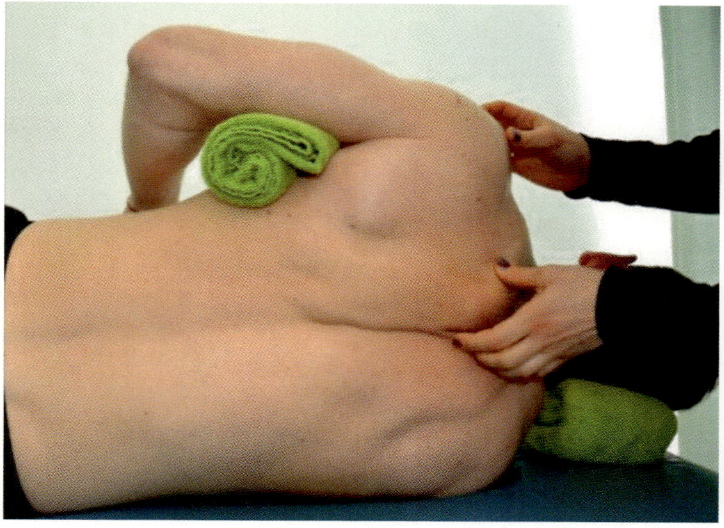

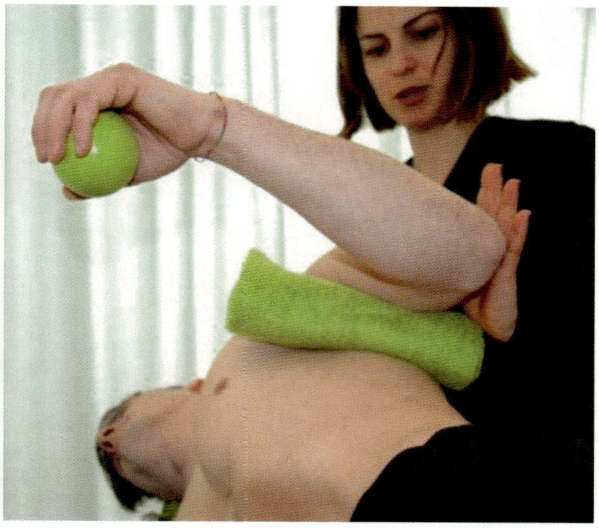

Figs. 3.87 and 3.88 Side-lying position with selective activation of the lower and middle trapezius (Fig. 3.87); subsequently combined with external rotation (Fig. 3.88)

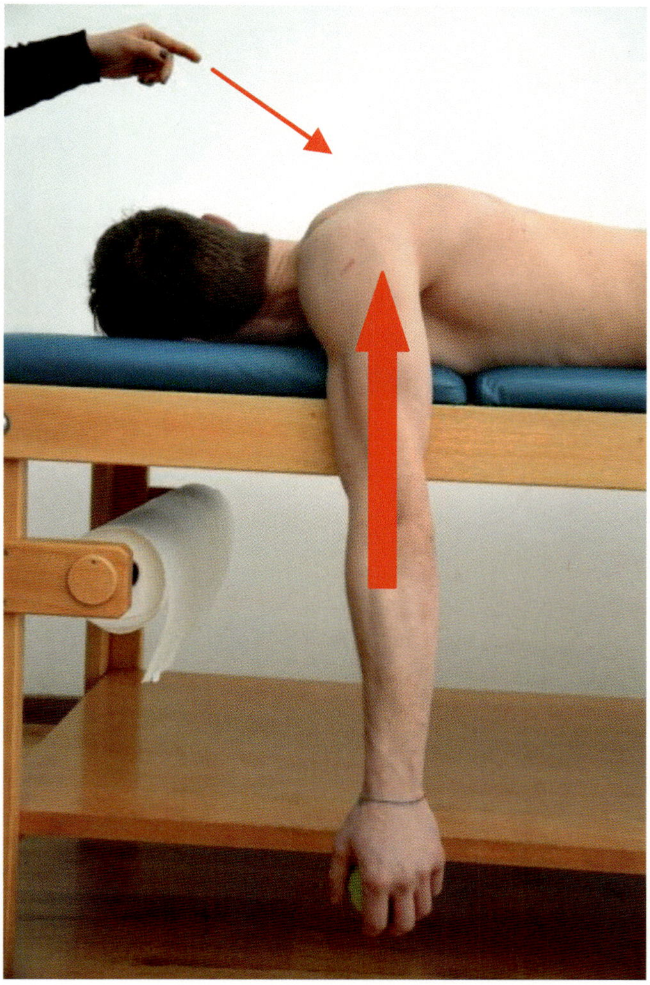

Fig. 3.89 Full lower and middle trapezius activation

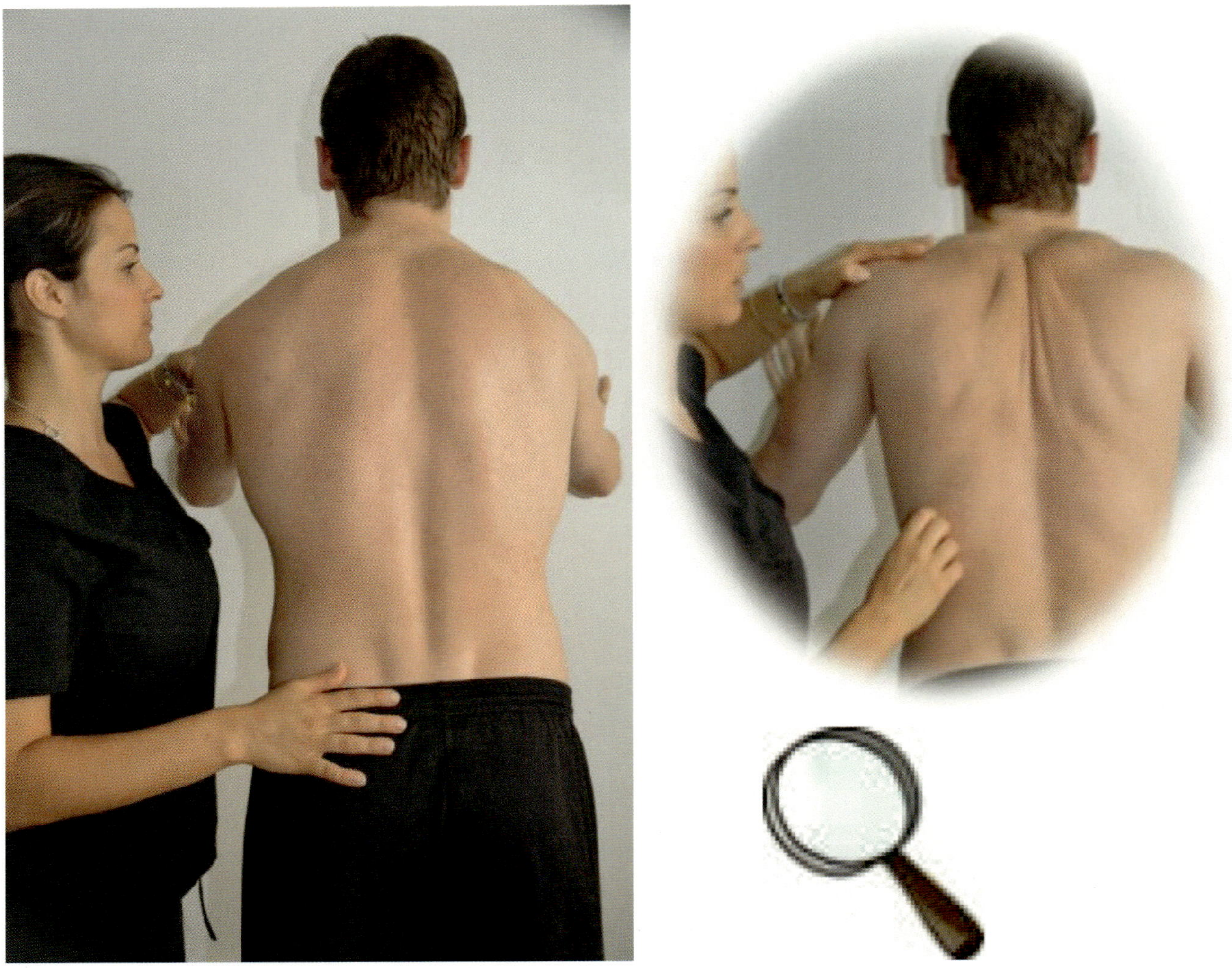

Fig. 3.90 Wall push-up plus

Phase III: 12 Weeks to Sports Integration

The third clinical check-up is carried out at the outset of phase 3. The physiotherapist should take in consideration that bone-to-bone healing takes place in the third month. The surgeon must verify that full ROM is no less than 90 % of the contralateral side before authorizing gradual and progressive return to the specific athletic movement. In fact the shoulder must not be considered as a single isolated muscle set but as an integral part of a kinetic chain activated by a simple but sophisticated system of concentric rings that are activated distally and subsequently recruit all – even the smallest – proximal muscle fibers [149, 150]. It follows that this phase should only be initiated in patients who have developed good neuromuscular control and have completed the CKC exercises, together with other simple OKC movements like lawnmower and robbery (Figs. 3.81a, b and 3.82a, b) before passing to the OKC exercises of phase 3.

Goals	How to do
Improve range of motion and regain Full ROM	Active stretching assisted by physiotherapist and self-assisted (Fig. 3.91)
	Sleeper stretch exercise (Fig. 3.92)
	Stretch of the anterior structure to avoid stiffness
	Wall slide exercise (Fig. 3.93)
Improve muscular balance	Wall push-up plus (Fig. 3.90)
	Unilateral serratus anterior punch (Fig. 3.94)
Improve proprioception and muscular stability	Integrated elastic exercises
	Integrated weight exercises

- *Enhance/Ensure Adequate Scapular Function*: In phase 3 the patient is free to move his arm on any plane. Having regained ROM (90°), the goal is now to allow the patient to return to his particular sports activity, which will only be possible, however, if muscle strength and neuro-proprioceptive control has been reinstated completely during the previous phases. Hardwick et al. show how certain exercises can specifically activate the fibers of the serratus anterior in positions over 90° ROM.

  A perfect example of a closed kinetic chain exercise involving maximum activation of the serratus anterior is the wall slide (Fig. 3.93). With arms in the scapular plane, the patient slides his hands slightly outward against the wall. Hardwick et al. [162] have shown how this exercise is completely painless because carried out in CKC and has the advantage of especially activating the lower trapezius.
- *Progressive Return to Sports Activity and Final Clinical Check-Up at 6 Months*: The final rehabilitation period includes sports-specific activity involving more intense strengthening of pertinent districts, to be decided by the specialist training team, taking into account the surgery undergone by the athlete and the resultant strength and neuromuscular deficit.

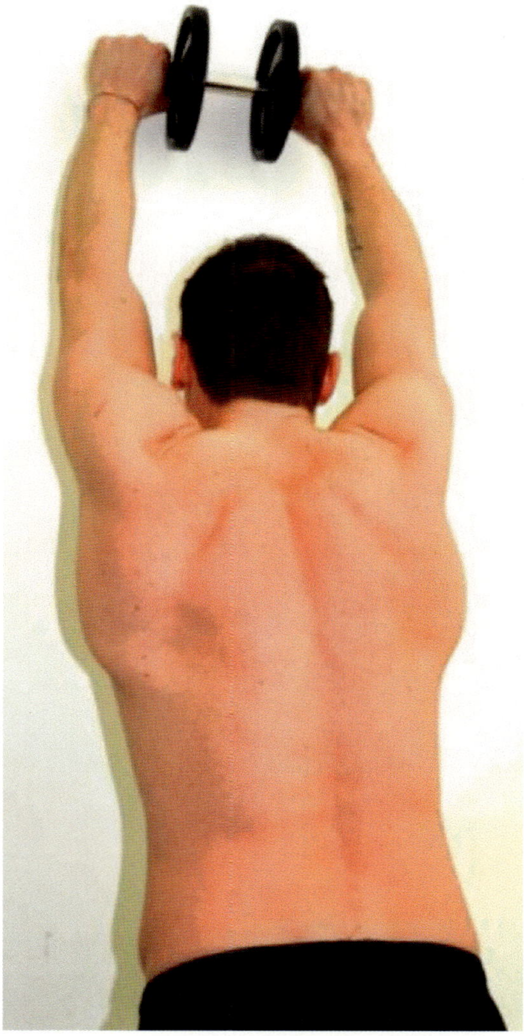

Fig. 3.91 Improve stretching

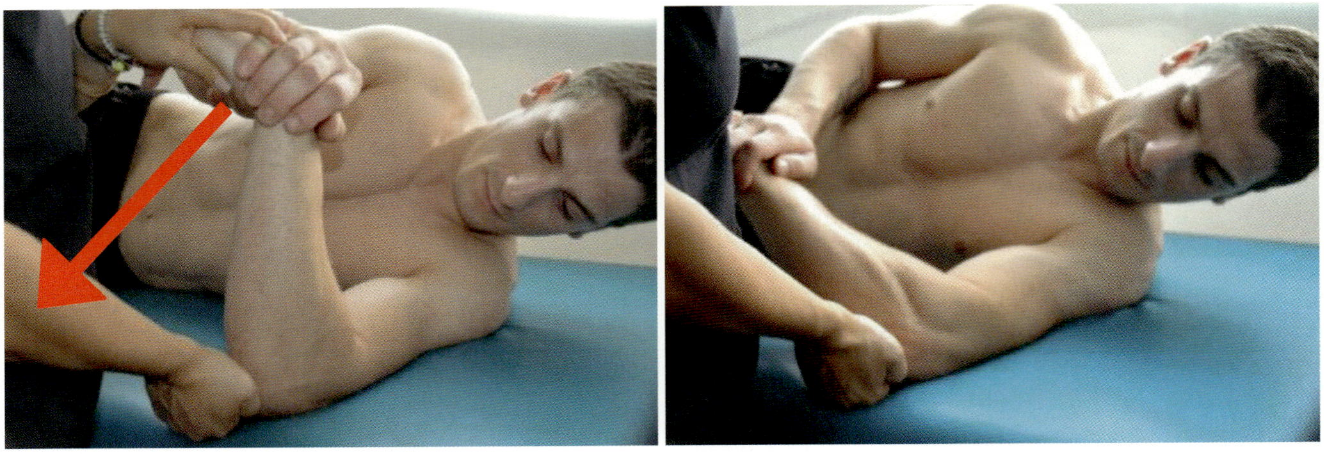

Fig. 3.92 Sleeper stretch

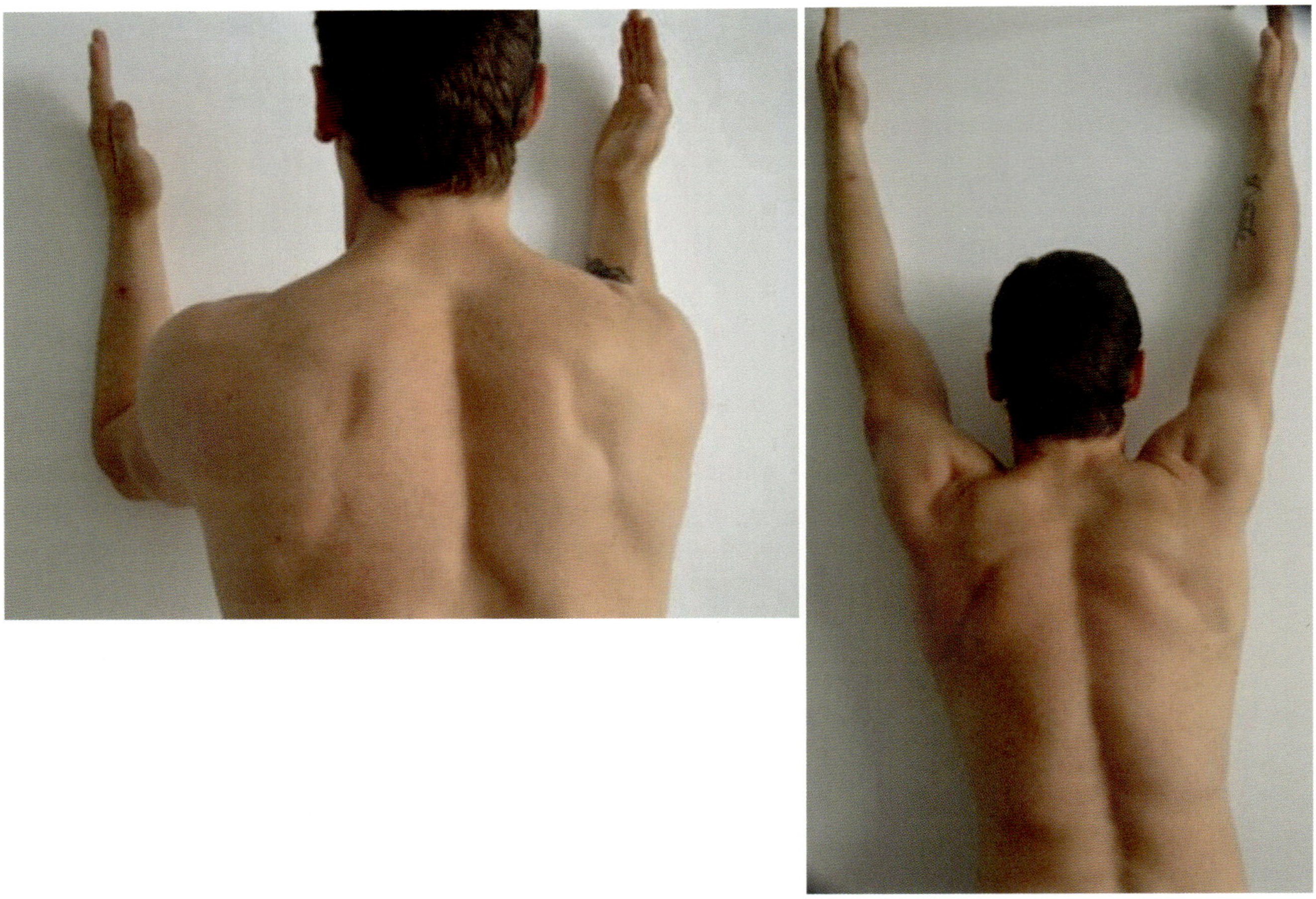

Fig. 3.93 Wall Slide

Fig. 3.94 Variation of the bilateral serratus anterior punch as proposed by Reinold

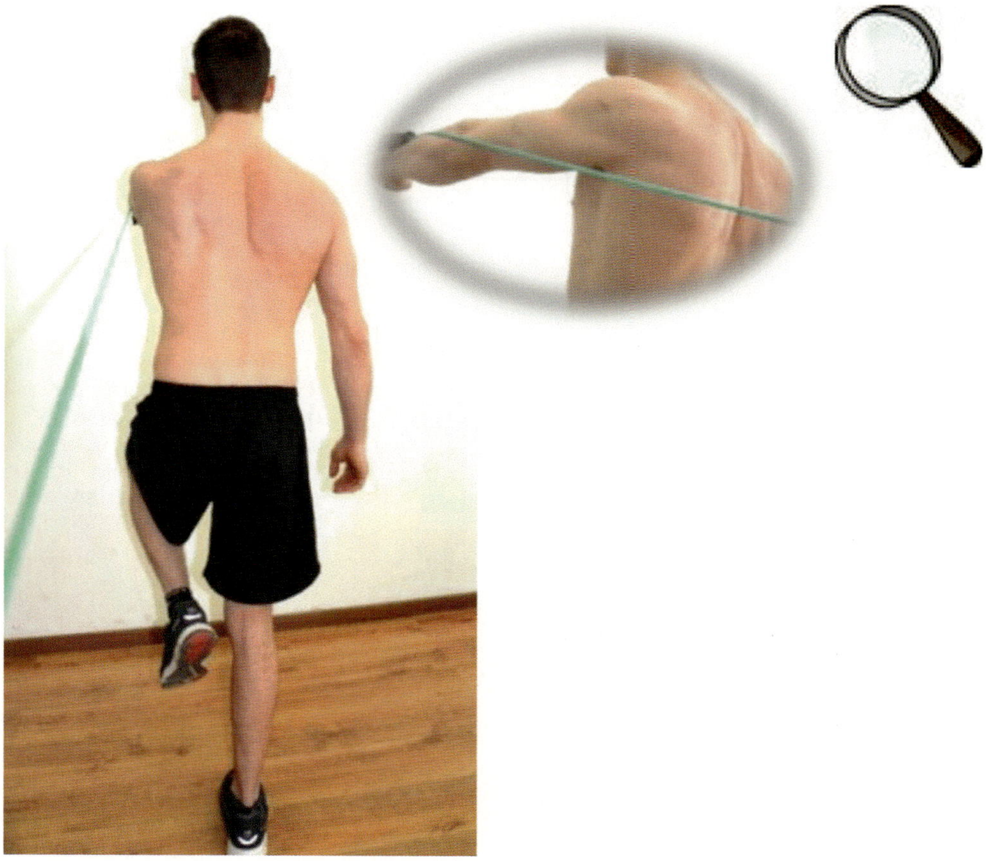

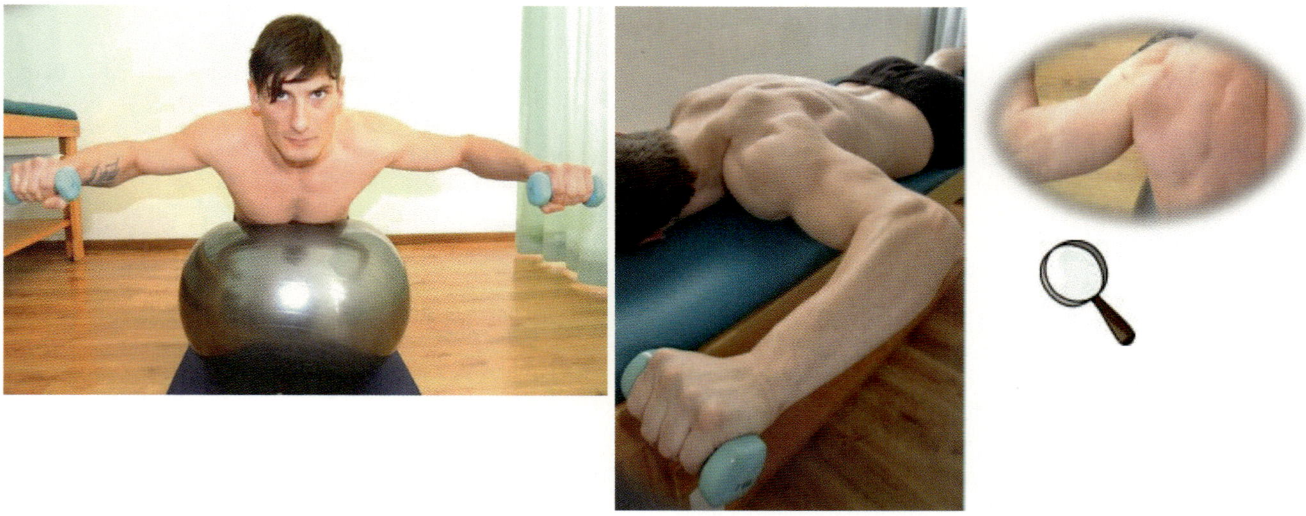

Fig. 3.95 Prone position on the ball to activate the scapular muscles thanks to neuromuscular activation on account of ball-induced core instability

References

1. Saha AK (1983) Mechanism of shoulder movements and a plea for the recognition of "zero position" of glenohumeral joint. Clin Orthop 173:3–10
2. Neumann DA (2002) Kinesiology of the musculoskeletal system: foundations for physical rehabilitation. Mosby, St Louis
3. Kapandji IA (1985) The physiology of the joints. Upper extremity. Churchill Livingstone, Philadelphia
4. Ellenbecker TS (2006) Shoulder rehabilitation: non-operative treatment. Thieme, New York
5. Inman VT, Saunders JB, Abbott LC (1944) Observations on the function of the shoulder joint. J Bone Joint Surg 26(1):1–30
6. Weiner DS, MacNab I (1970) Superior migration of the humeral head. J Bone Joint Surg Br 52:524–527
7. Burkhart SS, Morgan CD, Kibler WB (2003) The disabled throwing shoulder: spectrum of pathology Part I: pathoanatomy and biomechanics. Arthroscopy 19(4):404–420
8. Bagg SD, Forrest WJ (1988) A biomechanical analysis of scapular rotation during arm abduction in the scapular plane. Arch Phys Med Rehabil 67:238–245
9. Hsu AT, Chang JH, Chang CH (2002) Determining the resting position of the glenohumeral joint: a cadaver study. J Orthop Sports Phys Ther 32(12):605–612
10. Kaltenborn FM (1989) Manual mobilization of the extremity joints. Olaf Norlis Bokhandel, Oslo
11. Magee DJ (2009) Orthopaedic physical assessment, 5th edn. Saunders, St Louis
12. Abboud JA, Soslowsky LJ (2002) Interplay of the static and dynamic restraints in glenohumeral instability. Clin Orthop Relat Res 400:48–57
13. Itoi E, Morrey BF, An KN (2009) Biomechanics of the shoulder. In: Rockwood C Jr, Matsen FA III, Wirth MA, Lippitt SB (eds) The shoulder, 4th edn. Saunders/Elsevier, Philadelphia, pp 213–265
14. Itoi E (2004) Pathophysiology and treatment of a traumatic instability of the shoulder. J Orthop Sci 9(2):208–213
15. Boileau P, Villalba M, Héry JY, Balg F, Ahrens P, Neyton L (2006) Risk factors for recurrence of shoulder instability after arthroscopic Bankart repair. J Bone Joint Surg Am 88:1755–1763
16. Mologne TS, McBride MT, Lapoint JM (1997) Assessment of failed arthroscopic anterior labral repairs. Findings at open surgery. Am J Sports Med 25:813–817
17. Calandra JJ, Baker CL, Uribe J (1989) The incidence of Hill-Sachs lesions in initial anterior shoulder dislocations. Arthroscopy 5(4):254–257
18. Rowe CR, Zarins B, Ciullo JV (1984) Recurrent anterior dislocation of the shoulder after surgical repair. Apparent causes of failure and treatment. J Bone Joint Surg Am 66:159–168
19. Hill HA, Sachs MD (1940) The groove defect of the humeral head. A frequently unrecognized complication of dislocations of the shoulder joint. Radiology 35:690–700
20. Bigliani LU, Newton PM, Steinmann SP, Connor PM, McIlveen SJ (1998) Glenoid rim lesions associated with recurrent anterior dislocation of the shoulder. Am J Sports Med 26:41–45
21. Rowe CR, Patel D, Southmayd WW (1978) The Bankart procedure: a long-term end-result study. J Bone Joint Surg Am 60:1–16
22. Ungersböck A, Michel M, Hertel R (1995) Factors influencing the results of a modified Bankart procedure. J Shoulder Elbow Surg 4:365–369
23. Richards RD, Sartoris DJ, Pathria MN, Resnick D (1994) Hill-Sachs lesion and normal humeral groove: MR imaging features allowing their differentiation. Radiology 190(3):665–668
24. Armitage MS, Faber KJ, Drosdowech DS, Litchfield RB, Athwal GS (2010) Humeral head bone defects: remplissage, allograft, and arthroplasty. Orthop Clin North Am 41(3):417–425
25. Bankart ASB (1923) Recurrent or habitual dislocation of the shoulder joint. BMJ 2:1132–1133
26. Henry JH, Genung JA (1982) Natural history of glenohumeral dislocation: revisited. Am J Sports Med 10:135–137
27. Hovelius L, Eriksson K, Fredin H et al (1983) Recurrences after initial dislocation of the shoulder: results of a prospective study of treatment. J Bone Joint Surg Am 65:343–349
28. Kralinger FS, Golser K, Wischatta R, Wambacher M, Sperner G (2002) Predicting recurrence after primary anterior shoulder dislocation. Am J Sports Med 30:116–120
29. Norlin R (1994) Use of Mitek anchoring for Bankart repair: a comparable, randomized, prospective study with traditional bone sutures. J Shoulder Elbow Surg 3:381–385
30. Townley CO (1950) The capsular mechanism in recurrent dislocation of the shoulder. J Bone Joint Surg Am 32:370–380
31. Burkhart SS, De Beer JF (2000) Traumatic glenohumeral bone defects and their relationship to failure of arthroscopic Bankart repairs: significance of the inverted-pear glenoid and the humeral engaging Hill-Sachs lesion. Arthroscopy 16:677–694
32. Griffith JF, Antonio GE, Tong CWC, Ming CK (2003) Anterior shoulder dislocation: quantification of glenoid bone loss with CT. AJR Am J Roentgenol 180:1423–1430
33. Singson RD, Feldman F, Bigliani L (1987) CT arthrographic patterns in recurrent glenohumeral instability. AJR Am J Roentgenol 149:749–753
34. Fujii Y, Yoneda M, Wakitani S et al (2006) Histologic analysis of bony Bankart lesions in recurrent anterior instability of the shoulder. J Shoulder Elbow Surg 15:218–223
35. Baudi P, Righi P, Bolognesi D et al (2005) How to identify and calculate glenoid bone deficit. Chir Organi Mov 90:145–152
36. Sugaya H, Moriishi J, Dohi M et al (2003) Glenoid rim morphology in recurrent anterior glenohumeral instability. J Bone Joint Surg Am 85:878–884
37. d'Elia G, Di Giacomo A, D'Alessandro P et al (2008) Traumatic anterior glenohumeral instability: quantification of glenoid bone loss by spiral CT. Radiol Med 113:496–503
38. Flower WH (1861) On the pathological changes produced in the shoulder-joint by traumatic dislocation, as derived from an examination of all the specimens illustrating this injury in the museums of London. Trans Pathol Soc London 12:17–201
39. Eve FS (1880) A case of sub-coracoid dislocation of the humerus, with the formation of an indentation on the posterior surface of the head, the joint being unopened; with remarks on the mode of production of fracture of the anatomical neck, with dislocation. Med Chir Trans 63:317–321
40. Hermodsson I (1934) Rontgenologischestudienuber die traumatischen und habituellen schultergelenkverrenkungen nach vom und nach unten. Acta Radiol Suppl 20:1–173
41. Neer CS, Rockwood CA (1984) Fracture;-and dislocations of the shoulder. In: Rockwood CA, Green EP (eds) Fractures in adults. J.B. Lippincott, Philadelphia, pp 675–985
42. Čičak N, Bilić R, Delimar D (1998) Hill-Sachs lesion in recurrent shoulder dislocation: sonographic detection. J Ultrasound Med 17:557–560
43. Itoi E, Yamamoto N, Kurokawa D, Sano H (2013) Bone loss in anterior instability. Curr Rev Musculoskelet Med 6(1):88–94
44. Owens BD, Nelson BJ, Duffey ML, Mountcastle SB, Taylor DC, Cameron KL, Campbell S, DeBerardino TM (2010) Pathoanatomy of first-time, traumatic, anterior glenohumeral subluxation events. J Bone Joint Surg Am 92(7):1605–1611
45. Cetik O, Uslu M, Ozsar BK (2007) The relationship between Hill-Sachs lesion and recurrent anterior shoulder dislocation. Acta Orthop Belg 73(2):175–178
46. Yamamoto N, Itoi E, Abe H et al (2007) Contact between the glenoid and the humeral head in abduction, external rotation, and

horizontal extension: a new concept of glenoid track. J Shoulder Elbow Surg 16:649–656
47. Di Giacomo G, Itoi E, Burkhart S (2014) Evolving concept of bipolar bone loss and the Hill-Sachs lesion: from "engaging/non-engaging" lesion to "on-track/off-track" lesion. Arthroscopy 30(1):90–98
48. Metzger PD, Barlow B, Leonardelli D, Peace W, Solomon DJ, Provencher MT (2013) Clinical application of the "glenoid track" concept for defining humeral head engagement in anterior shoulder instability. Orthop J Sports Med 1(2):1–7
49. Kaar SG, Fening SD, Jones MH, Colbrunn RW, Miniaci A (2010) Effect of humeral head defect size on glenohumeral stability: a cadaveric study of simulated Hill-Sachs defects. Am J Sports Med 38:594–599
50. Sekiya JK, Wickwire AC, Stehle JH, Debski RE (2009) Hill-Sachs defects and repair using osteoarticular allograft transplantation: biomechanical analysis using a joint compression model. Am J Sports Med 37:2459–2466
51. Cho SH, Cho NS, Rhee YG (2011) Preoperative analysis of the Hill-Sachs lesion in anterior shoulder instability: how to predict engagement of the lesion. Am J Sports Med 39:2389
52. Warner JJP, Gerber C, Itoi E, Lafosse L (2013) Shoulder instability: an international perspective on treatment. ICL 107. Presented at the 2013 annual meeting of the American Academy of Orthopaedic Surgeons, Chicago, March 2013
53. Provencher MT, Abrams JS, Boileau P, Ryu RKN, Tokish JM (2013) Challenging problems in shoulder instability: how to get it right the first time and what to do if you don't. ICL 282. Presented at the 2013 annual meeting of the American Academy of Orthopaedic Surgeons, Chicago, March 2013
54. Kurokawa D, Yamamoto N, Nagamoto H et al (2013) The prevalence of a large Hill-Sachs lesion that needs to be treated. J Shoulder Elbow Surg 22:1285–1289
55. Kelkar R, Wang VM, Flatow EL et al (2001) Glenohumeral mechanics. A study of articular geometry, contact, and kinematics. J Shoulder Elbow Surg 10:73–84
56. Kirkley A, Werstine R, Ratjek A, Griffin S (2005) Prospective randomized clinical trial comparing the effectiveness of immediate arthroscopic stabilization versus immobilization and rehabilitation in first traumatic anterior dislocations of the shoulder: long-term evaluation. Arthroscopy 21(1):55–63
57. Bottoni CR, Wilckens JH, DeBerardino TM et al (2002) A prospective, randomized evaluation of arthroscopic stabilization versus nonoperative treatment in patients with acute, traumatic, first-time shoulder dislocations. Am J Sports Med 30:576–580
58. Jones KJ, Wiesel B, Ganley TJ, Wells L (2007) Functional outcomes of early arthroscopic Bankart repair in adolescents aged 11 to 18 years. J Pediatr Orthop 27:209–213
59. Hovelius L, Augustini BG, Fredin H, Johansson O, Norlin R, Thorling J (1996) Primary anterior dislocation of the shoulder in young patients. A ten year prospective study. J Bone Joint Surg Am 78:1677–1684
60. Aronen JG, Regan K (1984) Decreasing the incidence of recurrence of first time anterior shoulder dislocations with rehabilitation. Am J Sports Med 12:283–291
61. Deitch J, Mehlman CT, Foad SL, Obbehat A, Mallory M (2003) Traumatic anterior shoulder dislocation in adolescents. Am J Sports Med 31:758–763
62. Rowe CR (1980) Acute and recurrent anterior dislocation of the shoulder. Orthop Clin North Am 11:253–270
63. Simonet WT, Melton LJ, Cofield RH, Iltrup DM (1984) Incidence of anterior shoulder dislocation in Olmsted County, Minn. Clin Orthop Relat Res 186:186
64. Kim D-S, Yoon Y-S, Yi CH (2010) Prevalence comparison of accompanying lesions between primary and recurrent anterior dislocation in the shoulder. Am J Sports Med 38:2071
65. Balg F, Boileau P (2007) The instability severity index score. A simple pre-operative score to select patients for arthroscopic or open shoulder stabilisation. J Bone Joint Surg Br 89-B:1470–1477
66. Broca A, Hartmann H (1890) Contribution a l'étude des luxations d'épaule (luxations dites incomplětes, décollements périostiques, luxations directes et luxations indirectes). Bull Soc Anat 4:312–336
67. Delorme DHD (1910) Die Hemmungsbaender des Schultergelenks und ihre Bedeutung fuer die Schulterluxationen. Arch Klein Chir 92:72–101
68. Taylor DC, Arciero RA (1997) Pathologic changes associated with shoulder dislocations: arthroscopic and physical examination findings in first time, traumatic anterior dislocations. Am J Sports Med 25(3):306–311
69. Purchase RJ, Wolf EM, Hobgood ER, Pollock ME, Smalley CC (2008) Hill-Sachs "remplissage": an arthroscopic solution for the engaging Hill-Sachs lesion. Arthroscopy 24:723–726
70. Boileau P, O'Shea K, Vargas P, Pinedo M, Old J, Zumstein M (2012) Anatomical and functional results after arthroscopic Hill-Sachs remplissage. J Bone Joint Surg Am 94:618–626
71. Haviv B, Mayo L, Biggs D (2011) Outcomes of arthroscopic "remplissage": capsulotenodesis of the engaging large Hill-Sachs lesion. J Orthop Surg Res 6:29
72. Koo SS, Burkhart SS, Ochoa E (2009) Arthroscopic double pulley remplissage technique for engaging Hill-Sachs lesions in anterior shoulder instability repairs. Arthroscopy 25:1343–1348
73. Nourissat G, Kilinc AS, Werther JR, Doursounian L (2011) A prospective, comparative, radiological, and clinical study of the influence of the "remplissage" procedure on shoulder range of motion after stabilization by arthroscopic Bankart repair. Am J Sports Med 39:2147–2152
74. Park MJ, Garcia G, Malhotra A, Major N, Tjoumakaris FP, Kelly JDIV (2012) The evaluation of arthroscopic remplissage by high-resolution magnetic resonance imaging. Am J Sports Med 40:2331–2336
75. Park MJ, Tjoumakaris FP, Garcia G, Patel A, Kelly JD IV (2011) Arthroscopic remplissage with Bankart repair for the treatment of glenohumeral instability with Hill-Sachs defects. Arthroscopy 27:1187–1194
76. Zhu YM, Lu Y, Zhang J, Shen JW, Jiang CY (2011) Arthroscopic Bankart repair combined with remplissage technique for the treatment of anterior shoulder instability with engaging Hill-Sachs lesion: a report of 49 cases with a minimum 2-year follow-up. Am J Sports Med 39:1640–1647
77. Priest JD, Nagel DA (1976) Tennis shoulder. Am J Sports Med 4(1):28–42
78. Young SW, Dakic J, Stroia K, Nguyen NL, Harris AHS, Safran MR (2004) High incidence of infraspinatus muscle atrophy in elite professional female tennis players. Am J Sports Med 43(8):1989–1993
79. Safran M (2004) Nerve injury about the shoulder in athletes, part 1. Am J Sports Med 32(3):803–819
80. Piatt BE, Hawkins RJ, Fritz RC, Ho CP, Wolf E, Schickendantz M (2002) Clinical evaluation and treatment of spinoglenoid notch ganglion cysts. J Shoulder Elbow Surg 11:600–604
81. Kibler WB, Uhl TL, Maddux JW, Brooks PV, Zeller B, McMullen J (2002) Qualitative clinical evaluation of scapular dysfunction: a reliability study. J Shoulder Elbow Surg 11:550–556
82. McMahon PJ, Jobe FW, Pink MM, Brault JR, Perry J (1996) Comparative electromyographic analysis of shoulder muscles during planar motions: anterior instability versus normal. J Shoulder Elbow Surg 5:118–123
83. Kibler WB (1998) The role of the scapula in athletic shoulder function. Am J Sports Med 26:325–337
84. Wilk KE, Reinold MM, Macrina LC, Porterfield R, Devine KM, Suarez K, Andrews JR (2009) Glenohumeral internal rotation measurements differ depending on stabilization techniques. Sports Health 1(2):131–136

85. Ellenbecker TS, Roetert EP, Piorkowski PA, Schulz DA (1996) Glenohumeral joint internal and external rotation range of motion in elite junior tennis players. J Orthop Sports Phys Ther 24:336–341
86. McFarland EG, Torpey BM, Carl LA (1996) Evaluation of shoulder laxity. Sports Med 22:264–272
87. Pagnani MJ, Warren RF (1994) Stabilizers of the glenohumeral joint. J Shoulder Elbow Surg 3:73–90
88. O'Brien SJ, Neves MC, Arnvoczky SP et al (1990) The anatomy and histology of the inferior glenohumeral ligament complex of the shoulder. Am J Sports Med 18:449–456
89. Hawkins RJ, Mohtadi NGH (1991) Clinical evaluation of shoulder instability. Clin J Sports Med 1:59–64
90. Gerber C, Ganz R (1984) Clinical assessment of instability of the shoulder with special reference to anterior and posterior drawer tests. J Bone Joint Surg Br 66(4):551–556
91. Altchek DW, Dines DW (1993) The surgical treatment of anterior instability: selective capsular repair. Oper Tech Sports Med 1:285–292
92. Hawkins RJ, Schulte JP, Janda DH, Huckell GH (1996) Translation of the glenohumeral joint with the patient under anesthesia. J Shoulder Elbow Surg 5:286–292
93. Ellenbecker TS, Bailie DS, Mattalino AJ et al (2002) Intrarater and interrater reliability of a manual technique to assess anterior humeral head translation of the glenohumeral joint. J Shoulder Elbow Surg 11(5):470–475
94. Carter C, Wilkinson J (1964) Persistent joint laxity and congenital dislocation of the hip. J Bone Joint Surg Br 46:40–45
95. Beighton P, Horan F (1969) Orthopaedic aspects of the Ehlers-Danlos syndrome. J Bone Joint Surg Br 51(3):444–453
96. Juul-Kristensen B, Rogind H, Jensen DV, Remvig L (2007) Inter-examiner reproducibility of tests and critera for generalized joint hypermobility and benign joint hypermobility syndrome. Rheumatology (Oxford) 46(12):1835–1841
97. Cameron KL, Duffey ML, DeBerardino TM, Stoneman PD, Jones CJ, Owens BD (2010) Association of generalized joint hypermobility with a history of glenohumeral joint instability. J Athl Train 45(3):253–258
98. Ellenbecker TS & Davies GJ (2016) Current Concepts in Rehabilitation of Rotator Cuff Pathology: Non-Operative and Post-Operative Considerations Orthopaedic Knowledge Update: Sports Medicine 5, Miller M (ed): American Academy of Orthopaedic Surgeons, Rosemont, IL
99. Ellenbecker TS, Manske RC, Kelley MJ (2011) The shoulder: physical therapy patient management utilizing current evidence. In: Current concepts of orthopaedic physical therapy, 3rd edn. Orthopaedic Section APTA, LaCrosse
100. Black KP, Lim TH, McGrady LM, Raasch W (1997) In vitro evaluation of shoulder external rotation after a Bankart reconstruction. Am J Sports Med 25:449–453
101. Penna J, Deramo D, Nelson CO, Sileo MJ, Levin SM, Tompkins B, Ianuzzi A (2008) Determination of anterior labral repair stress during passive arm motion in a cadaveric model. Arthroscopy 24(8):930–935
102. Fleck SJ, Kraemer WJ (1987) Designing resistance training programs. Human Kinetics Publishers, Champaign
103. Moseley JB Jr, Jobe FW, Pink M, Perry J, Tibone J (1992) EMG analysis of the scapular muscles during a shoulder rehabilitation program. Am J Sports Med 20(2):128–134
104. Decker MJ, Hintermeister RA, Faber KJ, Hawkins RJ (1999) Serratus anterior muscle activity during selected rehabilitation exercises. Am J Sports Med 27:784–791
105. Kibler WB, Sciascia AD, Uhl TL, Tambay N, Cunningham T (2008) Electromyographic analysis of specific exercise for the scapular control in early phases of shoulder rehabilitation. Am J Sports Med 36(9):1789–1798. Epub 9 May 2008
106. Tsuruike M, Ellenbecker TS (2015) Serratus anterior and lower trapezius muscle activities during multi-joint isotonic scapular exercises and isometric contractions. J Athl Train 50(2):199–210
107. Ekstrom RA, Donatelli RA, Soderberg GL (2003) Surface electromyographic analysis of exercises and serraturs anterior muscles. J Orthop Sports Phys Ther 33(5):247–258
108. Ellenbecker TS, Davies GJ (2000) The application of isokinetics in testing and rehabilitation of the shoulder complex. J Athl Train 35:338–350
109. Jensen BR, Sjogaard G, Bornmyr S, Arborelius M, Jørgensen K (1995) Intramuscular laser-Doppler flowmetry in the supraspinatus muscle during isometric contractions. Eur J Appl Physiol Occup Physiol 71:373–378
110. Rathbun JB, Macnab I (1970) The microvascular pattern of the rotator cuff. J Bone Joint Surg Br 52(3):540–553
111. Ellenbecker TS, Cools A (2010) Rehabilitation of shoulder impingement syndrome and rotator cuff injuries: an evidence based review. Br J Sports Med 44(55):319–327
112. Sakita K, Seeley MK, Myrer JW, Hopkins JT (2015) Shoulder-muscle electromyography during shoulder external rotation exercise with and without slight abduction. J Sport Rehabil 24:109–115
113. Malanga GA, Jenp YN, Growney ES, An KN (1996) EMG analysis of shoulder positioning in testing and strengthening the supraspinatus. Med Sci Sports Exerc 28(6):661–664
114. Ballantyne BT, O'Hare SJ, Paschall JL et al (1993) Electromyographic activity of selected shoulder muscles in commonly used therapeutic exercises. Phys Ther 73:668–677
115. Blackburn TA, McLeod WD, White B, Wofford L (1990) EMG analysis of posterior rotator cuff exercises. J Athl Train 25:40–45
116. Reinold MM, Wilk KE, Fleisig GS, Zheng N, Barrentine SW, Chmielewski T et al (2004) Electomyographic analysis of the rotator cuff and deltoid musculature during common shoulder external rotation exercises. J Orthop Sports Phys Ther 34(7):385–394
117. Townsend H, Jobe FW, Pink M, Perry J (1991) Electromyography analysis of glenohumeral muscles during a baseball rehabilitation program. Am J Sports Med 19(3):264–272
118. Wuelker N, Plitz W, Roetman B (1994) Biomechanical data concerning the shoulder impingement syndrome. Clin Orthop 303:242–249
119. Carter AB, Kaminsky TW, Douex AT Jr, Knight CA, Richards JG (2007) Effects of high volume upper extremity plyometric training on throwing velocity and functional strength ratios of the shoulder rotators in collegiate baseball players. J Strength Cond Res 21(1):208–215
120. Niederbracht Y, Shim AL, Sloniger MA, Paternostro-Bayles M, Short TH (2008) Effects of a shoulder injury prevention strength training program on eccentric external rotation muscle strength and glenohumeral joint imbalance in female overhead activity athletes. J Strength Cond Res 22(1):140–145
121. Moncrief SA, Lau JD, Gale JR, Scott SA (2002) Effect of rotator exercise on humeral rotation torque in healthy individuals. J Strength Cond Res 16(2):262–270
122. Ellenbecker TS, Davies GJ, Rowinski MJ (1988) Concentric versus eccentric isokinetic strengthening of the rotator cuff. Objective data versus functional test. Am J Sports Med 16(1):64–69
123. Graichen H, Hinterwimmer S, von Eisenhart-Rothe R, Vogl T, Englmeir K-H, Eckstein F (2005) Effect of abduction and adducting muscle activity on glenohumeral translation, scapular kinematics and subacromial space width in vivo. J Biomech 38(4): 755–760

124. Bitter NL, Clisby EF, Jones MA, Magarey ME, Jaberzadeh S, Sandow MJ (2007) Relative contributions of infraspinatous and deltoid during external rotation in healthy shoulders. J Shoulder Elbow Surg 16(5):563–568
125. Burkhart SS, Morgan CD (1998) The peel-back mechanism: its role in producing and extending posterior type II SLAP lesions and its effect on SLAP repair rehabilitation. Arthroscopy 14:637–640
126. Harryman DT, Sidles JA, Clark JM, Mcquade KJ, Gibb TD, Matsen FA (1990) Translation of the humeral head on the glenoid with passive glenohumeral joint motion. J Bone Joint Surg 72A(9):1334–1343
127. Matsen FA, Lippitt SB, Sidles JA, Harryman DT (1994) Practical evaluation and management of the shoulder. W.B. Saunders, Philadelphia
128. McCabe RA, Orishimo KF, McHugh MP, Nicholas SJ (2007) Surface electromyographic analysis of the lower trapezius muscle during exercises performed below ninety degrees of shoulder elevation in healthy subject. N Am J Sports Phys Ther 2(1):34–43
129. Chen SK, Simonian PT, Wickeiwicz TL, Otis JC, Warren RF (1999) Radiographic evaluation of glenohumeral kinematics: a muscle fatigue model. J Shoulder Elbow Surg 8(1):49–52
130. Ebaugh DD, McClure PW, Karduna AR (2006) Scapulothoracic and glenohumeral kinematics following an external rotation fatigue protocol. J Orthop Sports Phys Ther 36(8):557–571
131. Cain PR, Mutschler TA, Fu FH, Lee SK (1987) Anterior stability of the glenohumeral joint. A dynamic model. Am J Sports Med 15(2):144–148
132. Byram IR, Bushnell BD, Dugger K, Charron K, Harrell FE, Noonan TJ (2010) Preseason shoulder strength measurements in professional baseball pitchers: identifying players at risk for injury. Am J Sports Med 38(7):1375–1382
133. Riemann BL, Davies GJ, Ludwig L, Gardenhour H (2010) Hand-held dynamometer testing of the internal and external rotator musculature based on selected positions to establish normative data and unilateral ratios. J Shoulder Elbow Surg 19(8):1175–1183
134. Ellenbecker TS, Sueyoshi T, Bailie DS (2015) Muscular activity during plyometric exercises in 90 degrees of glenohumeral joint abduction. Sports Health 7(1):75–79
135. Davies GJ (1992) A compendium of isokinetics in clinical usage and rehabilitation techniques, 4th edn. S & S Publishing, Onalaska
136. Wilk KE, Andrews JR, Arrigo CA, Keirns MA, Erber DJ (1993) The strength characteristics of internal and external rotator muscles in professional baseball pitchers. Am J Sports Med 21:61–66
137. Ellenbecker TS, Mattalino AJ (1999) Concentric isokinetic shoulder internal and external rotation strength in professional baseball pitchers. J Orthop Sports Phys Ther 25:323–328
138. Ellenbecker TS, Roetert EP (2003) Age specific isokinetic glenohumeral internal and external rotation strength in elite junior tennis players. J Sci Med Sport 6(1):63–70
139. Mont MA, Cohen DB, Campbell KR, Gravare K, Mathur SK (1994) Isokinetic concentric versus eccentric training of shoulder rotators with functional evaluation of performance enhancement in elite tennis players. Am J Sports Med 22(4):513–517
140. Quincy RI, Davies GJ, Kolbeck KJ, Szymanski JL (2000) Isokinetic exercise: the effects of training specificity on shoulder strength development. J Athl Train 35:S64
141. Bleacher J, Ellenbecker TS (2006) Modification of traditional exercises for shoulder rehabilitation and a return to lifting program. In: Ellenbecker TS (ed) Shoulder rehabilitation: non-operative treatment. Thieme, New York
142. Gross ML, Brenner SL, Sonogni JJ (1993) Anterior shoulder instability in weight lifters. Am J Sports Med 21:599–603
143. Ellenbecker TS, Reinold M, Nelson CO (2010) Clinical concepts for treatment of the elbow in the adolescent overhead athlete. Clin Sports Med 29(4):705–724
144. Kim SH, Ha KI, Jung MW, Lim MS, Kim YM, Park JH (2003) Accelerated rehabilitation after arthroscopic Bankart repair for selected cases: a prospective randomized clinical study. Arthroscopy 19(7):722–731
145. Lenters TR, Franta AK, Wolf FM, Leopold SS, Matsen FA 3rd (2007) Arthroscopic compared with open repairs for recurrent anterior shoulder instability. A systematic review and meta-analysis of the literature. J Bone Joint Surg Am 89(2):244–254
146. Petrera M, Patella V, Patella S, Theodoropoulos J (2010) A meta-analysis of open versus arthroscopic Bankart repair using suture anchors. Knee Surg Sports Traumatol Arthrosc 18(12):1742–1747
147. Castagna A, Markopoulos N, Conti M, Delle Rose G, Papadakou E, Garofalo R (2010) Arthroscopic bankart suture-anchor repair: radiological and clinical outcome at minimum 10 years of follow-up. Am J Sports Med 38(10):2012–2016
148. Jankauskas L, Rüdiger HA, Pfirrmann CW, Jost B, Gerber C (2010) Loss of the sclerotic line of the glenoid on anteroposterior radiographs of the shoulder: a diagnostic sign for an osseous defect of the anterior glenoid rim. J Shoulder Elbow Surg 19(1):151–156
149. McMullen J, Uhl TL (2000) A kinetic chain approach for shoulder rehabilitation. J Athl Train 35(3):329–337
150. Kibler WB, McMullen J, Uhl T (2001) Shoulder rehabilitation strategies, guidelines, and practice. Orthop Clin North Am 32(3):527–538
151. Smith J, Dahm DL, Kaufman KR, Boon AJ, Laskowski ER, Katajarvi BR, Jacofsky DJ (2006) Eletromyographic activity in the immobilized shoulder girdle musculature during scapulothoracic exercise. Arch Phys Med Rehabil 87(7):923–927
152. Burkhart SS, Morgan CD, Kibler WB (2003) The disabled throwing shoulder: spectrum of pathology Part III: the SICK scapula, scapular duskiness, the kinetic chain, and rehabilitation. Arthroscopy 19(6):641–661
153. Warner JJ, Lephart S, Fu FH (1996) Role of proprioception in pathoetiology of shoulder instability. Clin Orthop Relat Res 330:35–39
154. Myers JB, Lephart SM (2002) Sensorimotor deficits contributing to glenohumeral instability. Clin Orthop Relat Res 400:98–104
155. Fuchs E, Holmes P, David I, Ayali A (2012) Proprioceptive feedback reinforces centrally generated stepping patterns in the Cockroach. J Exp Biol 215:1884–1891, Published by The Company of Biologists Ltd
156. Sciascia A, Kibler WB (2011) Alterations in the kinetic chain are found in a high percentage of patients. Conducting the "nonshoulder" shoulder examination. J Musculoskelet Med 28:61–2
157. Kibler WB, Press J, Sciascia A (2006) The role of core stability in athletic function. Sports Med 36:189–198
158. Maenhout A, VanPraet K, Pizzi L, Van Herzeele M, Cools A (2010) Electromyographic analysis of knee push up variations: what is the influence of the kinetic chain on scapular muscle activity? Br J Sports Med 44:1010–1015
159. Cools AM, Dewitte V, Lanszweert F, Notebaert D, Roets A, Soetens B, Cagnie B, Witvrouw EE (2007) Rehabilitation of scapular muscle balance: which exercise to prescribe? Am J Sports Med 35(10):1744–1751. Epub 2 Jul 2007
160. De Mey K, Cagnie B, Danneels LA, Cools AM, Van de Velde A (2009) Trapezius muscle timing during selected shoulder rehabilitation exercise. J Orthop Sports Phys Ther 39(10):743–752
161. Ludewig PM, Hoff MS, Osowski EE, Meschke SA, Rundquist PJ (2004) Relative balance of serratus anterior and upper trapezius

muscle activity during push-up exercise. Am J Sports Med 32(2):484–493
162. Hardwick DH, Beebe JA, McDonnell MK, Lang CE (2006) A comparison of serratus anterior muscle activation during a wall slide exercise and other traditional exercises. J Orthop Sports Phys Ther 36(12):903–910

Further Reading

163. Ogston JB, Ludwig PM (2007) Differences in 3-dimensional shoulder kinematics between persons with multi-directional instability and asymptomatic controls. Am J Sports Med 35(8):1361–1370
164. Kibler WB (1991) The role of the scapula in the overhead throwing motion. Cont Orthop 22:525–532
165. DeMey K, Danneels LA, Cagnie B, Huyghe L, Seyns E, Cools AM (2013) Conscious correction of scapular orientation in overhead athletes performing selected shoulder rehabilitation exercises: the effect on trapezius muscle activation measured by surface electromyography. J Orthop Sports Phys Ther 43(1):3–10
166. Wilk KE, Voight ML, Keirns MA et al (1993) Stretch-shortening drills for the upper extremities: theory and clinical application. J Orthop Sports Phys Ther 17:225–239
167. Flesing GS, Jameson GG, Cody KE, et al (1998) Muscle activity during shoulder rehabilitation exercise. In: Proceedings of NACOB '98, the Third North American Congress on biomechanics. Waterloo, 14 Aug 1998, pp. 223–234
168. Hintermeister RA, Lange GW, Schultheis JM et al (1998) Electromyographic activity and applied load during shoulder rehabilitation exercises using elastic resistance. Am J Sports Med 26:210–220
169. Jobe FW, Moynes DR, Tibone JE et al (1984) An EMG analysis of the shoulder in pitching: a second report. Am J Sports Med 12:218–220
170. Jobe FW, Tibone JE, Jobe CM et al (1990) The shoulder in sport. In: Rockwood CA Jr, Matsen FA III (eds) The shoulder. W. B. Saunders, Philadelphia, pp 961–990
171. Litchfield R, Hawkins R, Dillman CJ et al (1993) Rehabilitation for the overhead athlete. J Orthop Sports Phys Ther 18: 433–441
172. Meister K, Andrews JR (1993) Classification and treatment of rotator cuff injuries in the overhead athlete. J Orthop Sports Phys Ther 18:413–421
173. Pappas AM, Zawacki RM, McCarthy CF (1985) Rehabilitation of the pitching shoulder. Am J Sports Med 13:223–235

Rehabilitation Following Rotator Cuff Repair

4

W. Ben Kibler and Aaron Sciascia

Contents

W.B. Kibler, MD (✉) • A. Sciascia, MS, ATC, PES
Lexington Clinic, Shoulder Center of Kentucky,
1221 South Broadway, Lexington, KY 40504, USA
e-mail: wkibler@aol.com

G. Di Giacomo, S. Bellachioma (eds.), *Shoulder Surgery Rehabilitation: A Teamwork Approach*,
DOI 10.1007/978-3-319-24856-1_4

4.1 Introduction

The goal of rehabilitation following rotator cuff repair is to restore the functional capability of the shoulder. It requires integrated input from both the surgeon and the rehabilitation clinician (physical therapist, occupational therapist, and/or athletic trainer). It is based on the restoration of the anatomy, but requires restoration of the physiology. It requires adherence to basic principles of tissue healing, muscle flexibility, muscle strength, and progression through rehabilitation stages and demands attention to several aspects of functional restoration. This chapter will discuss the role of the surgeon and basic principles of the rehabilitation protocol and will present guidelines and progressions for physical therapists and other rehabilitation clinicians through the protocols.

4.2 The Role of the Orthopedic Surgeon in Rotator Cuff Rehabilitation

The orthopedic surgeon usually does not prescribe specific exercises, does not supervise the exercise sessions, does not provide modalities, and does not see the patient weekly during the rehabilitation process following rotator cuff repair. However, the orthopedic surgeon plays several key roles that have large effects on the outcomes of the rehabilitation process. They relate to:

1. Optimizing the tissue anatomy as a basis for repair integrity
2. Knowing the phases of the rehabilitation sequence
3. Controlling repair loading during the key 6–8-week time period when the repair is most likely to be disrupted
4. Communicating effectively with the rehabilitation clinicians

4.2.1 Optimizing Tissue Anatomy

Many factors that are not under the surgeon's direct control affect the healing capability of the rotator cuff repair. However, the surgeon does control the technical aspects of how the rotator cuff tissue is mobilized, aligned on the humerus, repaired within the tendon, and attached to the bone. The goal of surgery is to create a repair that is properly mobilized, reduced in an anatomic alignment, and firmly attached across the footprint with minimal tension or shear force. This repair heals more frequently and can be rehabilitated relatively quickly in a standardized protocol. The majority of symptomatic full-thickness rotator cuff tears are what is considered U-shaped tears [1]. The "U" is most commonly an L-shaped tear that has undergone some retraction under tension. The apex of the "L" can be either anterior or posterior. The surgeon must grasp and manipulate both edges of the "U" to discover which the more mobile segment is and determine the exact apex of the "L" [2].

The apex can then be reduced to the footprint to start the repair under minimal tension [2]. Frequently, the tissues at the medial and posterior extents of the "U" will have been plastically deformed or stretched in the gradual progressions of the tear, and these areas can be incised and debrided in order to get better quality tissue for the repair and to allow more complete mobilization and reduction which create minimal tension on the entire repair. "Dog ears," the excess tissue on the edges of the repair, represent incomplete reduction of the tear, excessive tissue on one side of the repair, and create nonuniform tension on the tissues [3]. If the surgical goal is to reproduce the rotator cuff anatomy, then "dog ears" demonstrate that the goal has not been reached.

Once the type of tear is established, and the tear is mobilized to be reduced, there are multiple techniques for attachment to the footprint. Single-row repair, many variations of double-row repair, and margin convergence repairs have all been demonstrated to have adequate fixation and healing rates [4–8].

Other more complex rotator cuff patterns include multi-tendon tears, widely retracted tears, chronic tears with poor tissue quality, and tears associated with muscle atrophy. Surgical goals and techniques may need to be modified to address these issues, and the optimal anatomy obtained from these procedures may be less than ideal. Rehabilitation will need to be individually modified in these cases.

In summary, the surgical repair that creates the optimal anatomy, as close to "normal" in alignment and tension, allows rehabilitation to proceed at a physiological pace under normal physiological constraints.

4.2.2 Stages of Healing and Rehabilitation Progression

There are several methods to organize the stages of rehabilitation. This protocol uses *three stages* based on healing of the repair, baseline preparation of all of the tissues to return to function, and a sport- or activity-specific return to function. There are *specific goals*, activity progressions, and criteria for progression to the next phase. The surgeon has input into the decisions regarding how rapidly to move through each stage and when it is appropriate to move to the next stage.

1. The *ACUTE STAGE* involves the surgical repair and the early postoperative period, usually 6–8 weeks. The objective of this stage is to protect the repair sufficiently to create stable, healing local tissues, and optimal joint health and also to start early restoration of proximal kinetic chain function.

2. The *RECOVERY PHASE* involves a relatively long period of time starting around 6–8 weeks postoperatively during which the repair is completely healed. The kinetic chain is restored, and the local tissue inflexibilities, strength, and strength balance are restored. Entry into this phase assumes the tissues can be safely loaded in tension and compression. Force couple restoration, full range of motion, and scapular stability are also addressed.
3. The *FUNCTIONAL STAGE* will focus on restoring any further biomechanical deficits or strength imbalances and include exercises that relate to optimal function in the desired activities. They should simulate the motions, forces, loads, and durations of the activity. The functional stage will allow the return to activity or play and should also include a maintenance program to condition the shoulder after return to activity.

4.2.3 Control of Loading

Repair healing can be affected by the amount of mechanical load placed on the repair construct [9]. This is especially true in the first 6–8 weeks, when inflammation and tissue healing stages of the tendon process are predominant [9–13]. Excessive loading can alter the tissue properties, decrease the volume of healing tissue, and alter expression of growth factors for healing [9, 13]. The orthopedic surgeon, by overseeing the timing of exercises and exercise progressions, by limiting the ranges of allowable motion, by limiting the types of exercises, and by regulating the placement of the scapula and humerus, can affect both tensile and compression loading of the repair.

Excessive tensile loading is a known risk factor for failure of tendon healing [9]. It can create either a complete re-tear or an elongation of the healing tissue, both resulting in an incompetent repair. Excessive tensile loading can occur from a weight in an outstretched hand, gravity on an outstretched hand, ranges of motion greater than tissue repair flexibility, continued muscle activation after muscle fatigue, and excessive eccentric activations [9, 11, 12]. Surgeons should be cautious about prescribing these activities in the first 4–6 weeks:

1. Active or passive range of motion greater than 90° in any plane
2. Unsupported pendulum (Codman) exercises (hand should be supported on a ball or other object)
3. Active or passive exercises that involve a long lever arm (exercises performed with the elbow extended)
4. Exercises to muscle fatigue
5. Open-chain exercises with a weight in the hand

Compressive loading is also deleterious to tendon repair healing. Animal studies have shown tissue quality, tissue volume, and tissue mechanics are all decreased with resulting decrease in healing rates in repairs subject to excessive compression during early healing [10, 14]. Excessive compression occurs from dynamic downward and forward tilt of the acromion, which occurs during scapular protraction [15, 16]. This mainly occurs in the presence of scapular dyskinesis, which can occur from multiple causes, including excessive sling use; tight pectoralis major and/or minor, upper trapezius, and latissimus dorsi muscles; weak serratus anterior or lower trapezius muscles; and weak core muscles.

The surgeon should evaluate the patient for scapular dyskinesis by clinical observation of the medial scapular border [15] and examination for periscapular muscle tightness or weakness. Exercises to correct the dyskinesis and place the scapula in stable retraction and the acromion in posterior tilt should be instituted both preoperatively and in the early postoperative stages. Care must be taken to keep passive range of motion below 90° of elevation or abduction because higher angles of arm motion are associated with decreased acromial upward rotation, leading to more compression [16].

4.2.4 Communication with Physical Therapists and Other Rehabilitation Clinicians

The basis for integrated functional rehabilitation of rotator cuff repair is effective communication between the surgeon and rehabilitation clinician. It is good to establish a general agreement regarding expectations of rehabilitation progress, patterns of exercises, types of motions and positions, and exercise content in each stage. An information sheet covering these areas of concern should be given to each patient and the treating clinician. There are various methods through which the ongoing communication regarding rehabilitation progress could go, including telephone communication, mobile text messaging, website literature, and face-to-face discussion, but the most common method is the exercise prescription either completed by hand or electronic copy. The prescription should include as appropriate:

1. Pertinent information about the repair anatomy (number of tendons, tissue quality, security of the repair, etc.)
2. Allowable ranges of motion (below 60° flexion and flexion, up to 90°, less than 30° external rotation)
3. Types of exercises (closed chain, Codman's on ball or other supportive device. humeral head depression)
4. Mechanics of exercises (short lever arm, plyometric, slow speed, horizontal/diagonal)
5. Exercises for other body areas (core stability/strengthening, scapular retraction)
6. Any specific limits or progressions including advancements to the next stages of rehabilitation

4.3 Rehabilitation following Rotator Cuff Repair

The physical therapist and other rehabilitation clinicians are responsible for arranging and applying the content of the exercises and modalities to fulfill the goals of the prescription, providing feedback regarding progress or limitations, readying the patient for progression to the next stage, and overseeing the functional progressions to allow return to activity or play. The object of rehabilitation following rotator cuff repair is to restore the deltoid/rotator cuff force couple to dynamically center the humeral head in the glenoid socket throughout all the ranges of arm motion. The following protocol contains goals, guidelines, and suggestions for exercises that can be used.

4.3.1 Acute Stage

The acute stage is concerned with protecting the healing tissues while maintaining general body function. Passive arm motions should be monitored and should stay below 90°. Scapular retraction should be emphasized to avoid excessive compression loading in this vulnerable time. Closed chain exercises, by supporting the hand and emphasizing proximal co-contractions, are effective at decreasing tensile loading. Immobilization may be useful in the first 4–6 weeks, but many studies demonstrate that short-term immobilization (2–3 weeks) and controlled passive motion (less than 90°) are more effective than longer-term immobilization in regaining motion with no difference in healing rates [17–19].

Stage I: Acute stage (weeks 1–3)

Pearls	Goals
Acquire motion Upper extremity: Table slides (Fig. 4.1a, b) Physioball progression (Fig. 4.2a–d) Lower extremity: Hip rotation Hip extension Hip flexors Other maneuvers as needed	Decrease stiffness while protecting repair Establish trunk/hip motion and strength for quality scapular motion later
Establish core strength and stability Lower extremity strengthening *focusing on hip abduction and extension recommended*: Lateral step Step downs Lunge progression	

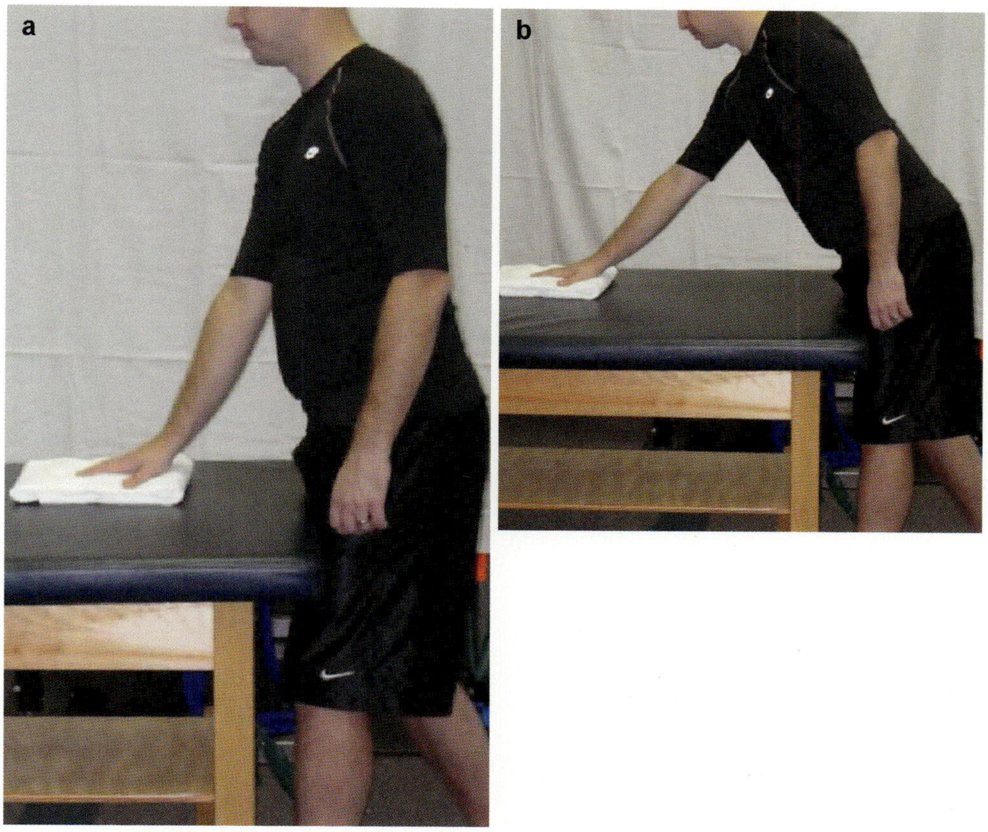

Fig. 4.1 (**a**, **b**) Table slides for early closed-chain motion. The patient should be instructed to flex (**a**) and extend (**b**) the trunk in order to facilitate arm motion. Both flexion and abduction (not pictured) can be performed

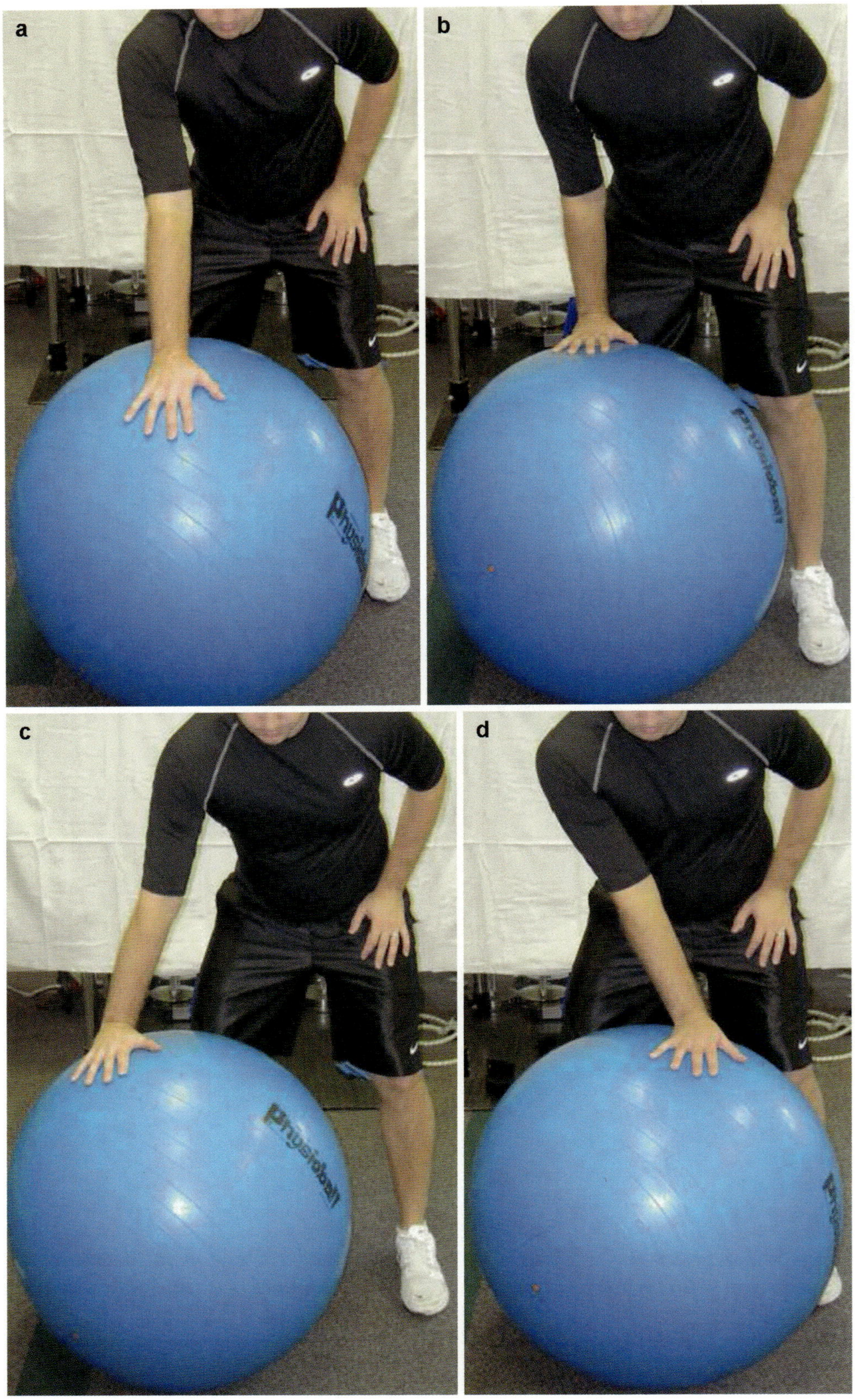

Fig. 4.2 (**a–d**) Physioball motion program. The program requires use of the larger kinetic chain muscles (legs/trunk) to initiate the restoration of arm motion using the directions of flexion (**a**), extension (**b**), abduction (**c**), adduction (**d**), and rotation (not pictured)

4.3.2 Recovery Stage

The recovery stage is concerned with restoring the full range of motion and strength capability of the rotator cuff and integrating it with the kinetic chain functional capability. Ranges of motion can be extended above 90° and can be assisted actively. Integration of scapular control and rotator cuff strengthening exercises reestablishes the stable scapular base for maximal rotator cuff activation. Proprioceptive neuromuscular facilitation and closed-chain exercises are effective early in the stage, and open-chain exercises can be added as strength increases.

Stage II: Recovery stage (weeks 4–6)

Pearls	Goals

Facilitate critical kinetic chain links
  Facilitate retraction with arm close to body
    Lawn mower (Fig. 4.3a, b)
    Robbery (Fig. 4.4a, b)
	Lower extremity driving upper extremity motion
	Full active range of motion
	Adequate scapular control to progress to longer lever exercise maneuvers

Utilize closed- to open-chain exercise
  Closed chain
    Table slides (for integrated motion)
    Low row (Fig. 4.5a, b)
    Inferior glide (Fig. 4.6)
  Open chain
    Low row with step back (Fig. 4.7a, b)
    Lawn mower with step back (Fig. 4.8a, b)
    Robbery with step back (Fig. 4.9a, b)	

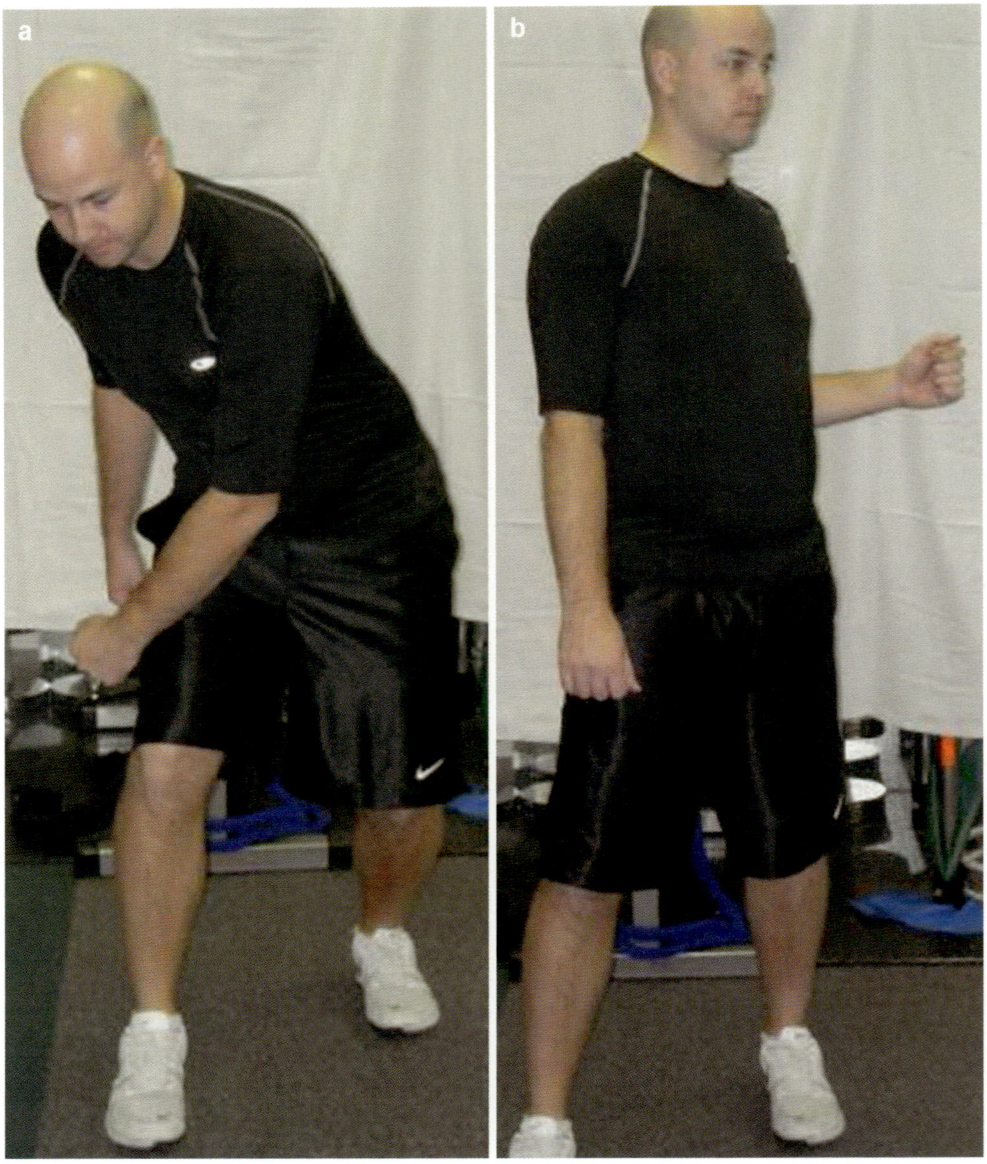

Fig. 4.3 (**a**, **b**) Lawn mower exercise. The lawn mower begins with the hip and the trunk flexed and the arm slightly forward elevated (**a**). The patient instructed to extend the hips and trunk and to "place elbows in the back pockets," holding this final position for 5 s (**b**)

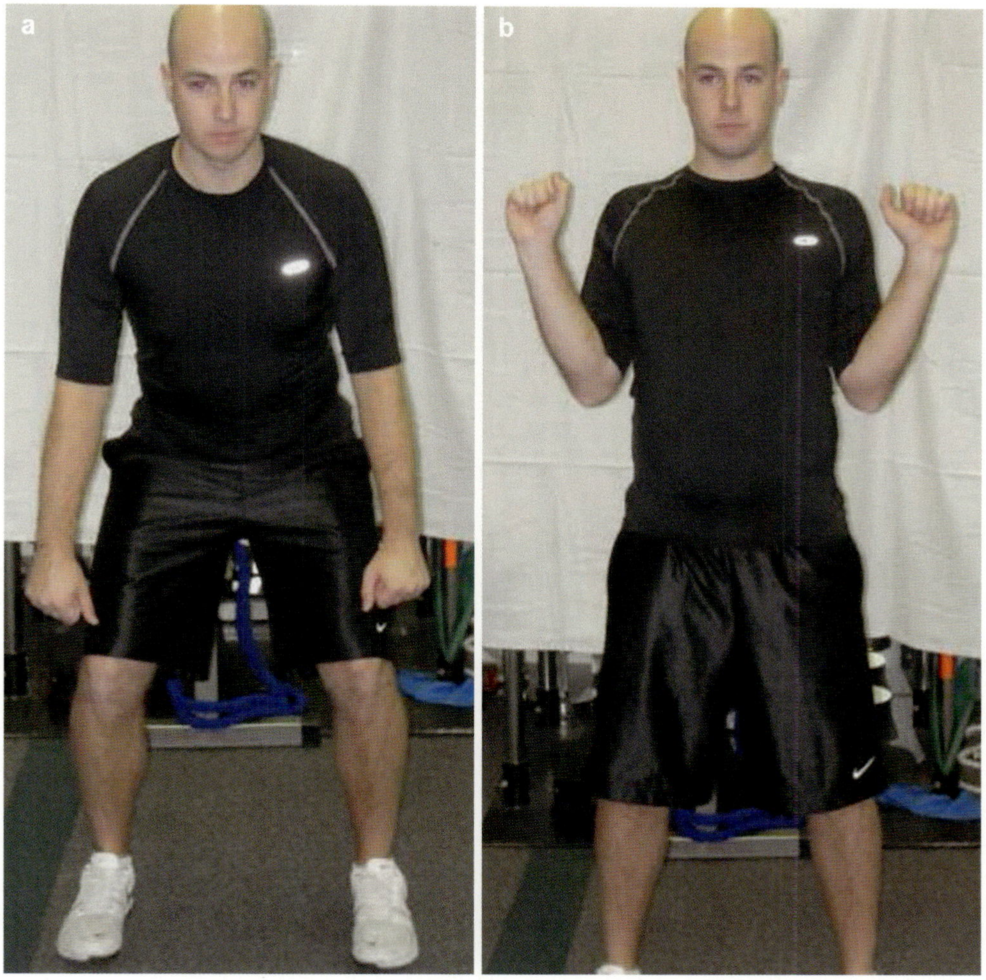

Fig. 4.4 (**a**, **b**) Robbery exercise. The robbery maneuver begins with the knees and trunk flexed and the arms held away from the body (**a**). The patient is instructed to extend the hips and trunk and to "place the elbows in the back pockets," holding this final position for 5 s (**b**)

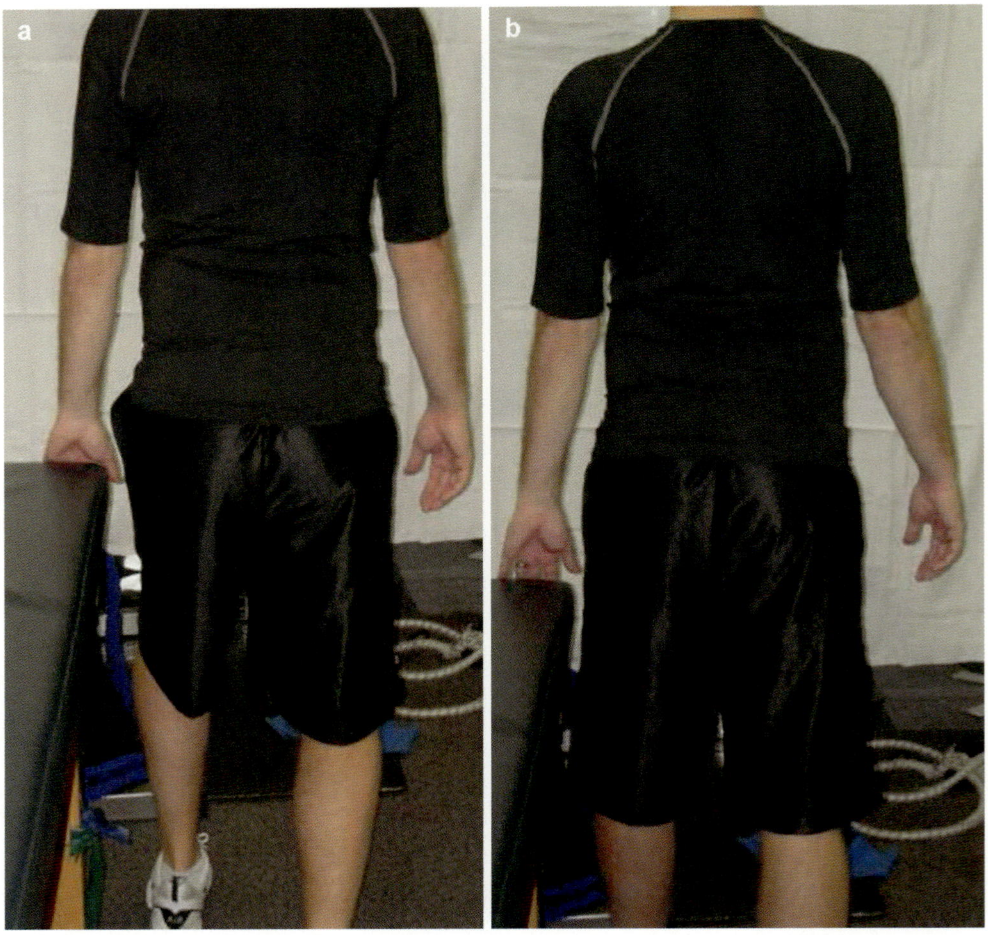

Fig. 4.5 (**a**, **b**) Low-row exercise. The patient is positioned standing with the hand of the involved arm against the side of a firm surface and legs slightly flexed (**a**). The patient should be instructed to extend the hips and trunk to facilitate scapular retraction and hold the contraction for 5 s (**b**)

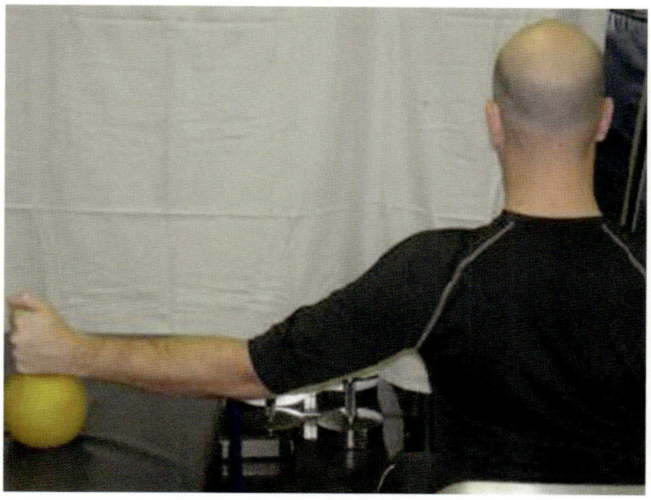

Fig. 4.6 Inferior glide. This maneuver encourages co-contraction of local and global muscles resulting in depression of the humeral head

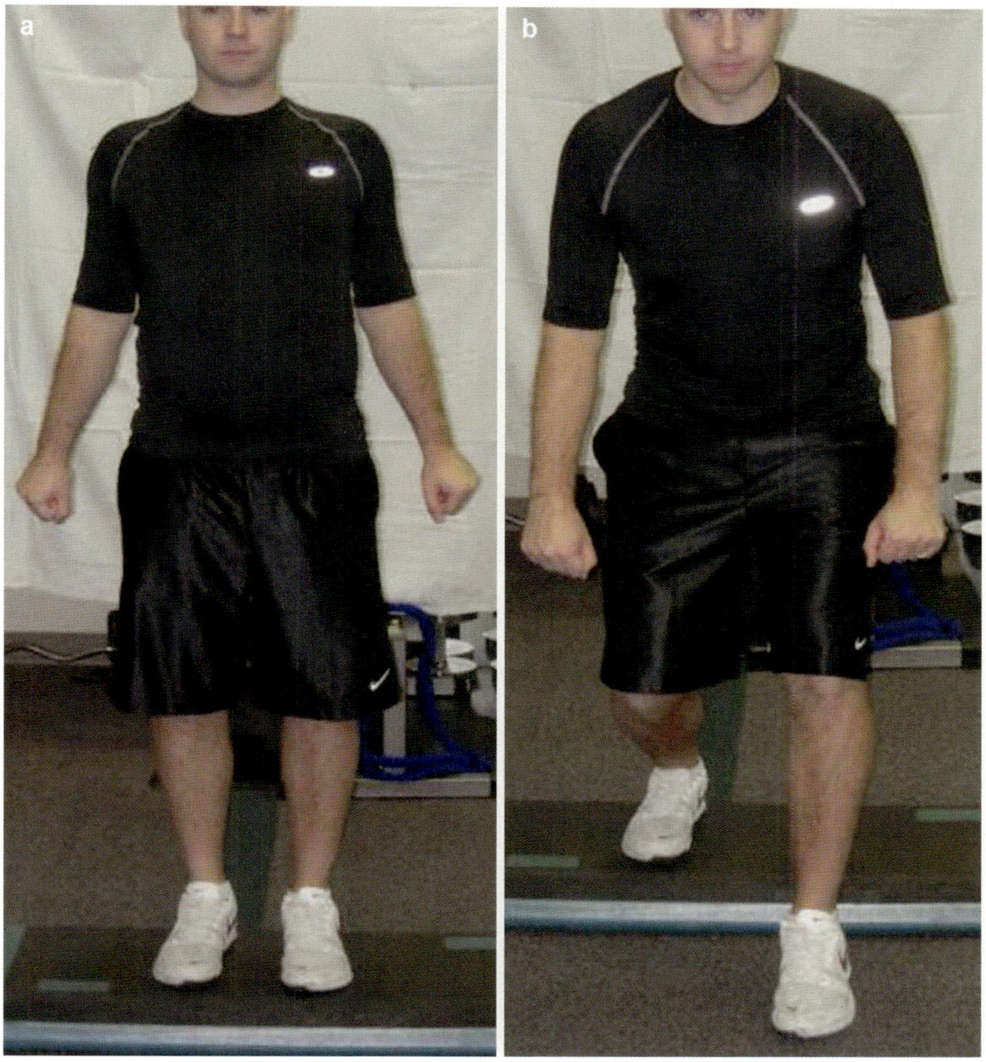

Fig. 4.7 (**a**, **b**) Low row with posterior step. The posterior step back requires hip and trunk extension which facilitates scapular retraction and depression

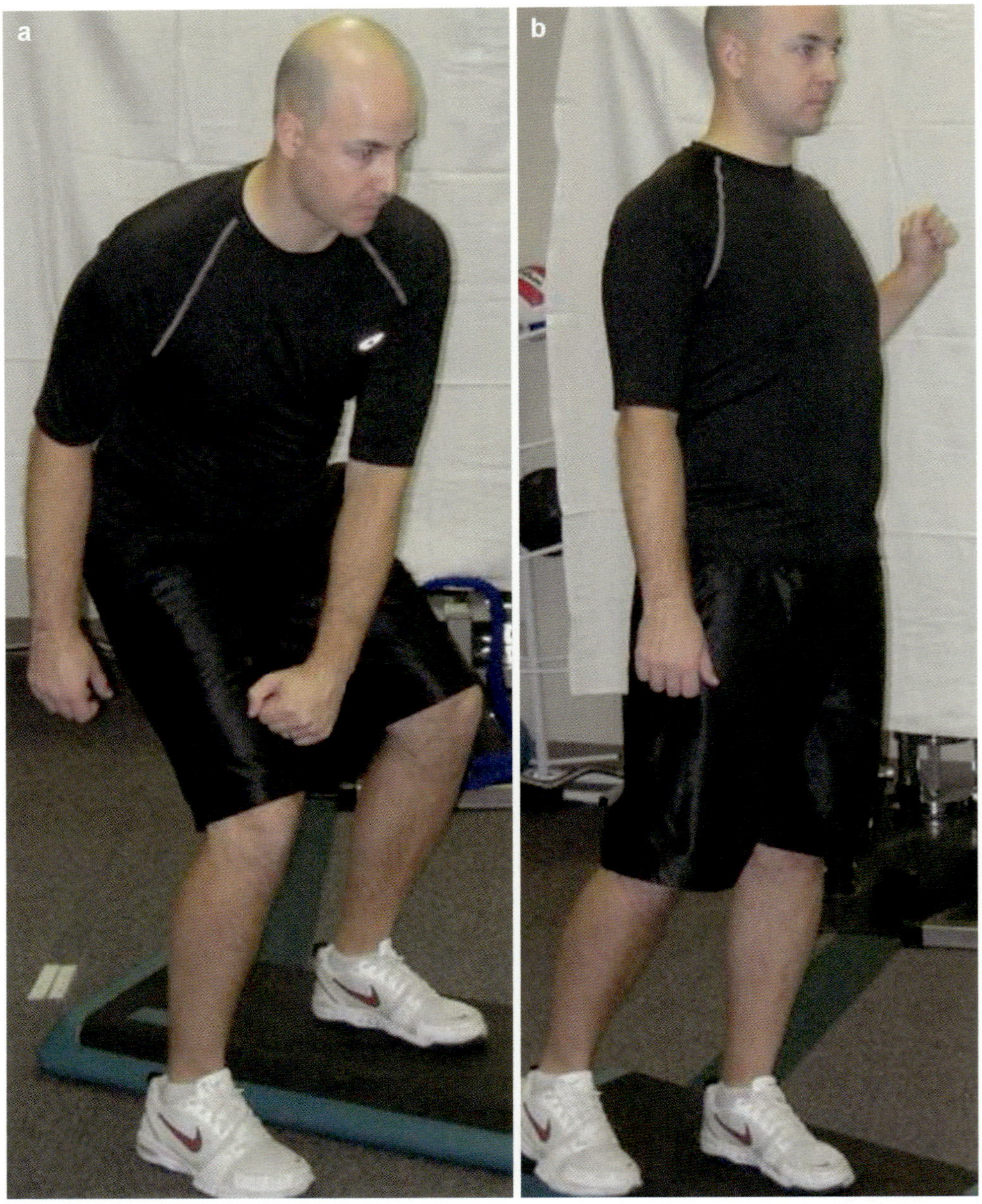

Fig. 4.8 (**a**, **b**) Lawn mower with lateral step. By adding the step, the patient is forced to utilize the hip abductors making the exercise more functional

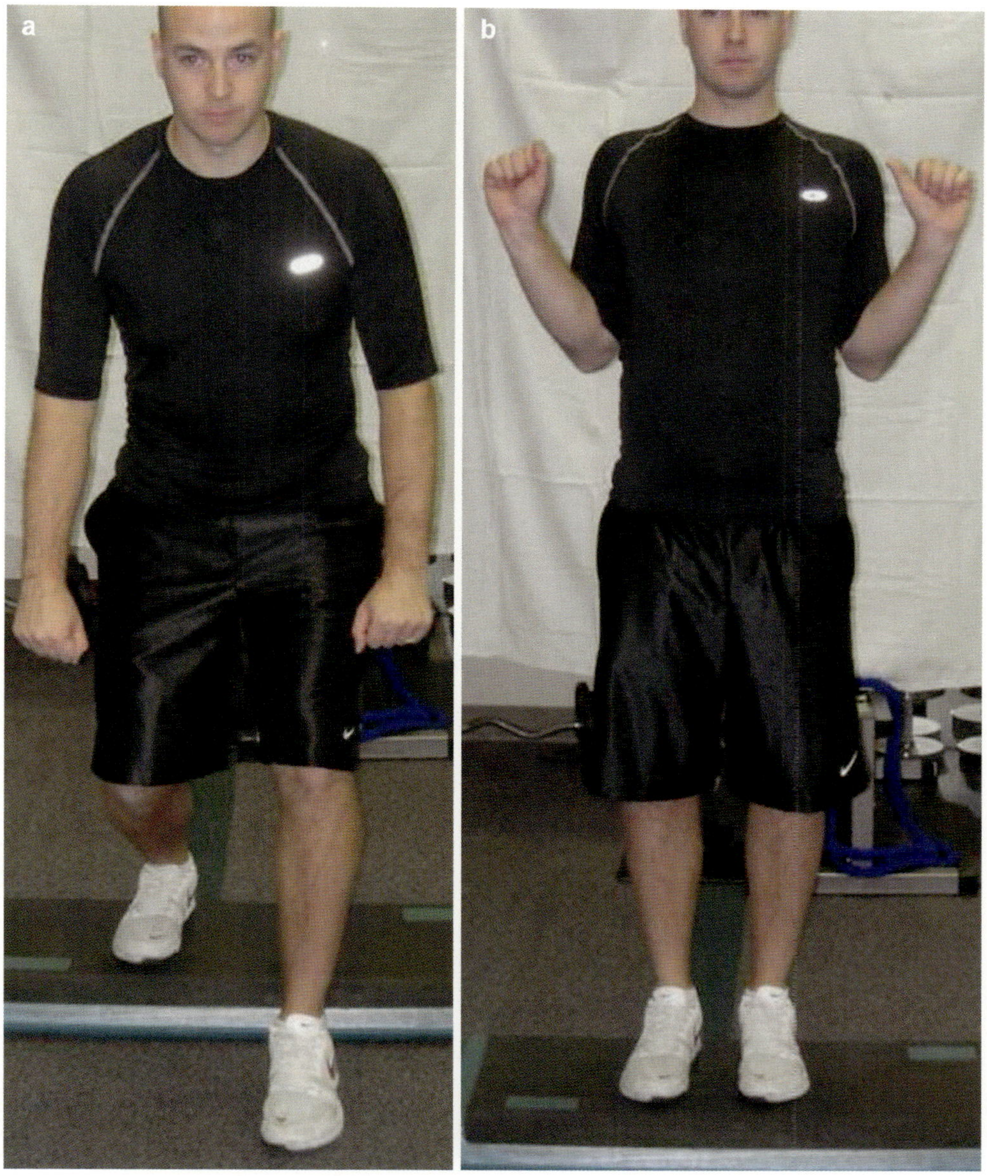

Fig. 4.9 (**a**, **b**) Robbery exercise with posterior step. Utilizing the step allows the lower extremity to drive the upper extremity

4.3.3 Functional Stage

The functional stage is concerned with establishing the capabilities to respond to the specific activity demands of the patient, whether it be work, recreation, or athletic play. Maximal ranges of motion, dynamic muscle strength balance, and generation of power and endurance are the key goals. As the patient acquires these capabilities, maintenance conditioning for the activity should be included. Functional progression testing may be done to simulate the body's ability to withstand the sport- or activity-specific demands.

Stage III: Functional activity stage (weeks 7±)

Pearls	Goals

Work in multiple planes
  Integrated motion
    Punching
    Power position (Fig. 4.10)
    Power position with step back (Fig. 4.11)
  Traditional rotator cuff exercises
    Scaption
    Horizontal abduction
    Internal and external rotation
	Fine-tune scapular motion to alleviate all dyskinesis
	Increase strength and endurance of rotator cuff and scapular-stabilizing muscles

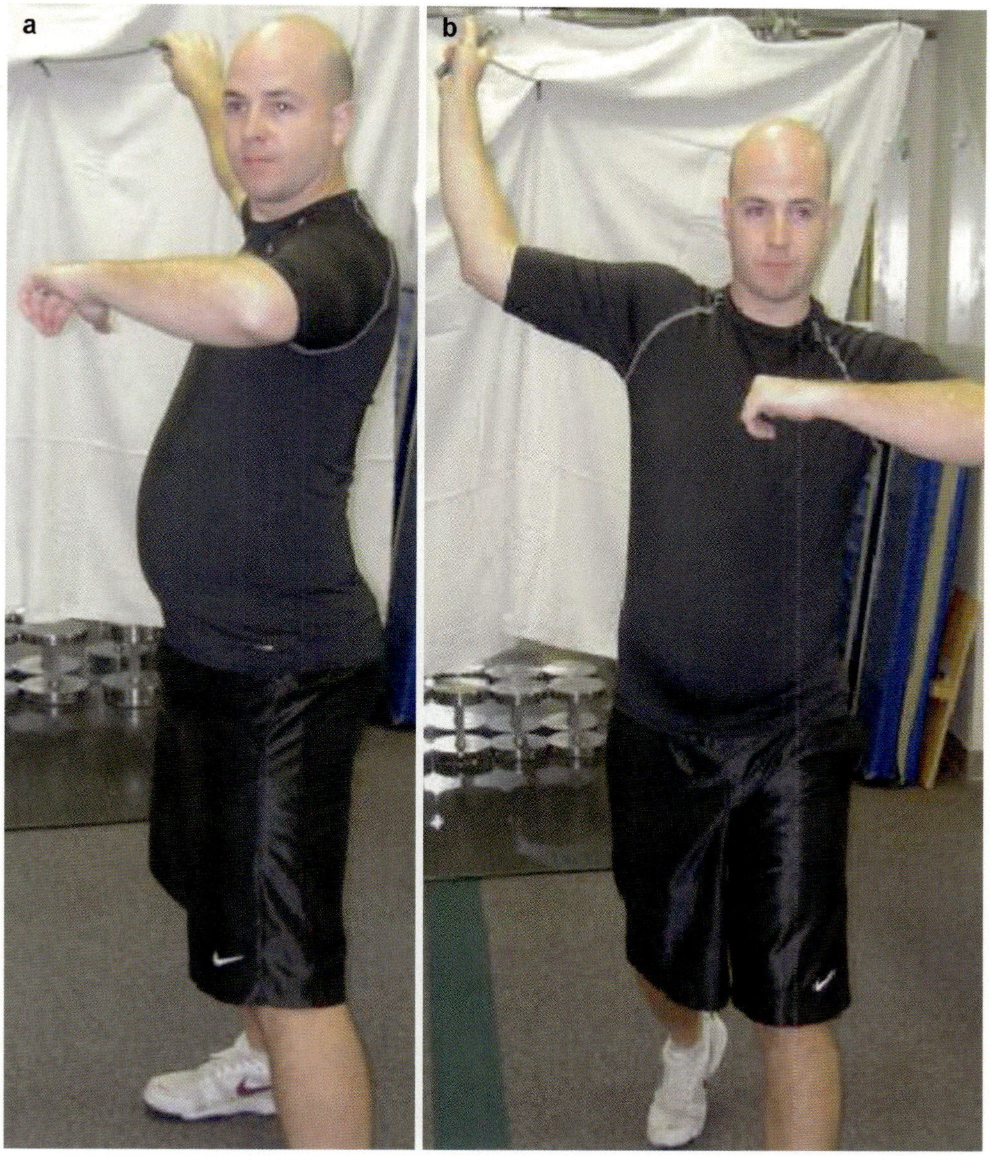

Fig. 4.10 (**a**, **b**) Power position. The athlete is positioned standing with dominant arm in 90/90 position and forearm pronated (**a**). The athlete is instructed to rotate the trunk without moving the feet while maintaining the 90/90 position of the arm (**b**). The forearm should be allowed to supinate to imitate the act of the overhead throwing

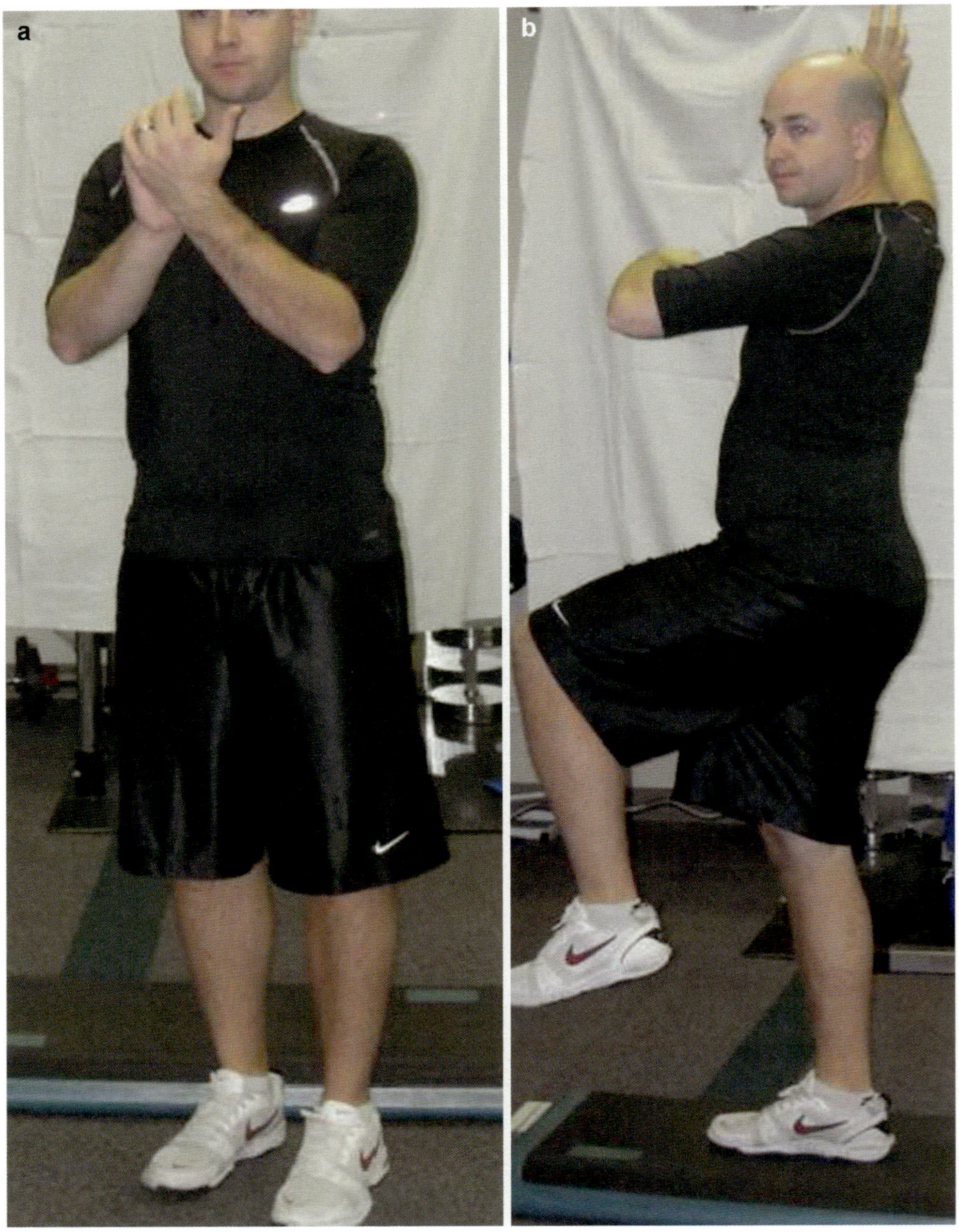

Fig. 4.11 (**a**, **b**) Power position with step back. This maneuver requires stability of the lower extremity in order for the upper extremity positioning to be achieved

4.3.4 Return-to-Activity Stage

Specific criteria should be established to return to activity [20]. This should involve restoration of functional capability, objectively demonstrated through range of motion and strength measurement and by physical performance testing [21], rather than by time or imaging.

Stage IV: Return-to-activity stage (weeks 10±)

Pearls	Goals
High repetition exercises designed to increase lower extremity muscle endurance Utilize *integrated sport-specific exercise* to encourage use of the improved lower extremity muscle strength and endurance to help facilitate upper extremity muscle activation Address upper extremity power and endurance via high repetition, *long lever exercises* performed in standing and prone positions	Optimal kinetic chain links (pelvis control over planted leg, effective hip, and trunk extension) Scapular retraction achievement while controlling scapular protraction Proper flexibility of upper and lower extremity Advancement through functional progressions without regression of prior deficits/symptoms

Conclusion

Rehabilitation after rotator cuff repair can only be accomplished by an integrated approach involving the skills and participation of surgeons and rehabilitation clinicians. Each has specific roles to play, each must understand the anatomy and physiology underlying the whole process, and each must communicate well so the central focus of the process, the patient, will obtain the best functional result.

References

1. Sallay PI, Hunker PJ, Lim JK (2007) Frequency of various tear patterns in full-thickness tears of the rotator cuff. Arthroscopy 23(10):1052–1059
2. Burkhart SS, Lo IK, Brady PC (2006) Burkhart's view of the shoulder: a cowboy's guide to advanced shoulder arthroscopy. Lippincott Williams and Wilkins, Philadelphia
3. Ryu KJ, Kim BH, Lee Y, Lee YS, Kim JH (2014) Modified suture-bridge technique to prevent a marginal dog-ear deformity improves structural integrity after rotator cuff repair. Am J Sports Med 43(3):597–605
4. Boyer P, Bouthors C, Delcourt T, Stewart O, Hamida F, Mylle G et al (2015) Arthroscopic double-row cuff repair with suture-bridging: a structural and functional comparison of two techniques. Knee Surg Sports Traumatol Arthrosc 23:478–486
5. Freehill MT, Rogers JP, Mannava S (2015) Shoulder and rotator cuff repair: single vs double row. Oper Tech Orthop 25:23–32
6. Lapner PLC, Sabri E, Rakhra K, McRae S, Leiter J, Bell K et al (2012) A multicenter randomized controlled trial comparing single-row with double-row fixation in arthroscopic rotator cuff repair. J Bone Joint Surg Am 94:1249–1257
7. Mascarenhas R, Chalmers PN, Sayegh ET, Bhandari M, Verma NN, Cole BJ et al (2014) Is double-row rotator cuff repair clinically superior to single-row rotator cuff repair: a systematic review of overlapping meta-analyses. Arthroscopy 30(9):1156–1165
8. Millett PJ, Warth RJ, Dornan GJ, Lee JT, Spiegl UJ (2014) Clinical and structural outcomes after arthroscopic single-row versus double-row rotator cuff repair: a systematic review and meta-analysis of level I randomized clinical trials. J Shoulder Elbow Surg 23:586–597
9. Thomopoulos S, Williams GR, Soslowsky LJ (2003) Tendon to bone healing: differences in biomechanical, structural, and compositional properties due to a range of activity levels. J Biomech Eng 125:106–113
10. Carpenter JE, Thomopoulos S, Flanagan CL, DeBano CM, Soslowsky LJ (1998) Rotator cuff defect healing: a biomechanical and histologic analysis in an animal model. J Shoulder Elbow Surg 7(6):599–605
11. Galatz LM, Charlton N, Das R, Kim M, Havlioglu N, Thomopoulos S (2009) Complete removal of load is detrimental to rotator cuff healing. J Shoulder Elbow Surg 18:669–675
12. Killian ML, Cavinatto L, Galatz LM, Thomopoulos S (2012) The role of mechanobiology in tendon healing. J Shoulder Elbow Surg 21:228–237
13. Reuther KE, Thomas SJ, Tucker JJ, Yannascoli SM, Caro AC, Vafa RP et al (2014) Scapular dyskinesis is detrimental to shoulder tendon properties and joint mechanics in a rat model. J Orthop Res 32(11):1436–1443
14. Hettrich CM, Gasinu S, Beamer BS, Stasiak M, Fox A, Birmingham P et al (2014) The effect of mechanical load on tendon-to-bone healing in a rat model. Am J Sports Med 42(5):1233–1241
15. Kibler WB, Ludewig PM, McClure PW, Michener LA, Bak K, Sciascia AD (2013) Clinical implications of scapular dyskinesis in shoulder injury: the 2013 consensus statement from the "scapula summit". Br J Sports Med 47:877–885
16. Ludewig PM, Reynolds JF (2009) The association of scapular kinematics and glenohumeral joint pathologies. J Orthop Sports Phys Ther 39(2):90–104
17. Chang KV, Hung CY, Han DS, Chen WS, Wang TG, Chien KL (2015) Early versus delayed passive range of motion exercise for arthroscopic rotator cuff repair: a meta-analysis of randomized controlled trials. Am J Sports Med 43(5):1265–1273
18. Huisstede BMA, Koes BW, Gebremariam L, Keijsers E, Verhaar JAN (2011) Current evidence for effectiveness of interventions to treat rotator cuff tears. Man Ther 16:217–230
19. Lee BG, Cho NS, Rhee YG (2012) Effect of two rehabilitation protocols on range of motion and healing rates after arthroscopic rotator cuff repair: aggressive versus limited early passive exercises. Arthroscopy 28(1):34–42
20. Sciascia A, Cromwell R (2012) Kinetic chain rehabilitation: a theoretical framework. Rehabil Res Pract 2012:1–9
21. Reiman MP, Manske RC (2011) The assessment of function: how is it measured? A clinical perspective. J Man Manipulative Ther 19(2):91–99

The Athlete's Shoulder: Surgical Treatment and Rehabilitation

5

Kevin E. Wilk, Todd R. Hooks, and James R. Andrews

Contents

K.E. Wilk, PT, DPT, FAPTA (✉)
Champion Sports Medicine, Birmingham, AL, USA

Associate Clinical Professor, Marquette University, Programs in Physical Therapy, Milwaukee, WI, USA
e-mail: kwilkpt@hotmail.com

T.R. Hooks, PT, ATC, OCS, SCS, NREMT-1, CSCS
Assistant Athletic Trainer/Physical Therapist, New Orleans Pelicans Basketball Team, Metaire, LA, USA

J.R. Andrews, MD
Andrews Sports Medicine and Orthopaedic Center, AL, USA

G. Di Giacomo, S. Bellachioma (eds.), *Shoulder Surgery Rehabilitation: A Teamwork Approach*,
DOI 10.1007/978-3-319-24856-1_5

Overhead athletes are susceptible to shoulder joint pathology due to the repetitive nature of throwing activities and the unique and sports-specific pattern of the sporting activities. Extreme forces are placed upon the glenohumeral joint as a result of anterior shear forces that approach 50 % body weight that occur as a result of high angular velocities that reach 7250°/s during the throwing motion [1–3]. High levels of muscular activity are generated during the throwing motion that approaches 120 % maximal volitional isometric contraction (MVIC) [4]. A delicate balance between adequate mobility and inherent shoulder stability is required to effectively perform overhead activities and to minimize the potential for shoulder pathology.

Most shoulder injuries in athletes can be successfully treated nonoperatively to allow the athlete to return to competition. Although varying degrees of pathology can be present, the overhead athlete typically has involvement of the rotator cuff, glenohumeral joint capsule, and biceps brachii as a result of repetitive movements, whereas, athletes involved in contact sports have acute distributions of either the rotator cuff or glenohumeral capsule. When athletes have failed conservative measures and continued to have pain and inability to perform athletic activities, surgical intervention is often warranted. The specific surgical procedure indicated is dependent upon the nature and extent of the pathologies present to adequately address the athlete's condition.

5.1 Postoperative Rehabilitation

Rehabilitation plays a vital role in the functional outcome following shoulder injury for both the overhead and the contact sports athlete. The goal of the postoperative treatment is to restore the delicate balance between the mobility and stability that is required to perform athletic activities in the overhead-throwing athlete as they exhibit functional stability while allowing extreme motions necessary to throw effectively. The rehabilitation programs we utilized are a criteria-based treatment approach that are divided into four progressive phases with each phase consisting of specific goals and exercises that are designed to systematically introduce applied forces and loads to the healing tissues while avoiding overstressing these tissues. The rehabilitation programs for athletes with instability are based on several key factors (Table 5.1) and each athlete's unique characteristics (Table 5.2) that serve to classify each patient in order to minimize postoperative complications. It is the intent of these programs to serve as merely a guideline; therefore, based on both the athlete's presentation and the surgical intervention, the clinician will be able to make appropriate adjustments to each program. Additionally, the rehabilitation program should be continually modified based on tissue type, healing rate, and specific surgical procedure.

Table 5.1 Shoulder instability classification

Onset
Traumatic, atraumatic, repetitive microtrauma
Frequency
Acute, recurrent, chronic (fixed)
Direction
Anterior, posterior, multidirectional
Degree
Dislocation, subluxation, silent subluxation
Volition
Voluntary, involuntary

Table 5.2 Patient variables and factors

Patient's tissue status
Hyperelasticity ↔ hypermobility
Dynamic stabilizer status
Muscle – bone
Muscular strength and balance
Proprioceptive ability
Classification of instability
Previous activity level
Desired activity level (expectations)
Healing abilities
Rapid healers, slow healers

5.2 Factors Affecting the Rehabilitation Program

The clinician should consider several factors before designing and implementing a postsurgical rehabilitation program (Table 5.3). It is imperative the clinician understand the exact surgical procedure as well as the fixation method including any concomitant procedures to the supporting structures including the rotator cuff, glenoid fossa, and/or the labrum. The progression of ROM, strengthening exercises, and closed-chain activities will be based upon the healing constraints of all tissues involved. The clinician should consider the type and degree of instability exhibited by the patient. Overhead athletes generally have an appreciable degree of congenital laxity that can be observed on examination of the contralateral shoulder; therefore, the greater the degree of congenital laxity the slower the progression of range of motion. It is the experience of the authors that individuals who exhibit a positive sulcus on their uninvolved shoulder rarely have difficulty gaining motion with their operative shoulder, whereas athletes that play contact sports often have traumatic injuries that can result in unidirectional instability. The patient's tissue status is the third factor that should be considered. We advocate progressing patients with congenital instability or acquired laxity (overhead athlete) slower than someone who forms collagen more rapidly after surgery (i.e., "fast healer") as they should be monitored and accelerated to prevent loss of motion.

The status of the athlete's dynamic stabilizers should be considered; therefore, an athlete who has good to excellent muscular development, strength, dynamic stability, and proprioceptive awareness will naturally progress more rapidly than someone who has an underdeveloped musculature and decreased dynamic stability. The athlete's particular sport/position and level of participation should be considered as well as the philosophical approach of the surgeon as this has often been shaped by his training and previous personal experiences. We institute all of these factors carefully before implementing a postsurgical rehabilitation program to allow the appropriate formulation of an appropriate treatment program for the progression of ROM, strengthening exercises, and the initiation of functional activities and interval sports programs.

Table 5.3 Factors affecting the rehabilitation program

Type of surgical procedure
(Exposure, specific procedure, tissue used)
Method of fixation
Type of instability
(Instability classification)
Patient's tissue status
(Hyperelasticity, normal, hypoelasticity)
Patient's response to surgery
Patient's dynamic stabilization
(Muscular strength, dynamic stability, proprioception)
Patient's activity level
(Past, present, desired goals)
Physician's philosophical approach

5.3 Principles of Rehabilitation

There are six basic principles that are employed when designing a postsurgical rehabilitation program (Table 5.4). First, healing tissues should never be overstressed; therefore, the program must be progressive and sequential with each phase progressing from the prior phase. Based upon the authors' experience of poorer outcomes following prolonged immobilization immediately followed by a rapid progression of ROM, we implement the immediate implementation of ROM in a gradual, systemic format with stretching precautions for the first 8–10 weeks following surgery. Second, the effects of immobilization must be minimized especially in the overhead athlete. Often after shoulder stabilization surgery, a short period of immobilization may be indicated to allow initial healing; however, the clinician can incorporate mild dynamic stabilization drills, gentle restricted passive motions, and submaximal isometrics to enhance dynamic stability, assist in collagen organization, and prevent loss of motion. The clinician should continually monitor the quality of end feel throughout the rehabilitation by applying a slight overpressure at the end range of passive ROM. If a firm or hard end feel is noted, the clinician may accelerate the rate of ROM progression, whereas with a soft or empty end feel, the patient's stretching program will be slowed. Third, the patient must fulfill specific criteria to progress from one phase to the next; this allows the rehabilitation program to be individualized based on the athlete's unique healing rate and constraints. Finally, a successful outcome is related to a team effort, with the physician, physiotherapist, and athlete all working together toward a common goal. The key to a team approach is communication; it is the role of the physician to communicate with the rehabilitation team, providing information regarding the type of surgical procedure, the method of fixation, the integrity and quality of the patient's tissue, and the expectations of the physician for that specific athlete. This information is invaluable in designing and implementing a rehabilitation program.

Table 5.4 Basic principles of rehabilitation

Healing tissue should never be overstressed
The effects of immobilization must be minimized
The patient must fulfill specific criteria to progress
The rehabilitation program should be based on current scientific and clinical research
The rehabilitation program must not be a cookbook
Team approach – physician, therapist, and patient

5.4 General Rehabilitation Guidelines after Surgery

The first phase, the immediate postoperative period, begins with immediate restricted motion that serves to prevent loss of motion and neurological complications, nourish cartilage, and assist in collagen synthesis, organization, alignment, and enhancement of tensile strength [5–12].

The primary goal of this phase is to prevent excessive scarring without the utilization of aggressive stretching to compromise the surgical repair. Therefore, following anterior stabilization, motions such as extension and ER are limited or restricted to minimize stress upon the anterior capsule, whereas scapular plane elevation as opposed to shoulder abduction. Submaximal and sub-painful isometric contractions are initiated during phase 1 to stimulate muscle training, neuromodulate pain, and prevent muscle atrophy that occur as a result of immobilization (Fig. 5.1) [13, 14].

Phase II, the intermediate phase, emphasizes the gradual progression of shoulder mobility. We utilize the incorporation of AAROM and PROM exercises into the treatment program to gradually increase the patient's ROM. The athlete's ROM and capsular end feel will be used to determine rate of progression; consequently, patients with sufficient ROM and a soft end feel will be progressed slower than a patient with restricted ROM and a hard end feel. If one side of the capsule is excessively tight, the humeral head will displace excessively in the opposite direction away from the tightness; thus, joint-mobilization techniques are used to restore normal motion and to correct asymmetric capsular tightness (Fig. 5.2). When treating an overhead athlete, the physiotherapist will progress the stretching exercises to allow the athlete to obtain "thrower's motion" of approximately $115° \pm 5°$ ER to allow the athlete to return to throwing. During this phase, we usually initiate the "Thrower's Ten exercise" program that includes isolated rotator cuff and scapular exercises that are based upon EMG data to ensure restoration of muscle balance in the treatment of the overhead athlete [15–24]. The physiotherapist can progress treatment to include dynamic stabilization drills, manual resistance training, and PNF drills with rhythmic stabilizations that serve to enhance neuromuscular control aimed to reestablish muscular balance.

Phase III is intended to maintain shoulder ROM and mobility while improving strength, power, and endurance. Strengthening exercises are progressed to restore optimal sufficient muscle ratios (Table 5.5). Prior to initiating aggressive strengthening exercise such as plyometrics or functional activities, for example, throwing and swimming, the athlete should reestablish muscular balance, and dynamic joint stability should be achieved to allow adequate generation and dispersion of forces (Fig. 5.3). During this phase, eccentric muscle training and proprioceptive training are emphasized (Fig. 5.4). Plyometric training drills are utilized to increase the athlete's functional mobility and to gradually increase the functional stresses onto the shoulder joint. Wilk et al. [13, 25] have described a plyometric program that systematically introduces stresses upon the healing tissues beginning with two-handed drills such as chest pass, side-to-side throws, side throws, and overhead soccer throws. Upon successful completion of these two-handed drills, the athlete can progress to one-handed drills such as standing one-handed throws, wall dribbles, and plyometric step and throws [26]. Voight et al. [27] reported a relationship between diminished shoulder proprioception and muscle fatigue. Muscular endurance training is therefore performed to enhance dynamic functional joint stability and to prevent fatigue-induced instability [27]. This can be accomplished by progressing the athlete with the advanced Thrower's Ten program to improve strength, endurance, and posture (Fig. 5.5) [28]. An interval sports program is implemented during this phase of treatment [29]. Sports-specific programs (golf, tennis, football, baseball, softball, etc.) are intended to systematically introduce quantity, intensity, and duration of sporting activities to allow an athlete to return to sporting activities while minimizing the recurrence of injury and pain with activities.

Phase IV is the return-to-activity phase that is implemented to gradually and progressively increase the functional demands on the shoulder to prepare for the return to unrestricted sports or daily activities. Upon successful completion of the rehabilitation program and achieving the aforementioned goals, the athlete may initiate a gradual return to sports activity in a controlled manner. The physiotherapist should consider the healing constraints based on surgical intervention and the patient's tissue status before a functional program is initiated. The clinician should ensure the athlete maintains muscular strength, dynamic stability, and shoulder functional motion established in the previous phase; therefore, the patient is encouraged to maintain a stretching and strengthening program on an ongoing basis to maintain and continue to improve optimal shoulder function. Athletes are continued on the Thrower's Ten program to maintain flexibility and shoulder strength throughout this program to continue to ensure adequate postural awareness and shoulder function.

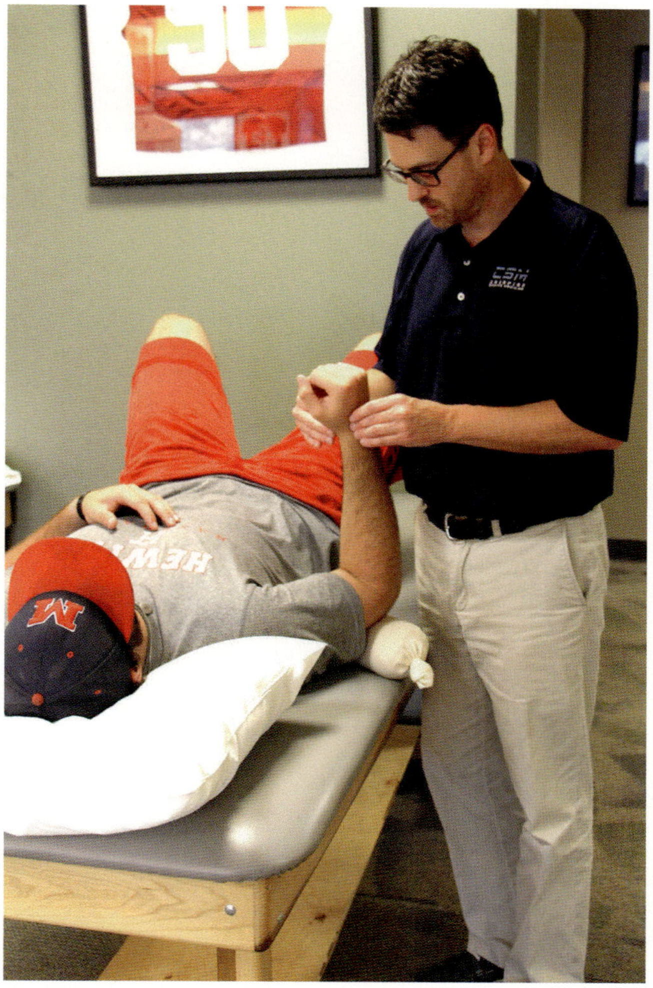

Fig. 5.1 Rhythmic stabilization drills for internal and external rotation to facilitate rotator cuff activation and neuromuscular control

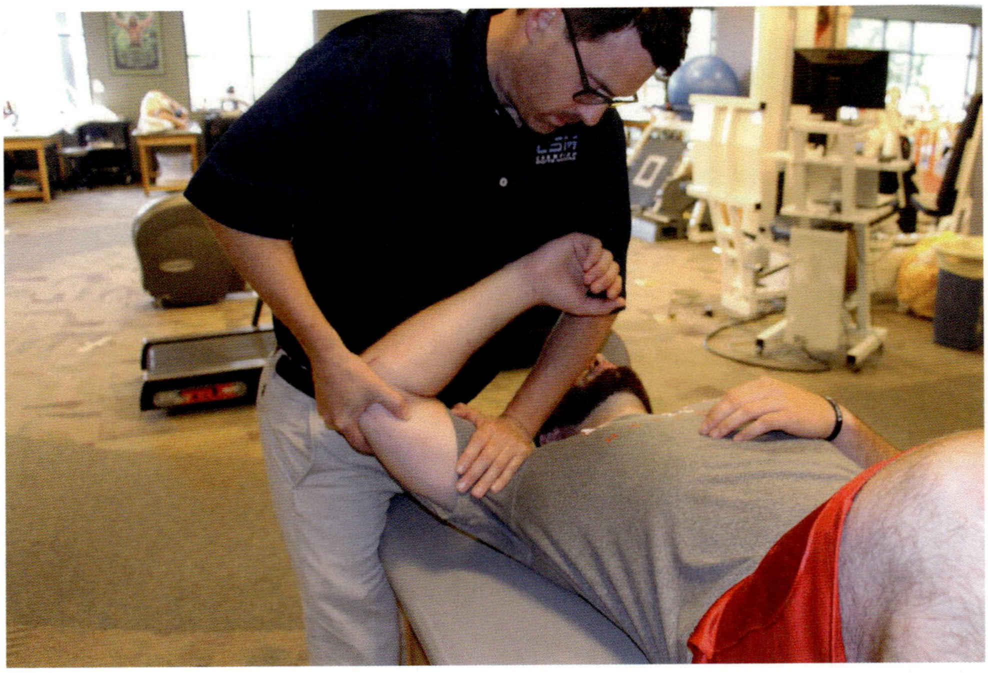

Fig. 5.2 Glenohumeral joint mobilizations performed for the posterior capsule performed in a posterior-lateral direction

Table 5.5 Isokinetic shoulder strength criteria for overhead athletes

Bilateral comparison (dominant arm versus nondominant arm)				
Velocity[a]	ER[b]	IR[c]	Abduction	Adduction
180	98–105 %	110–120 %	98–105 %	110–128 %
300	85–95 %	105–115 %	96–102 %	111–29 %
Peak torque (ft-lb)-to-body weight (lb) ratios				
Velocity[a]	ER[b]	IR[c]	Abduction	Adduction
180	18–23 %	28–33 %	26–33 %	32–38 %
300	12–20 %	25–30 %	20–25 %	28–34 %
Unilateral muscle ratios				
Velocity[a]		ER[b]/IR[c]	Abduction/adduction	ER[b]/abduction
180		66–76 %	78–84 %	67–75 %
300		61–71 %	88–94 %	60–70 %

[a]Degrees per second
[b]*ER* external rotation
[c]*IR* internal rotation

5.5 Rehabilitation following Arthroscopic Anterior Bankart Repair

Following surgery, the patient will don a sling during the day for 3–4 weeks while sleeping in an immobilizer brace for 4 weeks. Shoulder ROM will be monitored for elevation, ER, extension, and horizontal abduction limit motions as these can stress the anterior capsule. Passive and active-assisted ROM exercises for the shoulder begins on postoperative day within a prescribed motion permitting shoulder ER and IR ROM at 30° of abduction. The athlete will continue with a gradual restoration of glenohumeral ROM as ER and IR ROM is performed at 90° of abduction at week 7. Full functional ROM is achieved by week 8–9 allowing 160° of flexion, 90–100° of ER, and 70–75° of IR at 90° of abduction.

Therapeutic exercises are initiated with shoulder isometrics at 1–2 days following surgery while scapular isotonics and ER/IR strengthening exercises begin at postoperative week 4 and 6, respectively. The Thrower's Ten program which is progressed to include dynamic stabilization drills such as rhythmic stabilization drills concomitantly with tubing exercises and closed-chain stabilization ball on wall drills continues to augment the isotonic strengthening and dynamic stability program of the shoulder joint complex (Fig. 5.6). Sports-specific drills can begin during this phase to include plyoball throwing (Functional Integration Technologies, Watsonville, CA) for overhead athletes or swinging a golf club or tennis racket. A return-to-activity phase is usually initiated around 28 weeks following surgery that allows a gradual restoration to prior level of function and sports participation.

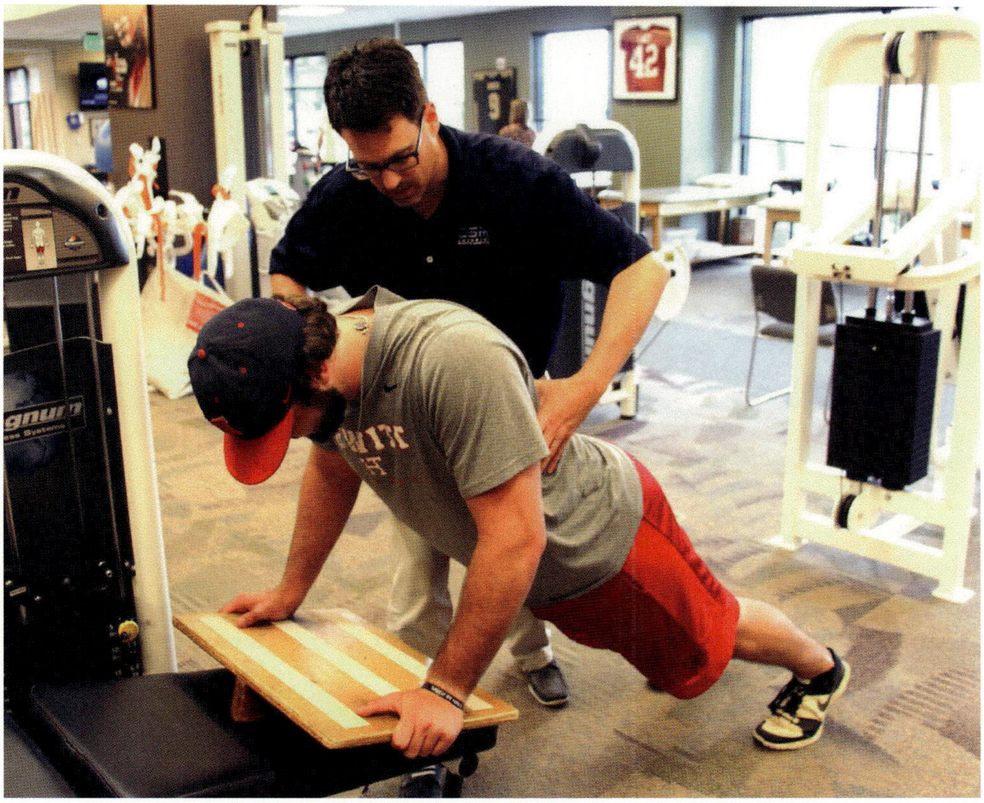

Fig. 5.3 Push-ups performed on an unstable surface with concomitant manual rhythmic stabilizations to facilitate dynamic stability of the shoulder and core musculature

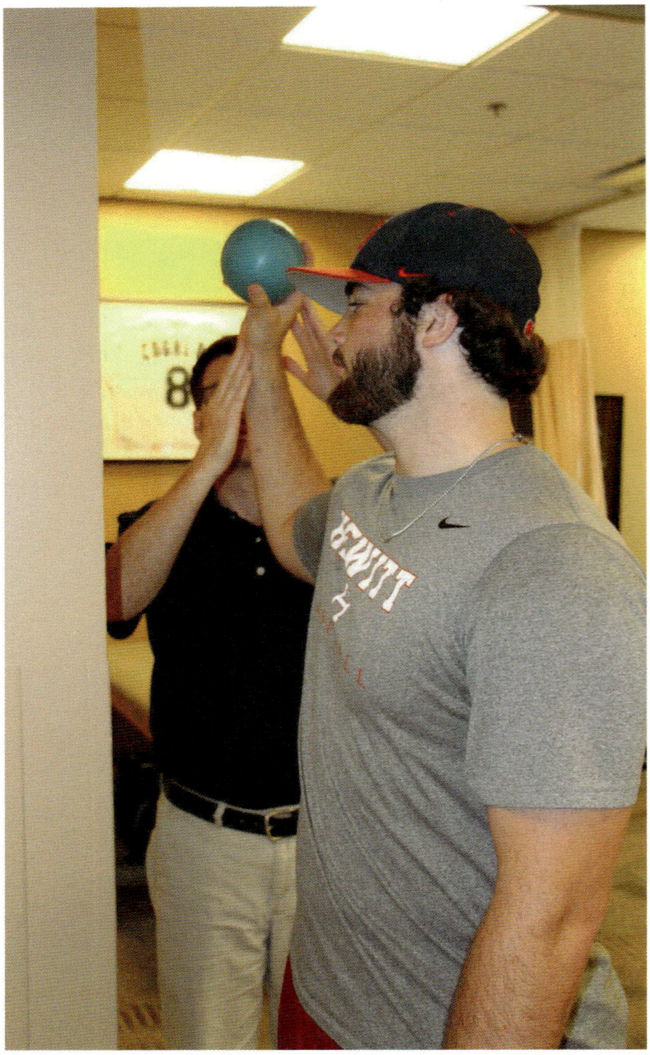

Fig. 5.4 Manual stabilizations performed as the athlete performs ball dribbles with the shoulder maintained at 90° abduction

5.6 Rehabilitation following Posterior Bankart

The rehabilitation following posterior capsular reconstruction is progressed relatively slower as compared to an anterior stabilization procedure due to the decreased thickness and tensile properties of the posterior capsule for restoration of glenohumeral ROM and return to function. In order to refrain from movements that place stress upon the posterior capsule, the athlete is instructed to strictly avoid internal rotation and horizontal adduction for the first 6–8 weeks following surgery, and these movements will continue to be controlled throughout the rehabilitation program. Following surgery, the athlete will be placed in an abduction immobilization sling that is maintained at approximately 30° of ER for 6 weeks in order to minimize stress on the posterior capsule. As a result of the detachment of the infraspinatus with open procedures, the initiation of ER strengthening exercises may be delayed as compared to an arthroscopic procedure.

Shoulder passive ROM is initiated week 2 after surgery with goals of 125° of shoulder flexion; external rotation is initiated at 90° of shoulder abduction to minimize stress upon the posterior capsule and is progressed to 90° of ER at 6 weeks postoperative. Range-of-motion exercises will continue as flexion is progressed to 165° by week 8 and IR at 90° of abduction is initiated at week 10 progressing to 60° by week 12. The mobility of the glenohumeral capsular mobility can be assessed beginning at 5–6 weeks following surgery, allowing anterior and inferior mobilizations as deemed appropriate; however, posterior glides should be cautioned as to not create deleterious stresses of the posterior capsule.

Shoulder isometrics are begun 2 weeks following surgery, progressing to isotonic strengthening for the rotator cuff and scapular musculature at week 4 with IR ROM limited to only neutral rotation. Muscle strength of the posterior rotator cuff and the scapular musculature is emphasized prior to the deltoid to increase dynamic stability of the posterior capsule. The clinician will avoid stressing the posterior capsule by delaying activities and exercises that create posterior translation upon the humerus (such as push-ups, bench press) for 12–14 weeks. Machine resistance training can begin weeks 13–20 following surgery; these exercises (lat pull, seated rows, seated bench press) are initiated within a monitored range of motion as to reduce both tensile stress on the posterior capsule and posterior humeral translation at end ranges of movement. Sports-specific training can begin at approximately 4–6 months following surgery and progressed to allow most athletes to return to full activity between 9 and 12 months postoperatively.

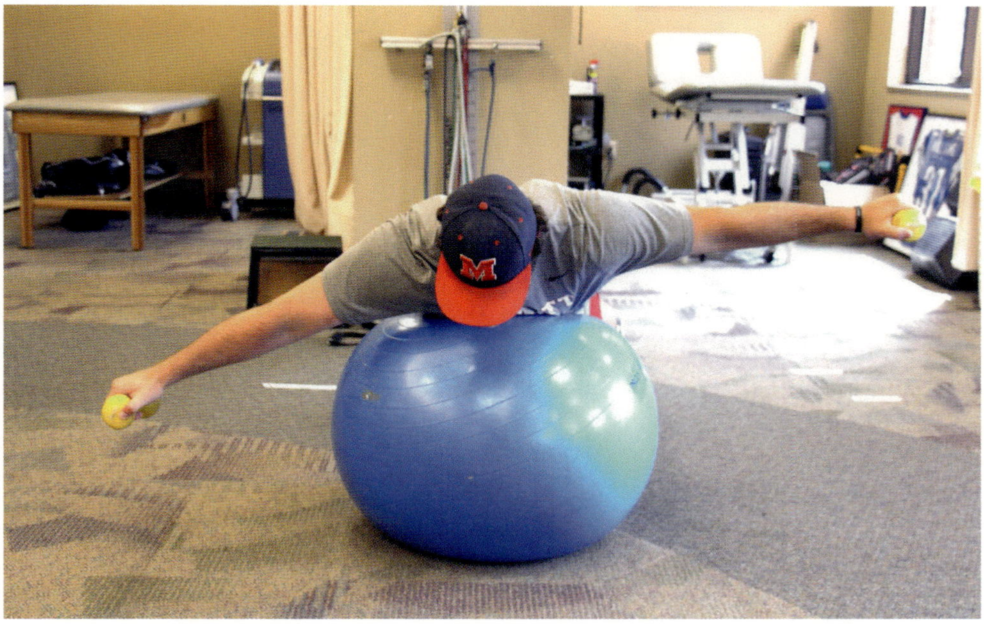

Fig. 5.5 Alternate sustained isometric holds performed on a stability ball to facilitate stabilization of the core musculature

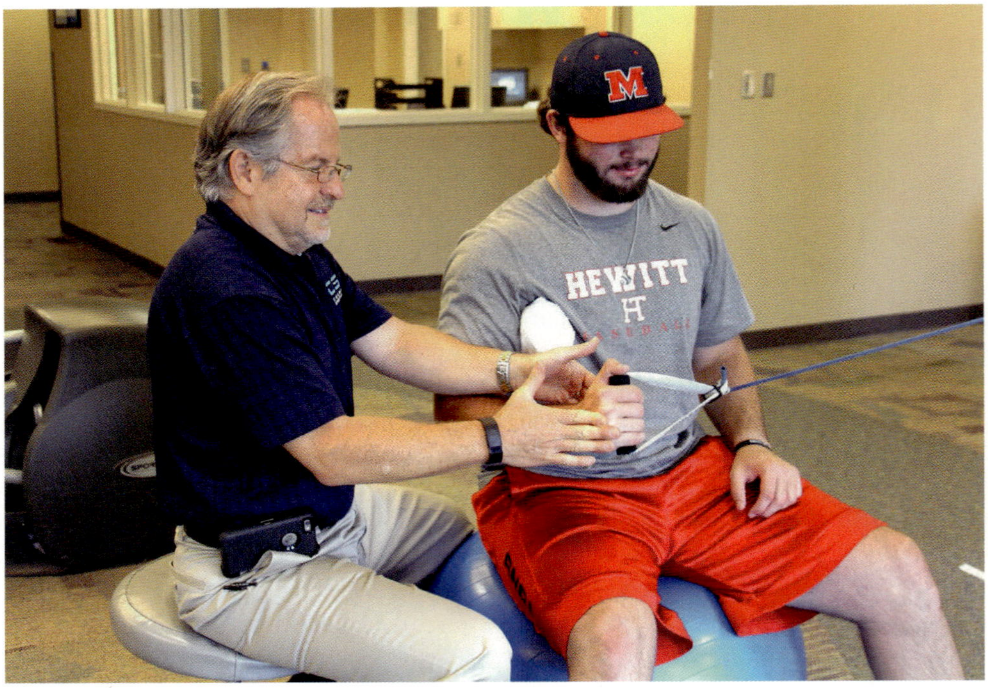

Fig. 5.6 External rotation tubing performed on a stability ball with concomitant rhythmic stabilizations to promote neuromuscular control, core, and dynamic stability

5.7 Rehabilitation following Arthroscopic Capsular Plication

The patient is instructed to sleep in an immobilizer and to avoid elevation and ER ROM for 6 weeks and limit overhead activities for 12 weeks following surgery. During the early stages of rehabilitation following capsular plication, an overall conservative approach in restoring glenohumeral ROM is taken due to the congenital laxity that is present, as limited ROM exercises will be delayed until 2 weeks following surgery. ROM is initiated at 2 weeks and is limited to 90° shoulder flexion and ER performed in the scapular plane to 0°. At 4 weeks following surgery, shoulder range of motion is gradually progressed to allow 145° of flexion and 45° of ER. ER ROM is performed at 90° of abduction to 70° at 6 weeks and flexion is performed to 160°. The restoration of ROM will be restored as needed based upon the patient's functional goals; therefore, overhead athletes will continue a gradual progression of motion allowing for thrower's motion at 10–12 weeks postsurgical, while the general MDI patient may discontinue ROM and stretching exercises.

Isometric exercises for the rotator cuff and scapula are integrated into the early stages of rehabilitation, while light isotonics can be initiated 4 weeks postoperatively as well as closed-chain rhythmic stabilization exercises to emphasize co-contraction of the rotator cuff. The athlete can continue to progress the strengthening program by initiating the Thrower's Ten program at week 7–8 that will be gradually progressed to incorporate overhead dynamic strengthening at week 12. Interval sporting activities below shoulder level can begin at week 14, whereas overhead activities are initiated at week 16. The athlete is usually able to return to contact sports 6–7 months following surgery, while overhead athletes may return 7–9 months following surgery.

5.8 Rehabilitation following Arthroscopic Glenoid Labrum Procedures

The specific rehabilitation program following surgical intervention of the superior glenoid labrum is dependent on the type and severity of the pathology.

Following a simple arthroscopic debridement of the frayed labrum, the rehabilitation program is somewhat aggressive in restoring motion and function with full range of motion expected by 10–14 days postoperatively. Internal and external rotation tubing exercises are initiated at day 10 and are gradually progressed to incorporate isotonic strengthening between weeks 2 and 8 and allowing the athlete to begin an ITP at week 8–12.

The rehabilitation following a type II SLAP lesion is more cautious for the first 4 weeks by having the athlete sleeping in an immobilizer and wearing a sling during the day and by not permitting isolated biceps strengthening for 6–8 weeks to allow adequate healing. Elevation range-of-motion activity is restricted for the first 4 weeks below 90°. Internal and external rotation is performed passively in the scapula plane to approximately 10–15° of external rotation and 45° of internal rotation for the first 2 weeks and is progressed to 90° of abduction at week 5–6. No excessive external rotation, extension, or abduction is allowed until week 5–6, when a light isotonic strengthening program is initiated. Motion is gradually increased to restore full range by 8–10 weeks and progressed to thrower's motion at week 10–12. Plyometric exercises are initiated at week 12 and the ITP at week 16. Return to play following surgical repair of a type II SLAP lesion occurs at approximately 9–11 months.

5.9 Rehabilitation following Proximal Biceps Tendon Procedures

Depending upon the extent of pathology and contributing factors, multiple surgical procedures can be performed to address the long head of the biceps. For partial tears including delamination and fraying of less than 25 % of the tendon in the athlete, debridement of the intra-articular portion of the biceps tendon maybe performed [30–32]. However, with extensive tendinopathy or gross instability, either a biceps tenotomy or tenodesis is performed. Biceps tenotomy is performed by sectioning the long head of the biceps tendon at its origin at the supraglenoid tubercle and superior labrum, as compared to a biceps tenodesis that also includes the distal anchoring of the surgically released tendon. The rehabilitation program following biceps debridement is progressed relatively quicker in regaining motion and function with full range of motion of the shoulder and elbow is expected by 10–14 days postoperatively. Shoulder isometrics are initiated immediately following surgery and allowed to begin internal and external rotation; tubing exercises are initiated at day 10 and are allowed to progress and incorporate isotonic strengthening at 2 weeks following surgery and progressed throughout week 8. The athlete is allowed to initiate an ITP at week 8–12.

The rehabilitation following either a tenodesis or tenotomy is similar, although a more cautious approach is utilized in following a biceps tenodesis. The rehabilitation following a tenotomy will be advanced more quickly due to a decreased protection required for the healing tissue. An overly aggressive approach could risk the athlete to a Popeye deformity that has been reported to be present in 62–70 % of patients following a tenotomy [33, 34]. Patients undergoing a biceps tenodesis will be progressed more slowly by utilizing a sling and refraining from isolated biceps activity for 8 weeks to allow soft tissue healing as the patient will be instructed to abstain from resisted biceps and forearm supination movements and activities. The athlete will begin shoulder passive range of motion with the elbow slightly bent to minimize strain upon the biceps tendon progressing to functional full range of motion at 6 weeks while minimizing movements that stress the biceps such as shoulder external rotation and extension. Shoulder isometrics can be initiated immediately following surgery and progressed to include rotator cuff training at weeks 2–3 following surgery. Shoulder elevation exercises can begin at week 4 and gradually progressed to the Thrower's Ten Program at week 6–8. The athlete can begin to perform plyometric activities at 12–14 weeks post-surgery with a gradual return to sporting activities following a return-to-activity phase.

References

1. Fleisig GS, Andrews JR, Dillman CJ, Escamilla RF (1995) Kinetics of baseball pitching with implications about injury mechanisms. Am J Sports Med 23(2):233–239
2. Fleisig GS, Barrentine SW, Escamilla RF, Andrews JR (1996) Biomechanics of overhand throwing with implications for injuries. Sports Med 21(6):421–437
3. Escamilla RF, Barrentine SW, Fleisig GS, Zheng N, Takada Y, Kingsley D, Andrews JR (2007) Pitching biomechanics as a pitcher approaches muscular fatigue during a simulated baseball game. Am J Sports Med 35(1):23–33
4. DiGiovine NM, Jobe FW, Pink M, Perry J (1992) An electromyographic analysis of the upper extremity in pitching. J Shoulder Elbow Surg 1(1):15–25
5. Coutts RD, Toth C, Kaita JH (1984) The role of continuous passive motion in the rehabilitation of the total knee patient. In: Hungerford DS, Krackow KA, Kenna RV (eds) Total knee arthroplasty: a comprehensive approach. Williams and Wilkins, Baltimore, pp 126–132
6. Dehne E, Torp RP (1971) Treatment of joint injuries by immediate mobilization. Based upon the spinal adaptation concept. Clin Orthop Relat Res 77:218–232
7. Haggmark T, Eriksson E (1979) Cylinder or mobile cast brace after knee ligament surgery. A clinical analysis and morphologic and enzymatic studies of changes in the quadriceps muscle. Am J Sports Med 7(1):48–56
8. Noyes FR, Mangine RE, Barber S (1987) Early knee motion after open and arthroscopic anterior cruciate ligament reconstruction. Am J Sports Med 15(2):149–160
9. Perkins G (1953) Rest and movement. J Bone Joint Surg Br 35-B(4):521–539
10. Salter RB, Hamilton HW, Wedge JH et al (1984) Clinical application of basic research on continuous passive motion for disorders and injuries of synovial joints: a preliminary report of a feasibility study. J Orthop Res 1(3):325–342
11. Salter RB, Simmonds DF, Malcolm BW, Rumble EJ, MacMichael D, Clements ND (1980) The biological effect of continuous passive motion on the healing of full-thickness defects in articular cartilage. An experimental investigation in the rabbit. J Bone Joint Surg Am 62(8):1232–1251
12. Wilk KE, Voight ML, Keirns MA, Gambetta V, Andrews JR, Dillman CJ (1993) Stretch-shortening drills for the upper extremities: theory and clinical application. J Orthop Sports Phys Ther 17(5):225–239
13. Wilk KE, Arrigo CA (1992) An integrated approach to upper extremity exercises. Orthop Phys Ther Clin North Am 1:337–360
14. Wilk KE, Arrigo CA, Andrews JR (1997) Current concepts: the stabilization structures of the glenohumeral joint. J Orthop Sports Phys Ther 25(6):364–379
15. Wilk KE, Andrews JR, Arrigo C (2001) Preventive and rehabilitative exercises for the shoulder and elbow, 6th edn. American Sports Medicine Institute, Birmingham
16. Blackburn TA, McLeod WD, White B et al (1990) EMG analysis of posterior rotator cuff exercises. Athl Train J Natl Athl Train Assoc 25:40–45
17. Decker MJ, Hintermeister RA, Faber KJ, Hawkins RJ (1992) Serratus anterior muscle activity during selected rehabilitation exercises. Am J Sports Med 7(6):784–791
18. Fleisig GS, Jameson GG, Cody KE et al (1998) Muscle activity during shoulder rehabilitation exercises. In: Proceedings of NACOB'98, The Third North American Congress on Biomechanics, Waterloo, 14 Aug 1998, pp 223–234.
19. Hintermeister RA, Lange GW, Schultheis JM et al (1998) Electromyographic activity and applied load during shoulder rehabilitation exercises using elastic resistance. Am J Sports Med 26:210–220
20. Jobe FW, Tibone JE, Jobe CM et al (1990) The shoulder in sports. In: Rockwood CA Jr, Matsen FA III (eds) The shoulder. WB Saunders, Philadelphia, pp 961–990
21. Jobe FW, Moynes DR, Tibone JE, Perry J (1984) An EMG analysis of the shoulder in pitching. A second report. Am J Sports Med 12(3):218–220
22. Moseley JB Jr, Jobe FW, Pink M, Perry J, Tibone J (1992) EMG analysis of the scapular muscles during a shoulder rehabilitation program. Am J Sports Med 29(2):128–134
23. Pappas AM, Zawacki RM, McCarthy CF (1985) Rehabilitation of the pitching shoulder. Am J Sports Med 13(4):223–235
24. Townsend H, Jobe FW, Pink M, Perry J (1991) Electromyographic analysis of the glenohumeral muscles during a baseball rehabilitation program. Am J Sports Med 19(3):264–272
25. Carpenter JE, Blasier RB, Pellizzon GG (1998) The effects of muscle fatigue on shoulder joint position sense. Am J Sports Med 26(2):262–265
26. Wilk KE (2000) Restoration of functional motor patterns and functional testing in the throwing athlete. In: Lephart SM, Fu FH (eds) Proprioception and neuromuscular control in joint stability. Human Kinetics, Champaign, pp 415–438
27. Voight ML, Hardin JA, Blackburn TA, Tippett S, Canner GC (1996) The effects of muscle fatigue on and the relationship of arm dominance to shoulder proprioception. J Orthop Sports Phys Ther 23(6):348–352
28. Wilk KE, Yenchak AJ, Arrigo CA, Andrews JR (2011) The Advanced Throwers Ten Exercise Program: a new exercise series for enhanced dynamic shoulder control in the overhead throwing athlete. Phys Sportsmed 39(4):90–97
29. Reinold MM, Wilk KE, Reed J, Crenshaw K, Andrews JR (2002) Interval sport programs: guidelines for baseball, tennis, and golf. J Orthop Sports Phys Ther 32(6):293–298
30. Barber FA, Byrd JW, Wolf EM, Burkhart SS (2001) How would you treat the partially torn biceps tendon? Arthroscopy 17:636–639
31. Barber FA, Field LD, Ryu R (2007) Biceps tendon and superior labrum injuries: decision-marking. J Bone Joint Surg Am 89:1844–1855
32. Sethi N, Wright R, Yamaguchi K (1999) Disorders of the long head of the biceps tendon. J Shoulder Elbow Surg 8:644–654
33. Boileau P, Baque F, Valerio L, Ahrens P, Chuinard C, Trojani C (2007) Isolated arthroscopic biceps tenotomy or tenodesis improves symptoms in patients with massive irreparable rotator cuff tears. J Bone Joint Surg Am 89:747–757
34. Kelly AM, Drakos MC, Fealy S, Taylor SA, O'Brien SJ (2005) Arthroscopic release of the long head of the biceps tendon: functional outcome and clinical results. Am J Sports Med 33:208–213

Index

G. Di Giacomo, S. Bellachioma (eds.), *Shoulder Surgery Rehabilitation: A Teamwork Approach*,
DOI 10.1007/978-3-319-24856-1

T

U

V

W